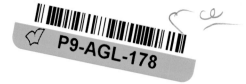

Quantity discounts are available, please contact the publisher.
Printed in the United States of America

Publisher: Parkinsons Creative Collective, Inc.
Email: Thebook@parkinsonscreativecollective.org
Website: www.Parkinsonscreativecollective.org
U.S. mail: P.O. Box 22416
Little Rock, Arkansas, 72211

ISBN 978-0-9893266-0-5 (paperback)
1.Parkinson's Disease 2.Chronic illness 3.Health care advocacy 4.Self-help 5.Personal narratives 6.Neurology
First Edition

Grateful acknowledgment is made for permission to reprint the following:
Epigraph: Reprinted by arrangement with the Heirs to the Estate of Martin Luther King Jr,
c/o Writers House as agent for the proprietor, New York, NY.
Copyright 1963 Martin Luther King, Jr., copyright renewed 1991 Coretta Scott King

Photo pg 58 Copyright The Naples News, reprinted with permission.

(Page 313 constitutes an extension of this copyright page.)

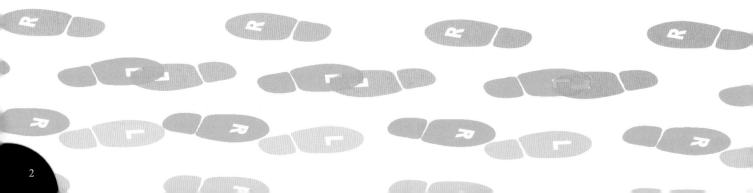

The NeuroWriters' Guide To

The Peripatetic Pursuit Of Parkinson Disease

Parkinsons Creative Collective

Lindy Ashford, Laura Brooks, Perry Cohen, Bob Cummings, May Griebel, Linda Herman,
Katherine Huseman, Pamela Kell, Girija Muralidhar, Peggy Willocks, Paula Wittekind,

and many contributors from the international Parkinson community.

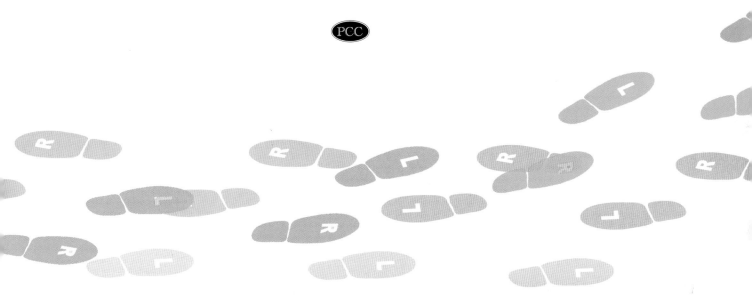

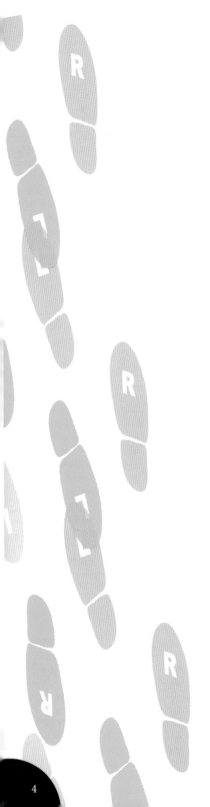

We dedicate this book, with love and thanks to

Bob Cummings
(1931 - 2012)

and

Paula Wittekind
(1950 - 2012)

who shared so much of their journey with us and the
wider Parkinson community.

Without them this book would not have been possible.
Their voices ring strong throughout its pages.

"THE FIERCE URGENCY OF NOW"

We are now faced with the fact, my friends, that tomorrow is today. We are confronted with the fierce urgency of now. In this unfolding conundrum of life and history, there is such a thing as being too late. Procrastination is still the thief of time. Life often leaves us standing bare, naked, and dejected with a lost opportunity. The tide in the affairs of men does not remain at flood - it ebbs. We may cry out desperately for time to pause in her passage, but time is adamant to every plea and rushes on. Over the bleached bones and jumbled residues of numerous civilizations are written the pathetic words, "Too late." There is an invisible book of life that faithfully records our vigilance or our neglect. Omar Khayyam is right: "The moving finger writes, and having writ moves on."

Dr. Martin Luther King, Jr.

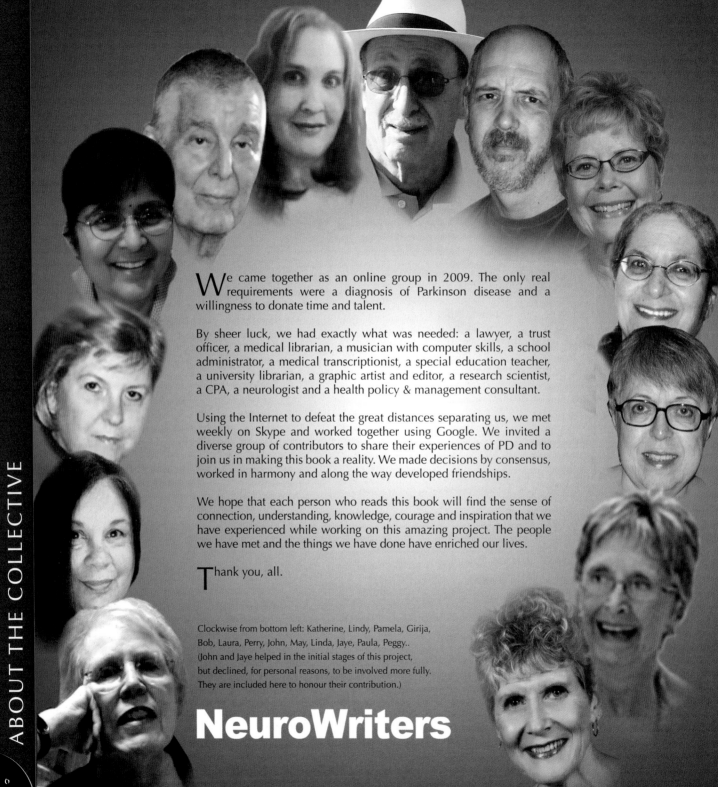

We came together as an online group in 2009. The only real requirements were a diagnosis of Parkinson disease and a willingness to donate time and talent.

By sheer luck, we had exactly what was needed: a lawyer, a trust officer, a medical librarian, a musician with computer skills, a school administrator, a medical transcriptionist, a special education teacher, a university librarian, a graphic artist and editor, a research scientist, a CPA, a neurologist and a health policy & management consultant.

Using the Internet to defeat the great distances separating us, we met weekly on Skype and worked together using Google. We invited a diverse group of contributors to share their experiences of PD and to join us in making this book a reality. We made decisions by consensus, worked in harmony and along the way developed friendships.

We hope that each person who reads this book will find the sense of connection, understanding, knowledge, courage and inspiration that we have experienced while working on this amazing project. The people we have met and the things we have done have enriched our lives.

Thank you, all.

Clockwise from bottom left: Katherine, Lindy, Pamela, Girija, Bob, Laura, Perry, John, May, Linda, Jaye, Paula, Peggy.. (John and Jaye helped in the initial stages of this project, but declined, for personal reasons, to be involved more fully. They are included here to honour their contribution.)

NeuroWriters

F O R E W O R D

In 2006, while hundreds of e-patients suffered at the unexpected and unexplained loss of their online community, I stepped up and offered what was meant to be a temporary home for them at a place we eventually called NeuroTalk. Today NeuroTalk is one of the premier online communities for neurological diseases (**http://neurotalk.psychcentral.com/**). The community offers a wide, diverse range of information, experiences and emotional support for individuals who have been diagnosed with diseases like amyotrophic lateral sclerosis (ALS, also known as Lou Gehrig's disease), multiple sclerosis, peripheral neuropathy and of course, Parkinson disease.

I'm not entirely certain that people always appreciate the value online communities bring to others. Some may think of an online support group as a place where people meet just to chat or talk about their "feelings." But online support communities like NeuroTalk are much more than that. They offer a place for people to learn about their disease first-hand from others who know what it's like to have it. What treatments are available and have been tried by others? Is one more effective than another? How will I know? What will I expect when I talk to my doctor or a specialist? Are there certain experts in the country I can go see to get the best care possible? How can I help my family learn about and better understand the disease?

Even more importantly, patient communities like NeuroTalk encourage patients to embrace participatory medicine -- to move from passive partners in their own care to active participants. Participatory medicine is a movement in which networked patients shift from being mere passengers to responsible drivers of their own health (see **http://participatorymedicine.org/** for more information). In the process, health care providers and doctors encourage and value patients as full partners in a patient's own healthcare decisions. Nowhere have I seen participatory medicine more embraced than within the Parkinson disease community and this group, the Parkinsons Creative Collective.

My time being involved with the Parkinson disease community online has been relatively short, compared to some individuals who have been actively involved in it for many years. What I do know is that we have provided a safe and secure community online for folks with Parkinson disease for four years now, and hope to do so for at least another forty.

It seems as though everybody's life is touched by tragedy or someone who has been affected by a life-threatening disease and my story is no different. In February 1999, my Dad was diagnosed with Parkinson disease. Eleven years later, he's still doing okay - not great, but he's still somewhat mobile - thanks to advances in our understanding of this disease and his never-ending optimistic take on life. In fact, the power of our minds to help heal our bodies is so often misunderstood or under-appreciated. While we cannot cure disease through pure willpower, our attitude and outlook on life has a direct impact not only on our health and wellbeing, but also on our ability to heal from disease more quickly and with less complications according to research. I attribute at least a part of my father's ongoing good health and ability to get around to his positive attitude. In early 2010, we went to Las Vegas together, a trip of a lifetime and something he immensely enjoyed. Advances in Parkinson disease understanding and treatments have made such trips possible, even 11 years into the disease.

But such advances don't only come through scientific research. They come through patient collaboration, outreach and advocacy. They come through a mutual collaboration and respectful discussion with our doctors, neurologists, and health care providers - and not a one-sided doctor directive, "Here's what we're going to do…"

Parkinson disease is perhaps all the more difficult and misunderstood because, unlike a lot of diseases, it is not an immediate death sentence. While there is no cure, there are many treatments available that help prolong an active and healthy life. But new treatments are slow in coming, and a cure still seems as improbable today as it did 20 years ago, despite the significant amount of resources and celebrity attention given to the disease.

It is with great hope that I see more patients embracing participatory medicine as a means of trying to further encourage new treatments, new ways of doing research (harnessing the power of Internet social media, for instance), to become activists in their own care and on behalf of those who cannot advocate for themselves. The Parkinsons Creative Collective is a prime example of a patient-empowered group working toward constructive change in the world of Parkinson.

The Parkinsons Creative Collective happened because of NeuroTalk, but I have no doubt that if NeuroTalk did not exist, this amazing, independent group of individuals would have found each other in some other way. The Internet simply enables people to do and learn things and meet one another more easily. NeuroTalk, and groups like it, are just tools to help people connect with one another to affect real change.

This book is just one example of what happens when you bring like-minded people together in an online community. The results of online communities like NeuroTalk are simply immeasurable, and I am both honored and humbled by enabling such communities. I hope you find some measure in this book - of comfort, of discovery, and of hope. The journey of Parkinson disease is long and sometimes lonely, but it is in no way a journey one has to make alone.

John M. Grohol, PsyD, CEO & founder PsychCentral.com

PERIPATETIC SCHOOL

An informal institution whose members conducted philosophical and scientific inquiries.

The school derived its name from the peripatoi (colonnades) of the Lyceum gymnasium in Athens.

A later legend claimed that the name came from Aristotle's alleged habit of walking while lecturing.

The word **peripatetic** comes from the ancient Greek word peripatêtikos meaning:

'of walking' or
'given to walking about'.

INTRODUCTION

This book was written by people with Parkinson disease, for people with Parkinson disease, their families, their friends and all who love and care for them. In other words, it's a book for the whole PD community. For someone with Parkinson, it is a support group between two covers. For others, it will be a window into the world of Parkinson. After reading a chapter, a nurse told us, "I never really knew what it was like from a patient's point of view."

We highlight the emergence of a worldwide Parkinson community, including the impact of the Internet, the education of patients and the rise of participation and advocacy. We invite all to become advocates and present many ways to do so; choose one that is comfortable for you and join in.

As you read, you'll discover this book is unique in several ways.

First, it is a collective project by people with Parkinson who are experts at living 24/7 with Parkinson disease. All of the editors, and most of the authors, have PD.

Second, it is an anthology of experiences. It contains articles by empowered and involved people with Parkinson - just open it anywhere and begin reading.

Third, the book reflects the international scope of the Parkinson community. The Internet connects us beyond geographic borders.

Fourth, as must be obvious, we don't think a book about a serious disease should be visually dull!

As with any book containing general information about medical, legal, financial and other important issues, please check with your medical team and appropriate professional advisors before you apply anything from this book to your own situation.

Finally, we all begin this trip in the deep, dark woods, alone. This book represents trails laid by those who have gone before to signpost possibilities. Others may find and extend the trails much further. Beyond that, we hope you will be inspired to become part of a more vocal, involved, international PD community. Walk with us on our journey - it might take you further than you could ever imagine.

Editor's Note: 1. There is a growing trend in the medical community to eliminate use of the possessive. Consistent with that position we will refer to Parkinson disease throughout, except when an organization retains the possessive as part of its corporate identity. 2. We have tried to retain the authors' original voice so you may notice variations in spelling and language conventions.

Learning about
Parkinson disease
the PwP way

The doctor diagnosed Parkinson disease with simple tests in his office. He asked her to walk, tap her fingers and a few more things. Then he said the words that changed her life forever, "You have Parkinson disease." If she's lucky, the doctor gave her a 5 minute description of what that means. She has so many questions: Just what is a progressive, degenerative, neurological disease? How much time does one have? What can one do? At this point nothing was clear. Information might help but the end result is the same: she has become a person with Parkinson (PwP).

She began to look for information on her new condition. She discovered that it is described as a "snowflake disease", because it is different in each person. That increased her discomfort with the diagnosis. So everything was still unclear, and she did what was necessary. She tried to live each day by staying in the present and hoped for a cure or better treatment options in her lifetime.

Welcome to the world of PD.

In this chapter you will find information and experiences from diagnosis to Deep Brain Stimulation - all from the patient's point of view. For any reader, a PwP, family member or even a medical professional, there will be something new.

If you're as strong as those living with PD, read on.

CHAPTER ONE
Parkinson basics and beyond

Levodopa   3   FDA Non-   Received

Medicinal Plant   3   3   0   0   Not Yet F

Anti Depressant   3   0   Not Yet F

Monoamine Oxidase Inhibitor   3   Approved

Anti Epileptic   3   0   Approved conditiona

Adenosine Re Antagonist   0   0   Not Yet F

Kinase Inhibitor   0   Not Yet F

Neurotrophic Fa   0   Not Yet F

Retinal Pi   0   Not Yet F

just learning how to deal with Parkinson can seem overwhelming

it helps to hear from people who have made this journey themselves

WHEN THE JOURNEY BEGINS

The real journey begins with diagnosis. For many, once the decision is made to seek professional help, the road to an actual diagnosis can be long and filled with obstacles. Misdiagnosis is common in both directions. If we are assured our symptoms do not fit Parkinson disease, we are often willing to suspend belief and accept it because the relief is so great. When PD is confirmed, many of us seek second and third opinions, hoping against hope for a dissent. Rarely is one obtained.

In the beginning we avoid the company of others who are further along. We keep our families sheltered from the realities of later stage PD for fear that they may grasp that it could be our future they see. The fear is not necessarily irrational. Families do sometimes dissolve under the strain of one partner having a progressive, debilitating, incurable neurological illness; at the same time other families are strengthened by it. Within the community there are stories of great failures - alongside stories of overwhelming triumphs.

We are as diverse as the human race itself. We are all colors, nationalities, religions and ages. We are men and we are women. We are educated and financially secure and we are poor and illiterate. We are everything and everyone and we have all come together to gain strength and courage from each other. The real difference in people with Parkinson and those without is the reason for this book. The neurologists can diagnose the disease, they can test us and they can medicate us, but they can't tell us how to live with PD. We can tell each other, because we are the experts at living with PD.

NeuroWriters

> "When my diagnosis came there were supportive people online who helped me understand what I was experiencing, not just in terms of my condition, but the medical and social responses to PD."
>
> **NeuroTalk comment**

I have Parkinson but Parkinson doesn't have me ....

Diagnosis was difficult for some and they were on a roller coaster emotionally trying to find out what was wrong.

The day you receive your diagnosis is the last day of your life as you know it. You were a lawyer; you were a teacher; you were a musician; you were a CEO. As soon as the words "Parkinson disease" are spoken over you, you become a patient. You are told what drugs to put in your body. You are told it's not a death sentence. You are told you probably have many more years of productivity left. The day before, you barely ever even took aspirin; having or not having a "death sentence" wasn't even a concept in your mind; why wouldn't you have years of productivity left? None of that was your concern before.

Regardless of what the neuro says about going along as if nothing had happened, your life is changed. You are told what to do and how to think. You are a patient, by etymology a passive creature. I know I am committing the cardinal sin of patients: I am "complaining." I have had PD for 14 years and I have known only a large handful of people who have died from it. But I know scores of people now dying from it, beloved friends, friends who have kept me going as I have kept them going, now fading, inexorably dying from the same disease that will claim - is daily claiming - my own life.`
Ann Wasson

We wish to share a snapshot of the many truths of PD, what it is to live with this weirdly paradoxical disease.

Charting this territory, we decided, is not just for PwP, it is also for the people who look after us; doctors - who decide what PD is and work towards better treatment and care, scientists looking at what is happening at cellular level. All those grappling with the indefinables; difficult diagnoses, ambiguous data, inconclusive studies. Parkinson disease is a slippery customer and does not like to be pinned down.

Those who understand the textbook definitions; have been taught about PD in a psychology lecture, know it in the abstract, but see, up close, that we rarely present as the median - underweight, 50 or 60-ish, slow, tremulous, male - with spidery writing, a shaky hand, an expressionless face. Please see that we come in all shapes and sizes, that our arrival at diagnosis, after a baffling, sometimes disheartening journey, is a beginning not an end.

Diagnosis brings questions. PD is rarely out of the news, it seems to be a focus of research. There are reports of new breakthroughs, new treatments. We read that treatments are problematic. Do we start the treatments, or wait? Do we know we have an option? Why did we start on this treatment? Are other people taking something else? Why is everything about PD elusive, intrusive, even when we've lived with it for years?

Promises of cures on the horizon arouse hopes that our own version of PD will one day be cured and life will be back on track. The truth is more economical. People in the PD community have lived with promises a long time, some are damaged beyond healing. They know that a cure is unlikely to come in time for them. They hope the next generation of people will see better treatments - and a cure.

The medical scientific community now says the fixes are unlikely to come as quickly as they had hoped: the task is complex, the treatments are hard to achieve. Parkinson disease is fragmenting into definable variants, differentiating into named conditions that are similar, requiring further research. We see it is unlikely that there will a 'one size fits all' cure.

The peripatetic path takes us in more directions than we imagined possible. We know what we have learned is incomplete. Witnessing the frustration of our medical 'partners' when the limited treatments have run their course, when what remains are treatments with distressing side effects, or none at all, we have to acknowledge that it is difficult for them too.

We can see their change of emphasis, they have gone beyond the polemic of 'a cure in five years'. We see medicine changing to recognize patient centrality in healthcare, supporting patients over venture capitalism. The democratizing of medicine is developing fast and likely to be inevitable.

Even the word 'patient' is less relevant. Medicine often refers to us as clients, consumers and sometimes even as partners. Pharmaceutical companies are moving in this direction too, we are now consumers, customers.

We ourselves are less patient than before, less passive, compliant. Faced with intolerable side-effects, we will complain. Wasteful prescribing is an issue for both privatized and socialized medicine. Treatments are expensive. We want to be partners with our doctors in deciding what is right for us. Impatient, with a need-to-know attitude, we come with the hopes and promises science and medicine offer.

An information revolution happened and it is not possible for us to close our minds. We want to be included in the processes of medicine, not just at the end-point. We want to contribute.

We hope our understanding of PD will help open minds to a bigger picture, with a wish that Parkinson disease will become more treatable, even curable, and that some day treatments will make diagnosis merely a blip in our health that can be wholly overcome.

Lindy Ashford

PAULA'S STORY

Those words, "You have Parkinson disease" left me initially numb, feeling like I was now without a future.

My outlook gradually changed, with more information, to a great deal of relief at finally having a name for it......... **Paula Wittekind**

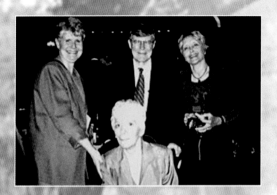

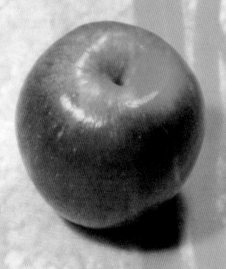

Top photo: Peg Willocks and Paula Wittekind with Mort and Milly Kondracke.

Lower photo: Paula with her students.

In the 1980s, I experienced a host of health problems that now could be considered the "usual PD suspects". The decade began with a pesticide poison, heptachlor, being discovered in the milk in Hawaii where I taught, at a private school for learning disabilities in Pearl Harbor. I had two children when in my 30s and then early menopause, gastrointestinal problems and a hypo-active thyroid. During the latter part of the 1980s, I wondered, even hoped, that I was becoming a hypochondriac.

By 1989 it was obvious to me that something was very wrong. My right hand was not fully functional; I couldn't wiggle my fingers. Showing others drew little reaction. An arthritis check was negative and the school nurse and my internist never suspected anything serious when I said my toes were curling. I stayed in denial. In 1992, I faced the enemy. The Encyclopedia Britannica confirmed which of my suspicions was correct. It was Parkinson disease. I was 42; my girls were elementary school students. After my diagnosis, other than my husband, I told just two people.

gradually changed, with more information, to a great deal of relief at finally having a name for it. I hid it for several years.

In 1989, I made a major change in my career and took a job teaching the physically impaired, undoubtedly the most enjoyable years of my career. These kids looked out for each other, didn't fight very often, were in pain, full of trust, but so very impaired.

Devastation: in spite of knowing I was going to hear those words, "You have Parkinson disease", it left me initially numb, feeling like I was now without a future. My outlook

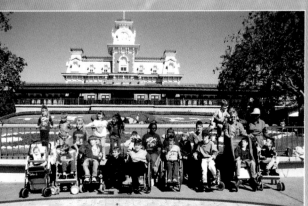

Working with these children, along with teaching those with learning disabilities, prepared me for understanding many of the physical and cognitive issues I am now experiencing.

15

What is Parkinson disease?

Newly diagnosed people and their families and friends will want to know what Parkinson disease is. It was first described by a 19th century doctor named James Parkinson. The condition, Idiopathic Parkinson disease (IPD) comes under an umbrella of movement disorders that includes several other conditions. Idiopathic Parkinson disease means 'a disease of unknown origin described by James Parkinson.'

There are several conditions that closely resemble IPD. Many people with one of these conditions were originally diagnosed with IPD, but when their symptoms became clearer the initial diagnosis was changed.

We ask; Why don't all these people slow down, and take a good look at us?

Parkinson described a condition that had four cardinal signs: Slowness, tremor, rigidity and postural instability. It is the canon by which diagnosis is still made, mainly but not exclusively by clinical observation. It is confirmed in some countries by use of DATScan, a special scanning technique that identifies neurons in the Substantia Nigra that have lost their ability to produce dopamine. Simple enough. Why, then, when patients compare notes, do they discover a disease that manifests itself in so many different ways that neurologists have difficulty diagnosing them? They are not all treated with the same medications. Even the 'gold standard' choice of medication, levodopa, is regarded by many as 'the drug you embrace as your best friend, and come to regard as your worst enemy'. **NeuroWriters**

PARKINSON RATING SCALES – TESTING MOTOR SKILLS OR MORE?

In your life with PD, at some time someone will mention PD rating scales. The most commonly used is the UPDRS, the Unified Parkinson's Disease Rating Scale. This and the Hoehn and Yahr, (H&Y) are the basic tests; some doctors add others for balance, depression, etc. on an as-needed basis. Even though PD is now recognized as more than a motor disorder, these tests, revised to include some other areas, still focus mainly on motor skills to evaluate PwP.

Even in the early stages as tested on the H&Y scale, many PwP have significant non-motor symptoms (NMS) and have greater discomfort from them than from their motor symptoms. The added irony is that NMS often can be effectively treated by physicians - if they know the PwP is troubled by NMS. Since current medical practice does not include assessment for NMS, many treatable symptoms are missed; further diminishing the PwP's quality of life.

The authors of the study listed below write that research has shown a need, "for a more complete assessment, of a specific method for classification of PD patients according to NMSB [NMS level of burden]."

The test they suggest,"**The Non-Motor Symptoms Scale** (NMSS) has 30 items, nine domains: cardiovascular (2 items), sleep/fatigue (4 items), mood/cognition (6 items), perceptual problems/hallucinations (3 items), attention/memory (3 items), gastrointestinal tract (3 items), urinary function (3 items), sexual function (2 items), and miscellaneous (4 items)."

A Proposal for a Comprehensive Grading of Parkinson's Disease Severity Combining Motor and Non-Motor Assessments: Meeting an Unmet Need. Kallol Ray Chaudhuri,1 Jose Manuel Rojo,2 Anthony H. V. Schapira,3 David J. Brooks,4 Fabrizio Stocchi,5 Per Odin,6 Angelo Antonini,7 Richard J. Brown,8 and Pablo Martinez-Martin9,*PLoS One. 2013; 8(2): e57221. Published online 2013 February 27. doi: 10.1371/journal.pone.005722

SYMPTOMS OF PARKINSON DISEASE

James Parkinson first described the disease named in his honor in 1817. Later in that century, the four cardinal motor signs, tremor, slowness of movement, rigidity and postural instability were identified. The original description of these signs remains the most commonly referred to measure of Parkinson disease. However, the list of motor symptoms is long and there is an additional list of non-motor symptoms that have been described more recently.

A hundred years ago the non-motor symptoms had not been observed, though today patients often place them top of the list when evaluating quality of life issues. The combination of symptoms makes for a very variable disease that is hard to diagnose.

Here are some of the motor and non-motor symptoms you may experience. It is important to note that very few people will have more than a fraction of these symptoms at any given time, let alone develop them all. There is no definitive list that describes when or if, in the course of the disease, symptoms may appear for any given patient because PD is such a variable condition.

Some of the symptoms listed may also appear as side effects of medication.

MOVEMENT
Shaky hands or feeling of shakiness (tremor), slowness, stiffness (rigidity), poor balance (postural instability), loss of arm swing, falling, stooped posture, walking with a shuffle, a dragging foot, an immobile 'masked' face, difficulty turning over in bed, walking with tiny fast steps, being suddenly unable to move, dystonia (can also be associated with medication 'wearing off' and 'wearing on'), dyskinesia (usually associated with medication).

COGNITION
Anxiety, apathy, depression, forgetting things, difficulties with multitasking, seeing things that are not there (visual hallucinations), hearing things that are not there (auditory hallucinations), believing in things that have not happened (delusions).

COMMUNICATION
Soft speech, speaking in a monotone, speaking slowly, mumbling, difficulty getting words out, stammering.

SLEEP
Inability to sleep at night (insomnia), daytime sleepiness, absence of dreams, waking up with cramps in legs, Restless Leg Syndrome, acting out dreams, drooling.

SIGHT
Persistent eye twitching, blurred vision, double vision, decreased blinking, dry or teary eyes, slow eye movements, sore eyes or styes.

ORAL & DIGESTIVE SYMPTOMS
Slow digestion and feelings of fullness, reflux, stomach or abdominal pain, swallowing difficulties, choking, poor dental health.

BLADDER AND BOWEL SYMPTOMS
Urinary incontinence, bowel incontinence, diarrhea (sometimes a side effect of specific medication), constipation, gastroparesis.

SEXUALITY (in men and women)
Loss of libido, increased libido, hypersexuality (sometimes a side effect of specific medications), difficulty achieving orgasm.

SKIN
Very dry skin, very oily skin, scaly scalp or excessive dandruff (seborrheic dermatitis).

BEHAVIOUR
Impulsive and compulsive disorders such as gambling, shopping, internet shopping, sex addiction, risk taking behaviours, (all are sometimes associated with specific types of PD medication).

AUTONOMIC NERVOUS SYSTEM
Orthostatic hypotension (can make you feel faint or giddy), sweating, heart rate changes.

PAIN
Pain in PD has many sources. Some of the most common are those due to rigidity, dystonia, dyskinesia.

FATIGUE
Fatigue in PD is very common.

We have come across many distressed people who have read about Parkinson and convinced themselves that not only are they or their loved ones in late stage disease, but also that it is one of the faster developing PD-like conditions.

Remember that PD usually progresses slowly. If you have concerns about your symptoms or those of a family member, you should discuss them with your neurologist, Movement Disorder Specialist, or Parkinson Nurse Specialist.

NeuroWriters

THE PARADOX OF PARKINSON

You come to Parkinson with little knowledge of the disease; the more you learn the more paradoxical it seems. The individual way it affects each person, the varying approaches of doctors, the bewildering array of treatments, can all seem perplexing. Once called the 'shaking palsy', not all patients shake; called a movement disorder, the non-motor symptoms can be the hardest to cope with. If you have it your lack of facial expression may make people's responses to you puzzling -you could be the last person to notice your Parkinson mask.

It is difficult to take a step forward or backwards. Turning takes a while. Choosing things in the supermarket stops you in your tracks. You are slow, slow, slow in nearly everything, but suddenly catch a ball. Walking is tedious and difficult, dancing a delightful freedom. Sometimes you're 'off' and sometimes you're 'on'. It's hard to get a word out, though you're an articulate person. You think you're smiling, they think you're grumpy. The world seems very fast, but you know it's you - going very slowly. Getting upstairs is no problem, coming down another matter. The stripe at the edge of the rug is like the edge of precipice. You sleep in the day, you're awake at night. Your handwriting is small and illegible. Your sense of smell has vanished. Your muscles seem firm, but don't do what you want them to do.

You are diagnosed by one doctor, another cannot see PD. You didn't ask the questions you prepared, you froze on the way out... Your medication works - for a few hours at a time - people think you are fine. When it doesn't they wonder what's wrong with you. You probably haven't told them anyway - what little people know of PD is that it strikes the old, infirm, and you are 30, or 40 or 50 - or a bit less or a bit more.

And while YOU know PD has neurological basis, there is a widespread misunderstanding that PD is a disease of the mind rather than the brain.
Lindy Ashford

Kinesia Paradoxica is the medical term for the phenomena observable in PD patients who are normally unable to move freely, but can suddenly overcome their immobility if shocked or scared.

The elephant in the room is Parkinson disease itself.....

IT HAD TO BE SOMEONE EXACTLY LIKE ME!

I was 34 years old, happily married to Mike for 16 years, two children aged 9 and 6, working part time and the future looked good.

But what was happening to the right side of my body? My fingers were not reaching the right keys on the keypad. My dad noticed I wasn't swinging my arm when I walked. My big toe would suddenly point straight up; it was painful and a friend noticed I walked with uneven steps, one normal and one short.

Repetitive Strain Injury, the first general practitioner (GP) said, but I didn't use my feet to key in!! I saw another GP who told me he didn't know what was wrong and sent me to see a Neurologist. After many tests there were still no answers. Possibly MS, but I was told get on with life and see what happens.

A couple of years later, after a car accident, my symptoms became worse. Again the tests were not conclusive. The Neurologist, not telling me what it was for, suggested I 'try' a 'tablet'. The internet gave me the diagnosis with the words 'TREATMENT FOR PARKINSON DISEASE'. I was devastated. I couldn't have Parkinson. I wasn't old enough. My life was over. What did the future hold? Would I be able to continue working? My mind was in a spin and I didn't know where to go to for help.

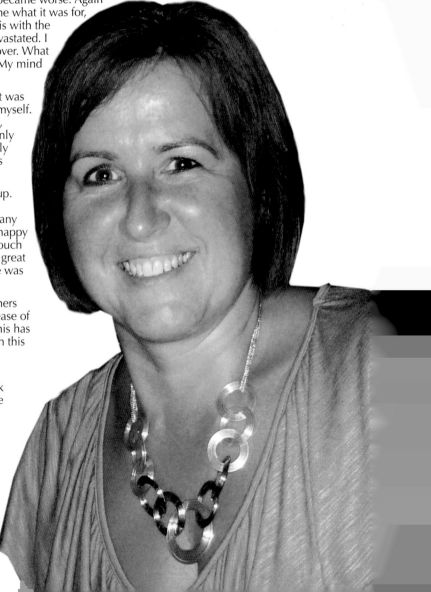

I was desperate to meet others who would understand what was happening to me. That person had to be a mirror image of myself. A lady my age, recently diagnosed with Parkinson, married, working and bringing up two children. She would be the only person who would fully understand. My husband and family were great but they could never fully understand how I was feeling.

The Parkinson Nurse suggested I visit the local support group. The first few visits were difficult. I cried all the way home. Was this my future? After a while I noticed that although many members had been diagnosed for a long time they were a happy bunch and most were living active lives. I was also put in touch with my 'mirror image'. We talked and talked and became great friends. I began to look forward and feel more positive. Life was worth living.

I became involved with the local support group helping others to cope and spreading the word that Parkinson is not a disease of old age but can affect people of any age, gender or race. This has helped me deal with my feelings after being diagnosed with this frustrating, fluctuating, progressive disease.

As a Young Onset Representative I organise social events where members with Parkinson have the opportunity to talk to others experiencing the same problems. Our partners are welcome too as they also need the support of others who live with Parkinson every day.

Parkinson did not mean my life was over. I am now 48 and coping. I have many new friends, have met many celebrities and have experienced opportunities I will never forget.

Karen Rose, UK

Karen has used the Wii Fit to help improve her Parkinson symptoms and to keep her mind active.

TYPES OF MEDICATIONS

Being diagnosed with Parkinson disease means that at some point a PwP will begin taking medicine. The particular combination of medication depends on our own special and individual form of Parkinson and its unique set of symptoms. The aim is to use our medication to give the best results over the longest possible time.

To protect ourselves, we must become aware of and informed, at the very least, about the medications we take or are planning to take. People are fallible and we all, from time to time, make mistakes. Remember we are our own best watch dogs.

Levodopa was the first treatment developed for PD. For a number of years, l-dopa has been combined with carbidopa which decreases the change in the liver of l-dopa to dopamine, thus allowing more l-dopa to get across the blood-brain barrier. The brain's enzymes can then convert l-dopa to dopamine, allowing a lower dose of l-dopa to be given and reducing risk of nausea. Entacapone, a COMT inhibitor, may be added to lengthen the time that dopamine is effective. Other medications may be added as the disease progresses. These include direct dopamine agonists.

Some doctors prefer starting with dopamine agonists, which are not dopamine but can act like it, "saving the gold standard" Sinemet (combined L-dopa plus carbidopa) for later, especially in younger patients. These medications include pramipaxole or ropinarole.

Other agonists include Apomorphine, an injectable form, Bromocriptine and Cabergoline. (Cabergoline is not available in the U.S.) All these types of drugs may also be added in the later stages to dopaminergic therapies to extend their effective time.

Another option to lengthen the effect of L-dopa is to add either selegeline or its newer relative, Azilect (rasagaline.) Both are MAO-B inhibitors and may have some direct DA agonist effect as well. Their use is complicated by potential interactions with

other medications. (The higher price of non-generic drugs may also influence the doctor and patient's decision to use a specific drug.)

One of the most troublesome side effects of long term dopaminergic therapy is dyskinesia, the uncontrollable movement so often associated with PD.

In its worst form dyskinesia can be debilitating. Antihistimines and anticholinergics such as Amantadine, or Diphenhydramine are often used to lessen those effects.

Since anxiety and depression often accompany Parkinson disease, we have included some of the drugs most commonly prescribed for persistent or long lasting episodes. For depression Effexor, Fluoxetine, Nortriptyline or Bupropion are frequently used and for anxiety, Alpraxolam and Diazepam. **NeuroWriters**

YOU AND YOUR MEDICATION
These are just some of the medications used in PD.

Knowing your medication and what it does is essential for PD patients. You should be able to discuss openly how you respond to your medications with your neurologist, prescribing physician and pharmacist.

A FEW OTHER TIPS
• Carry with you at all times a copy of all the medications including supplements and vitamins that you take.

• Make sure someone else knows your medication schedule.

• Be aware that supplements and other drugs may interact with your PD drugs

• Consult with your physican(s) and pharmacist before starting or stopping any new drug or supplement.

PD MEDICATION

TELLING THE PEOPLE YOU LOVE

It's final. You've been diagnosed. Some of your family knows, or perhaps they don't, either way there is still the rest of the world to be told. Just exactly how does one bring the subject up? There are endless methods, but here are three:

The Off-handed Casual Approach: **"Yes, I'll bring a cake to dinner on Friday, and by the way, I've just been diagnosed with Parkinson disease."**

The more formal approach: **"Now don't get all upset, I just found out I have an incurable, progressive, debilitating neurological disease."**

The dramatic approach: (my personal favorite), **"I probably won't be here in a few years so can we go to Europe this summer?"**

Kidding aside, giving the news to family and friends can be almost as difficult as getting the news was. There are children to be considered, how will they handle it? Will it frighten them? Will they look at you differently? Will they feel differently about you? Then there are parents, older, perhaps frail. Will hearing your diagnosis be more than they can bear? Finally there are friends, possibly the most difficult. At least with family there is a cushion of love that can blunt some of the ill thought-out comments, but friends, well that's another story.

I recall some statements to which the only response possible was a dumbfounded look of amazement at their insensitivity, ignorance and unbridled rudeness. *"Don't you lose your mind with that, like Alzheimer?" "I thought that was an old person's disease." "What did you do to get it?" "I thought only boxers got it." "Do you think your marriage will make it?" "How long do you have?"*

It isn't as though you have not asked yourself some of the same questions, it is hearing them said aloud that is so very jarring. What are the answers? Like everything else with Parkinson disease the answers are different for each of us. Do you lose your mind? Some do, some don't. The percentage is about twice that of those without PD. I thought it was an old person's disease? Partly true, most are over sixty when diagnosed but there are those younger than twenty. How long do you have?

Depends on how long you have had it, how old you are and how swiftly it progresses. When I was initially diagnosed I was obsessed with this question. I searched the internet for weeks trying to find any definitive answer. Finally there was one on a forum by an anonymous author. "You'll have five good years, five OK years, five bad years and then you'll die." By the time I found it I figured I had about fifteen months of good before I entered into the five OK years, a sobering realization. That was almost eight years ago and I'm still rocking along in the good years. Sometimes the answers we seek are to the wrong questions.

The reaction of family and friends can be a confirming experience, or it can be unexpectedly painful. For some of us our news was met with warm support and heart-felt expressions of concern, for others the response was less gratifying. For a few the response was devastating. Most of us have had experiences that span the spectrum and with the help of friends, both old and new and family we have survived and moved on.

Even the most supportive family and friends can fail to understand what is needed. In their efforts to console, sustain and boost our morale they can hover. In their zeal to make everything better they can be unintentionally dismissive of the feelings overwhelming us and understandably eager to change the subject.

Sometimes it is only those who have been through it who seem to actually understand what we are feeling and afford us the opportunity to vent those feelings without shame or fear of being labeled a complainer. Often it is only with the additional support of those in the same situation that we are able to learn to grapple with our new status.
Pamela Kell

It is, after all, only our own ability to accept and deal with our condition that determines the quality of the life we will live.

SUB-TYPES OF PARKINSON DISEASE

My first brush with Parkinson disease was in 1979 when my mother-in-law was diagnosed at age sixty. During the next five years she deteriorated to being a nonverbal, wheelchair-bound invalid unable to recognize her children or grandchildren and then she died.

By 1998 when my symptoms were so apparent I could no longer deceive myself, I was afraid that I too had Parkinson disease and saw my first neurologist. She diagnosed Benign Essential Tremor (BET) as I was so young (53) and not bilateral. A year later I sought a second opinion from a Movement Disorder Specialist (MDS) and he pronounced that I did indeed, have Idiopathic Parkinson disease (IPD).

When I asked if I too, like my mother-in-law, would be dead soon I was assured my mother-in-law had another disease entirely, probably Multiple System Atrophy (MSA) or perhaps Progressive Supranuclear Palsy (PSP). Such an alphabet soup of diseases. Those of us who have been around for a while have become familiar with these acronyms and rarely think of how clique-ish it once felt; after all it is a kind of selectivity none of us wishes for, yet no one wants to feel excluded either. So, much as it pains me, WELCOME TO THE CLUB.

Understanding the difficulty in sorting out the different forms of parkinsonism and distinguishing one from the other, we have included the following short explanations of some of the conditions that are similar to Parkinson disease, yet very different in their progression and treatment.
Pamela Kell

Denial or Resignation

After a year, with no discernible progress, I sought a second opinion from a Movement Disorders Specialist. He pronounced what I already knew to be true, I had Parkinson disease. I don't cry ordinarily, but upon hearing "Parkinson disease" said aloud, the tears began and grew and continued. I could not speak. My young doctor had the presence not to talk to me, or to reassure me, or try to diminish the effect of his news on me and for ten minutes his only act was to hand me a box of tissues. For this kind, understanding lack of action I will always be grateful.

• **IDIOPATHIC PARKINSON DISEASE** is the most familiar form of Parkinson disease. It is the form most of us have even though it may eventually be found to comprise many separate diseases. The confusion begins, but doesn't stop there. There are a number of other conditions that may initially appear to be PD. Through tests, imaging and observation our doctors may see differences that help them refine or change a diagnosis. While symptoms may be similar in the early stages these conditions progress at different rates, respond differently to medication and over time look clinically distinct.

• **BENIGN ESSENTIAL TREMOR** may be diagnosed if symptoms are mild or the patient is younger than usual. BET can be distinguished from IPD as it is usually bilateral from the onset and often familial. BET may be diagnosed if tremor is with intentional movement rather than at rest or diminishes with alcohol.

• **SECONDARY SYMPTOMATIC PARKINSONISM** is caused by the introduction of toxins such as MPTP, manganese and carbon monoxide.

• **POST ENCEPHALITIC PARKINSONISM** is caused by a viral infection. Following World War I five million people around the globe suffered the illness some subsequently developed a devastating form of parkinsonism. These patients were the subject of the book *Awakenings* by Dr. Oliver Sacks.

• **VASCULAR PARKINSONISM** is an atypical form that may be the result of vascular, arterial or cardiac problems and is sometimes called lower-body parkinsonism, which as its name suggests shows more in walking problems. Fewer people in this group respond well to levodopa treatment, though it can vary.

• **POST-TRAUMATIC PARKINSONISM** is a form that is the result of repeated head injuries.

Other forms of parkinsonism and definitions of conditions that present similarly to PD are in an ongoing state of revision as doctors and researchers find out more about them.

The Parkinson Plus Syndromes are a group of disorders that very often present as PD in the early stages. They are increasingly regarded as conditions in their own right, though doctors and patients organisations often group them together. The most common are:

- MULTIPLE SYSTEM ATROPHY (MSA)
- PROGRESSIVE SUPRANUCLEAR PALSY (PSP)
- LEWY BODY DISEASE

These conditions may respond less positively to Parkinson medications, have a faster rate of progress and a higher probability of dementia. It is hoped, as they become better understood, treatments for them will improve.

Parkinsonism can also be caused by drug use, medical and non-medical:

- TARDIVE DYSKINESIA Tardive dyskinesia is a neurological syndrome caused by the long-term use of neuroleptic drugs. Tardive dyskinesia is characterized by repetitive, involuntary, purposeless movements especially of the lip and tongue.

The majority of people with parkinsonism are classified as having idiopathic Parkinson disease (IPD). The other types account for around 15% of all parkinsonism diagnoses combined.

Confused yet? With a diagnosis of IPD there are many distinctive symptoms; these include the four cardinal signs, bradykinesia (slowness of movement), tremor, rigidity, and balance or instability problems, as well as a multitude of other symptoms that vary from person to person.

Until all the sub-types of Parkinsonism are identified and clinical trials designed accordingly, using medications will be a process of trial and error, with only so many to choose from . . . . .

Young Onset Parkinson & Late Onset Parkinson
Is there a difference?

Literature reviews seem to indicate that younger onset people tend to have more problems with dyskinesia and dystonia and it is thought they may have fewer incidences of dementia. Ages vary for identification of young onset; some define it as under age 50 and others under age 40. It is not uncommon for patients between 50-60 to be told that they are too young for PD. Patients themselves agree that the impact of the illness is greater on younger PwP in terms of employment and income, young families, psychosocial problems, possible premature retirement and longer disease duration.

Those diagnosed later in life may already be struggling with, among other things, conditions such as arthritis, cardiac problems, osteoporosis or deafness and poor vision and may have other complex needs. A perception that PD is a disease of aging can mean treatment options are narrower or that referral to a PD specialist may not happen.

Most who are diagnosed with Parkinson disease will present with at least one of the cardinal symptoms, though that symptom may not be the problem that is most troublesome. The list of symptoms is long, each person's list will be individual and it is rare for any one person to have every complaint on the list, so there can be considerable difficulty nailing down a definite diagnosis, especially early on. Time usually helps clarify things for PwP and doctors, but how much time? Sometimes it is a matter of months, sometimes years and occasionally, with an unusual presentation, a precise diagnosis is never made. These are a small sample of the ways in which Parkinson disease can differ. This has led to its being labeled a "designer disease." Many PwP believe that when the causes are finally identified idiopathic Parkinson disease will be seen as a spectrum of separate conditions all responsive to similar treatments. Until then we are in the same foxhole fighting the same enemy.

The good news is we are there together. Pamela Kell

Wow, what a ride!!

I have been diagnosed with Parkinson for a little over a month and the only appropriate description is "what a ride". I am only 32 years old and never imagined, that at this age, I would face such an ordeal. It is difficult to write about the emotions I've felt and equally hard to go through them. It started with confusion, led to anger, progressed to fear and then set in as reality.

Confusion

I went to the doctor with a right hand tremble I associated with stress. I had noticed it in stressful times but didn't think much about it. When things in my life improved, the tremble worsened. It was then my confusion began. I was confused about what to do, confused about the cause and confused by why it was occurring. My husband noticed the problem and called and made me a doctor appointment. The ride had just begun.

I was referred to a neurologist for a nerve study, maybe a nerve in my right arm had been damaged. Wrong. I was then sent for an MRI for the possibilities of stroke, MS or other vascular disease. Wrong again. After further discussion and tests on arm movement and leg movement, I began to take Parkinson medication as a diagnostic test on how I would respond. I wanted the medicine to work so I could type fast again, so I could put my daughter's hair in a ponytail, so I could eat normally, so I could put my makeup on normally and many other things. On the other hand, I didn't want it to indicate a diagnosis I didn't want. I responded to the medication with flying colors. I can do all those things normally now. At that point, confusion sets in. It is confusing with such a 'gray area' disease. I didn't have clear answers on why it happened, how, or how I could help myself.

Anger

After you struggle with the confusion of probably never having clarity, anger sets in. I was so mad at myself for letting it happen. Logically, I know that there is nothing that I could have done to prevent it. I was so mad because my family and friends were going to have to go through this battle with me. It's a disease that probably leads a lot of people over the edge with anger. It is not only anger at being diagnosed, but anger with the struggles you are faced with and knowing it is probably not ever going to be easy again.

After I was diagnosed, it was suggested I see a specialist. Specialists have the appropriate knowledge of the disease along with the most important thing, effective treatment. I thought this would be the easy task. If I am going to fight this disease for the rest of my life, I want the best specialist in the field who knows how to slow down the progression. I think I have the right to decide what is right for me. I am the one in this situation. I am still battling to get to the right specialist, but I am headed in the right direction on this uncertain road.

Fear

When I was first diagnosed, I was afraid my life was coming to an end. I imagined that I wouldn't be able to do so many things due to having Parkinson disease. I have a three year old little girl - I can't imagine not being involved in every aspect of her life. I was afraid that was about to be taken away. As for me, I didn't know much about the disease. The first thing that popped in my head was a mental image of a woman who could barely speak or move and was angry with the world. I was fearful that I was going to become that woman . . .

I have a wonderful husband who I, from the day I married him, knew that I would spend the rest of my life with and together we could dream about what the future holds for us. I was scared that PD would change that reality, not because he would be the kind of man to leave me, or give up, but because Parkinson was going to change who I was. Fear can do so many things to your mind that it makes you believe its going to happen. I also feared how I was going to tell people. I live in a small town and knew that is was inevitable that people were going to find out. It is very embarrassing to eat and have your right arm shake while you bring your fork to your mouth, or be talking and your arm shakes, or even write something down and only barely do it because of the tremor. I never know how people will respond or what they are thinking . . .

Reality

I have come to terms with my situation with help from my family and friends. I have realized that I am always going to be confused. There are always going to be battles with this disease that cause me anger; I will always fear how people are going to respond to me and what the future holds. Life is going to throw you curve balls. That's a given. You can stand there and do nothing, or you can swing at them and live life. I am determined to keep swinging at each and every curve ball that comes my way.

These bumps in the road of life are normal and expected. I am going to fasten my seat belt and be ready for the ride, no matter how many rough spots may be ahead.

Andrea Dickey

Andrea's diagnosis was changed to Dopamine Responsive Dystonia (DRD), which is similar to Parkinson disease in its symptoms, but has a better prognosis. Since then it has been changed yet again back to PD. We have included her eloquent descriptions of her emotional journey, so typical of people coming new to a long term disorder. The changes in diagnoses are evidence of how difficult PD is to diagnose.

SLICE OF LIFE
Jon the patient/Jon the neuroscientist

Bradykinesia, rigidity and tremor - the unholy trinity of Parkinsonian symptomatology. I had spent most of my research career looking at dopamine in the basal ganglia and for years I had drilled these cardinal symptoms into the medical students. So it shouldn't have been dificult to identify the same symptoms in myself, right? But somehow I missed them.

Bradykinesia - you never really notice yourself slowing down. It's just part of getting older, you tell yourself. Rigidity- just a little bit of rheumatism or arthritis surely. No big deal. And tremor? Well, it was probably no worse than the morning after a boozy dinner! It all seems obvious now but, like so many people with Parkinson I did not recognise the early symptoms for what they were.

So what drove me to the doctor? Initially it was a stiff shoulder, a surprisingly common presenting symptom, but mainly it was my handwriting. I had been marking scripts for the Open University in September 2006 (good old-fashioned pen and paper, none of this digital malarkey) and was struggling to find the right words of encouragement. Keen to avoid repetition, I turned to my March report. In six months my handwriting had changed from elegant copperplate to GP prescriptionese! It was a lightbulb moment and although neither my doctor nor I said the words, we were both thinking PD. The neurologist flirted briefly with other differential diagnoses before a DATscan removed all doubt and had me peeing radioactivity for a week. My kids called me 'Chernobyl Dad'. I am sure I fogged them.

Having worked on the basal ganglia for many years, I am only too aware of the irony of being diagnosed with PD. And in a particularly wry twist, I find myself being treated with a drug that I worked on some 20 years ago.

But what is it like being a patient and a neuroscientist? Whilst Jon the patient understandably resents the increasing disability and erosion of function, Jon the neuroscientist can't help but be fascinated by the tremor, dystonias and rigidity of the PD and the impulsivity and creativity induced by the drugs. You can take the scientist out of science but you can't take the science out of the scientist!

So while Jon the patient shakes enough that most of his spaghetti Bolognese lands on his shirt, Jon the scientist is fascinated by how the rhythm and amplitude of the tremors changes throughout the day as the thalamus and internal pallidum vie for the motor cortex's attention like squabbling siblings. Heading to the kitchen for a cloth, Jon the patient almost breaks into a run. Jon the scientist recognises festination instantly and adds another tick to his list of symptoms.

Exercise is increasingly recognised as a valuable means of delaying progression. But even there, the scientist does not switch off. While Jon the patient stiffly plays cricket, mentally calculating his score, Jon the scientist is totting up his UPDRS score. Hoehn and Yahr are to the scientist what Duckworth and Lewis are to the cricketer.

Diagnosed in late 2006, I started treatment at Easter 2007. Currently I take rotigotine and rasagiline each day, the dopamine agonist for symptomatic relief and the MAO-B inhibitor for neuroprotection. No levodopa yet. This regime seems to work best against rigidity. The tremors are remarkably recalcitrant little blighters.

Stupid though it may sound, I believe there has never been a better time to have Parkinson. 40 years on from the first use of levodopa, we have a battery of drug strategies. Moreover, the pipeline of potential new drug targets has never been richer. And then of course there are stem cells. Already talk is less about treatment and more about cure. These are optimistic times.

At the end of September the World Parkinson Congress came to Glasgow. Scientists and patients were present at the same conference and, to tell you the truth, I could hardly wait. By the end of the conference, I was so inspired that I wrote a blog entitled The Promised Land

Do I still work? Yes I do. Full-time and then some. Although I left academic neuroscience in 2003 when my lab closed, I have maintained a degree of involvement through teaching for the Open University and my ex-students here and abroad. I also work as a consultant for the Cure Parkinson's Trust.

> For my research life,
> I chose Parkinson.
> For my real life,
> Parkinson chose me.
> For better for worse,
> it's what you make of it.

Jon Stamford, PhD, is currently working on the international **Parkinson's Movement** initiative. designed to bring science, medicine and patients together to progress towards a cure

TREMOR

Tremor, one of the cardinal signs of PD, is described classically as a rhythmic to-and-fro, bidirectional oscillation, particularly of the upper limbs, which has a frequency of 4-6 cps, which occurs in a pill-rolling fashion at rest and which disappears with movement. It commonly is unilateral in its first appearance and may remain so for years. Initially it may be little more than an inconvenience. As its persistence and severity increase tremor can be debilitating, especially if it affects your dominant hand or if your job requires skilled use of both hands.

It is estimated that about 50% of people with PD don't present with the classic pill-rolling resting tremor but, in fact, have other types of tremor.

Tremor is a complex topic and may be approached in several different ways:

1. by cause (which are myriad, including substances like caffeine – either its use or withdrawal and other diseases such as hyperthyroidism. The list of possible causes for tremor is like a list of chapters in a medical text.)

2. by location (limb either one side or both, chin, head, tongue, voice, e.g.)

3. by the situation in which it occurs (stress, rest, with voluntary movement, with sustained postures)

4. by factors which improve or worsen it (for example, stress worsens many forms of tremor, alcohol intake may relieve benign essential tremor).

Most people have a physiologic tremor, that is a limb tremor that is increased with voluntary movements or with sustained postures, occurs at a frequency of 6-12 cps, is increased with stress or anxiety, and is finer in its range of oscillations than is the classic PD tremor. The movement may be hard to see because it is so fine. This type of tremor, because it is so fine and fast, is rarely confused with PD. Benign essential tremor which is slower in frequency, however, may be a PD patient's first misdiagnosis. Benign essential tremor, however, is usually bilateral, not unilateral and is not associated with the other symptoms which a PD patient manifests.

Because the PwP may have different types of tremor, they may find themselves on several of a variety of medications, including classic PD medicines, beta-blockers and others like amantadine.

May Griebel MD
Professor of Pediatrics and Neurology (ret.)
University of Arkansas for Medical Sciences
and the Arkansas Children's Hospital

BALANCE & FALLS

I was diagnosed ten years ago. During those ten years I have fallen about ten times. Each and every fall I have been able to analyze and determine that it could have happened to anyone.

Once I turned and stepped right in the middle of my old faithful dog, who was asleep at my feet. The fall came from trying not to kill her. Another time while walking across a parking lot the heel of my right shoe caught in the cuff of my left pant leg and because my hands were full of files, I fell like a tree.

The latest in the series happened at my daughter's new house on Christmas Eve when I failed to recall there was a short step down from her entry to her family room and fell, sprawling in to the floor in front of neighbors and in-laws without a hint of my usual grace.

Being assured by all witnesses that anyone under those circumstances could have fallen equally as flat and most likely would have broken something in the process, I began to feel a little better until I asked, "How many times have you hit the dirt in the last five years?" So far no one has given me any number save zero.

It appears there is but one conclusion to be drawn. My balance recovery abilities have been compromised by Parkinson disease.

This is far less a problem than that experienced by many whose equilibrium has fundamentally diminished and balance is a problem under all circumstances. So far, I fall as a result of specific causes, a fact for which I am profoundly grateful. Nevertheless, it is still a departure from others with brain cells intact, who may be able to stop their downward trajectory and recover without making complete spectacles of themselves.

Loss of balance is not a foregone conclusion and there are therapies to maintain and even improve the abilities we have. Exercise of course. is crucial and benefits a multitude of issues encountered with Parkinson disease. The best defense against falling, due to loss of balance is a good offence. Be proactive. Anticipate problems and train for them.

Always look where you are preparing to step, hold on to stair rails, learn to use a cane or a walker before you need to, wear supportive shoes and be careful of bifocals, they make the ground move. Being prepared is not the same as giving up. We prepare for all the important events in our lives so that we can handle the unexpected.

This is just one more thing that we have the ability to make less difficult by taking a common sense approach. Becoming cognizant of our surroundings is not a bad idea even for those without any physical impairment but for those of us who are challenged in one way or another, or are likely to be, it is mandatory.
Pamela Kell

Difficulty with balance occurs early in PD:
It isn't appreciated because it's not asked about nor tested.

Dr Lieberman et al. devised a questionnaire and simple tests to assess balance early, before patients fall and to assess it independently from walking difficulty and freezing of gait.

Balance difficulty resulting in falls is a well-recognized complication late in PD. It's not responsive to levodopa or other dopamine drugs or to deep brain stimulation (DBS). Less well known is that balance difficulty can occur early in PD. The reason it's not appreciated is that it's not asked about. The original Unified Parkinson Disease Rating Scale (UPDRS), the standard test for PD, contained a question on falling, not on balance. Falling is a late complication of balance difficulty. Asking about falling misses the people who have balance difficulty and are not falling. This group of patients may respond best to physical, occupational and balance therapy. Once a PD patient begins to fall the physical, occupational and balance therapy may not help because it's too late. The new UPDRS asks about gait and balance as though gait, walking and balance are the same. This is not so. Patients can have trouble walking, shuffling their feet and not have balance difficulty. And patients may have balance difficulty and not trouble walking. Think of balance and walking as the brake and accelerator on your car. If you have defective brakes, you will still be able to drive the car, but you are more likely to crash. And you can have good brakes and not be able to drive the car because the accelerator is defective.

To sort out the differences between balance and walking in addition to questions on walking we added a questionnaire about balance difficulty and in addition to the regular part of the UPDRS examination we added 3 simple tests: standing on one leg, turning 360 degrees, tandem walking and a balance score that's the sum of the 3 tests. We next examined balance in 102 consecutive PD patients.

Patients who reported difficulty with balance had PD longer 7.11 years (+4.5 years) versus patients who reported NO difficulty with balance 3.95 years (+1.79 years). This difference was significant. Additionally, 45% of 62 patients with PD for 1-5 years and 54% of 28 patients with PD for 6-10 years had balance difficulty indicating that balance difficulty is an early symptom of PD provided it is asked about. Patients who had balance difficulty had difficulty standing on one leg, turning and tandem walking. The tests enabled us to distinguish, early in PD, patients with balance difficulty utilizing a questionnaire that complements the questions on the UPDRS.

The balance questionnaire and the three balance tests provide a simple way of measuring balance difficulty early in PD before patients fall. This should allow testing of treatments, surgical and non-surgical, dopaminergic and non dopaminergic, before advanced balance difficulties (with falls) occur.

Dr. Abraham Lieberman is Director of the Muhammad Ali Parkinson Center, and Director of Movement Disorders at the Barrow Neurological Institute, Phoenix, Arizona, USA.

Bradykinesia and Parkinson Disease

Bradykinesia is a term derived from the Greek language meaning slow movement. Bradykinesia is a cardinal symptom of Parkinson that refers to the slowness of movement, difficulty initiating movement, and loss of automatic movement people living with Parkinson disease may experience. Bradykinesia is thought to occur when the brain fails to execute the command to move.

Although it is one of the most common features of Parkinson, bradykinesia may appear after tremors emerge. Yet subtle signs can be detected in the early stages of Parkinson. These include slowness of shrugging the shoulders, lack of gesturing, decreased arm swing and reduction in amplitude of movement, particularly with repetitive movements. It is because of this last symptom that a doctor may ask the person with Parkinson to perform a finger-tapping test.

Bradykinesia has many facets, depending on which part of the body is affected. Some people with Parkinson may lose spontaneous facial expression (also called masked facies, hypomimia) and experience a decrease in the frequency of blinking. For some, the loss of spontaneous movement is characterized by a lack of gesturing and a tendency to sit motionless.

Bradykinesia of an individual's dominant hand can result in small and slow handwriting (micrographia), in difficulty shaving, brushing teeth, combing hair, buttoning, applying make-up and other activities of daily living.

A person's walk may become slow with a shortened stride length, a tendency to shuffle and as mentioned, a decrease in arm swing. Bradykinesia not only affects the arms and legs but can also impair movement of the torso (truncal bradykinesia), leading to difficulty in rising from a deep chair, getting out of automobiles and turning in bed.

Fatigue, a common complaint in the mild stage of the disease, may be related to mild bradykinesia or rigidity. With advancing bradykinesia, slowness and difficulty in the execution of activities of daily living increase and can prevent a person with Parkinson from driving safely; the foot movement from the accelerator to the brake pedal is too slow.

Bradykinesia can cause soft speech (hypophonia) and lead the voice to develop a monotonous tone with a lack of inflection (aprosody). Many individuals living with Parkinson find they drool regularly. This results not from excessive production of saliva, but instead from failure to swallow spontaneously, a feature of bradykinesia. Swallowing may become impaired with advancing disease.

Levodopa is the gold standard treatment for easing the effects of bradykinesia and is very effective in doing so. Additionally for some individuals, reminders or cues can help. For example, arm swing may become normal if the person with Parkinson, with effort, reminds him or herself to have the arms swing when walking.

Stanley Fahn, M.D.,
Chair, Scientific Director, Parkinson Disease Foundation
Movement Disorders Division Chief
H. Houston Merritt Professor of Neurology
Division of Movement Disorders
Columbia University Medical Center

Bradykinesia makes the limbs feel rigid and almost impossible to move even though muscle tone when examined by the neurologist is normal. When one tries to move, it is as if the camera of life is set on extreme "slo-mo." Each movement is labored and takes exhausting extra effort, as if one were walking through the thickest "molasses in January."

The fatigue that results from attempting to move compounds the slowness. The length of a hallway can look as long as a marathon when one's movements are so slow and labored.

May Griebel

THE ROLE OF RIGIDITY IN PARKINSON DISEASE

The diagnosis of idiopathic Parkinson disease is based on the presence and recognition of the four cardinal motor features of the illness. These include tremor at rest, bradykinesia, rigidity and in the middle stages of the disease loss of postural reflexes (balance problems).

Rigidity is defined as resistance to the passive movement of a joint related to increased tone in the associated muscles.

The increase in muscle tone does not vary significantly regardless of which direction the muscles are moving and the velocity of the movement. This is an important point in discriminating rigidity arising from basal ganglia dysfunction (as in PD) from the spasticity that results from injury to another motor pathway (stroke, MS, trauma, tumors etc.) where the increase in tone is more specific to a particular group of muscles and is velocity-dependent.

Rigidity in PD is often accompanied by "cogwheeling," a ratchety movement of the joint probably related to underlying tremor.

Rigidity is commonly mistaken for arthritis or other rheumatological problems. Thus, rigidity can be the underlying cause of joint pain such as the very common shoulder pain noted in many newly diagnosed PD patients as well as the flexed posture seen in some PD patients.

Furthermore, bradykinesia and rigidity may combine to result in complaints such as difficulty turning in bed, loss of facial expression and gait and balance problems.

Notably, rigidity responds well to dopaminergic medications as well as to subthalamic nucleus and globus pallidus deep brain stimulation (DBS). In fact rigidity is the one of the most reliable clinical signs when we are assessing benefits for DBS.

There are certain measures that all PD patients should take upon themselves to improve their rigidity. I strongly encourage physical and occupational therapy, which has been documented to benefit rigidity. Furthermore, I have noted that in my own patients who perform daily stretching and range of motion exercises there is improvement in complaints of stiffness and joint discomfort and increased flexibility.

Michael Rezak, M.D., Ph.D.
Medical Director of the APDA National Young Onset Center as well as the Director of the Movement Disorders Center and Co-Director of the Deep Brain Stimulation Program of the Neurosciences Institute at Central DuPage Hospital in Winfield, IL.

FREEZING TIPS

Freezing is a very frustrating symptom of Parkinson and it doesn't mean we are cold all the time!! I approach a doorway and 'freeze' or stop dead in my tracks and then the problem is initiating movement again. There are some tricks to overcome this.

When approaching a doorway it is sometimes possible to 'walk yourself through the gap' mentally avoiding stopping in the first place. Unfortunately this rarely works with me so I find myself 'frozen' to the spot in the doorway. This is when I try a few other tricks.

Counting in my head helps as does marching. I lift my legs in a marching action which somehow seems to get movement going. If I am not working very well and already using my walking stick then I kick the stick and this initiates movement. The main thing is to avoid festination (taking lots of tiny steps but not moving forward much) as you become unbalanced and risk falling.

Paula Wittekind

The day I met Mister Park ......

You ask me, "Who is Mister Park?" He's a degenerative and progressive chronic disease! Since August 1994 I have struggled with this intruder in my life. It started in 1992. I was 44 years old, married for 28 years. My daughter was 22 years old. I had difficulties moving my right leg for several months. My writing had become small, irregular and semi-unreadable. My back was in pain all the time and painkillers gave me no relief. The doctors and nurses at work and I myself had never even thought of Parkinson. I had been a chief nurse in a department of internal diseases and oncology since 1972. After appointments with many different doctors, rheumatologists, psychotherapists, a diagnosis was made in ten minutes by a professor in Brussels. The doctors I had seen at the hospital where I worked for many years only spoke about depression. The verdict was PARKINSON DISEASE. I don't know what I felt at this moment. For me, even though I was a nurse, it was a disease of older people and I was only 44.

Once out of the office my husband said to me that with our love we would be able to battle against this disease. The announcement to the family was very difficult; amazement, disbelief and denial were the principal reactions. With their love, patience and devotion I was armed to attack the disease. My husband was always near me and at that time I could say life, even with Parkinson, was beautiful. It was, and still is, hard that I had to stop my job as a nurse. I loved helping others; now I was on the other side. I was the one who needed help.

Being active is one of the best drugs. We shouldn't live alone in a Parkinson world. Isolation is what many people do. They are afraid to be seen by others. We must say, 'We are normal people with less dopamine in our brains'. My daughter has always had difficulties accepting my disease. She would like the mother she had before. Her anger is a reflection of her anxiety and denial of the disease.

But Mister Park hadn't finished with my life. After 33 years of marriage my husband left me and asked for a divorce. But can I blame him? It is awful to see a beloved one with such a disease. Your spouse and friends can't do anything for you except watch the disease progress. I had to sell the house we had adapted for my disease, my father died that year and I lost my dog.

It took a few years for things to get better but now I can say that life is beautiful even with Parkinson. My daughter and I built a new house. The person who has helped me most is my little granddaughter Elise. She is now 5 years old. She is the sunshine in my life and gives me the strength to go on battling against Mister Park. For her it is normal that I have difficulties standing up, walking, picking up a paper, that I fall to the ground. Her little hand reaches out to me and with her lovely smile she says, "Mammy I will help you." She makes life much easier for me. The friends by my side are real friends but they are a small group; others went away the day they knew I had PD.

I have learned much as a result of PD: Here in Belgium the disease is not well known. Doctors need to adapt their way of caring for us and first have a good dialogue with their patients. Without patients who really know about PD they cannot develop good treatments. There is a lot to do. Tina

D on't look backward, or forward, live for the present day.

RANDOM THOUGHTS

EQUALITY

I am Iraqi
I have Parkinson disease
In this I am equal to you
My tremor has the same rhythm as yours
And I drag my leg just like you do
Our common suffering bonds us together
Like brothers

A SCENE FROM CHILDHOOD

The date: 1951
The place: My great aunt's house
in South Baghdad suburb,
about 200 meters from Tigris river

An extremely quiet boy of eight slips in,
no body notices him
Instead of playing carelessly as children do
He chooses to watch again a scene,
taking place in this house every day
He alone perceives and feels the drama
His eyes are fixed on his gentle great aunt
sitting in the mild winter sun,
Every part of her body shaking constantly
Her hands, arms, legs and lips shiver and shiver
She calls in her low voice
for her teenage daughter, Bushra
"Bushra, Bushra, please help me
to make my daily walk
(round the small open courtyard)"
Bushra is irritated and pretends not to hear.
The woman pleads again and again.
The boy thinks to himself:
"Don't worry Aunty, I will help you
when I grow up to be a man"

PRAYER FOR TEARS

The date: 1981
The place: Baghdad-UK-USA hospitals

The boy is now a man
He finds true love for the first time
But soon tragedy strikes
God takes away the one whom he loves most
He carries his sorrows patiently
But the pain digs in,
deeper and deeper inside his mind
And no longer can he feel it
As the memories fade away, his eyes cry for tears
He prays for tears like an arid earth cries for rain

COUNTRY LOST

Turmoil and tyranny in his country finally drive him out
The house he built brick by brick: abandoned!
The books he treasured: abandoned!
The little things and photos: abandoned!
Now the entire world is his country
Happy to carry his light bag
With identity card that proves he belongs
to the human race

MIRROR

I look in the mirror

I see a strange face
Whose face is this?
It isn't mine

EGO

Happy in his empty shell

Stars in heaven sooth his soul
Silence brings peace to his heart
But his ego plays games with him
Never gives up endless demands
Never stops seeking to see its self in the eyes of others
Oh! how much he wishes to devour this cursed enemy

PARKINSON DISEASE

My PD is my ever-present friend
I accept him even when he trespasses my territory
And plays havoc with my life
He demands full attention
And total devotion!
But I know he is the indispensable friend
Who came at the right time
To save me from worse calamities
And lift the veil that made me blind
And lost for direction
I know he will be with me when all others leave

Imad

JIN'S STORY

I was 46-years-old when I realized my gait was strange. My left foot was dragging and my left arm didn't move back and forwards. One year later, in 2007, I was diagnosed with Parkinson disease, but I was NOT ready to accept it. Why did this degenerative brain disease happen to me? Did I get punished for doing something wrong? To me everything had seemed easy in my life until then. I was married with two grown sons, but suddenly PD shook my whole life. Ironically I found that I really wanted to grasp my life more than ever since my diagnosis with Parkinson.

Whenever I meet difficulties I believe that at the other end a door will open for me. While surfing the Internet I read a webpage which attracted my interest. It was about the Parkinson's Disease Foundation's Quilt Project which was going to be displayed at the World Parkinson Congress in 2010. This inspired me to get involved and I felt at once that I had my own purpose in the PD community. The more stitches I put into my quilt piece, the closer I got to my Parkinson disease. I actively changed my perspective on PD. I took my first step into the WPC world with a quilt square and a video entry which took 2nd place. At the WPC I made many PwP friends and met qualified caregivers (I'd never heard about them before, as we do not have them in Korea) and people from medical teams and patient-centered organizations (they raise a lot of money, enough to manage big research projects!!) and now I have a greater confidence in myself as a PwP.

Korean people receive nation-wide medical insurance benefits and PD is classified as a rare disease, so PwP bear only around 10~20% of the cost of treatment. If PD symptoms don't allow you a normal daily life you can call a free caregiver, but this doesn't always come easy because PwP in early stages don't look that different when their drugs are working. Even doctors don't always understand our personal suffering unless we are hospitalized. In this regard I expect that medical staff can then come closer to PwP and see that we live real not 'laboratory' lives.

My PD friend Jung Hee told me that she would like to have more regional PwP communities, to share our PD sufferings and do art activities like music or drawing and sports. Yes, she's right. All Korean PwP have now are internet-based communities and of course we do share many things, but I'm not sure we can make much difference by complaining. We need to let people know more about PD and how we can help each other.

Jin Kyoung Choae

How a quilt brought one PwP half way round the world

Jin's quilt square below was part of the PDF sponsored Parkinson Quilt Project, which features quilt sqares made by PwP from around the world.

Her video, WALKING, was joint runner-up of the WPC 2010 video contest.

In 2013 Jin is an Ambassador for the 3rd WPC in Montreal.

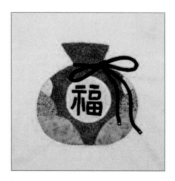

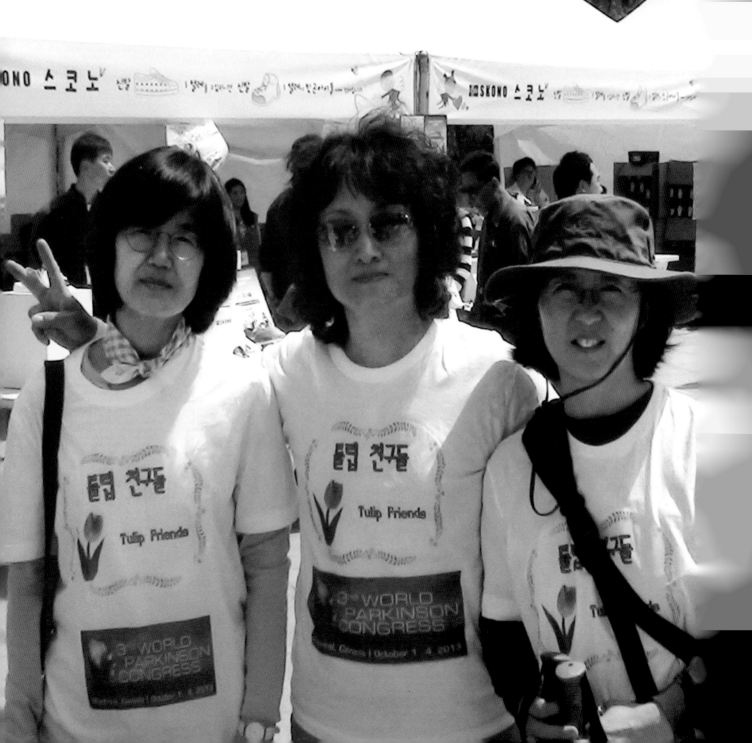

SIGNS & SYMPTOMS ETC. • DYSKINESIA • DYSTONIA

Signs, Symptoms & Side Effects

Deciding if something is a sign and symptom of PD versus a possible medication side effect can be confusing. The basic signs of PD are tremor, rigidity, slow movement or bradykinesia and postural instability. Medically, signs are those things that the doctor can see. Symptoms, on the other hand, are those things that are subjective and experienced by the patient. Those may or may not be taken into account by the physician at the time of diagnosis.

When a patient goes into treatment and is placed on medication, sometimes new movements develop. One wonders whether the new findings represent progression of the basic disease or relate to the medication.

Dyskinesias are medication-related and are not seen in PD patients who are not on medication. Dyskinesias occur often at peak dose times. However, people prone to dyskinesias may find that their movements are increased with stress or excitement. Even eating in a restaurant may bring out unwanted dyskinesias. Also they can occur suddenly in a rapid fashion alternating with dystonia, usually in later disease, in a process known as "on-off." Dystonia and dyskinesia are both terms that refer to abnormal movements based on basal ganglia dysfunction. Dyskinesias have been said to be a side-effect of L-dopa but not of dopamine agonists. However, with all things Parkinsonian, people differ and some PwP's movements have worsened when the dose of their dopamine agonist is increased.

Missed Diagnosis: A person will not be placed on medication appropriately if the PD diagnosis is missed. This happens most often if the person is younger or has atypical symptoms. Although the average age of patients is mid-fifties at diagnosis, there are significant numbers of " early onset" or "young onset" PD. Patients fifty and younger have been told that "they were too young to have PD."

The most effective way to be treated appropriately is to document your movements or tonal problems, describe their nature and the times of their occurrence and the times of your medication doses so that any relationship between the two can be assessed and then share that information with your physician.

May Griebel. MD

DYSKINESIA

"Dys" means faulty and "kinesia" means movement. Thus, the term dyskinesia could cover all abnormal or faulty movements in PD. However, "dyskinesia" is widely used in the PD community to mean the fast, twisting or jerky movements that can occur as a medication side effect. It may make a patient appear as if "they have ants in their pants". Dyskinesias occur usually at peak dose times. However, people prone to dyskinesias may find that their movements are increased with stress or excitement. They can also occur suddenly in a rapid fashion alternating with dystonia, in late stage PD in a process known as "on-off."

DYSTONIA

Dystonia is based on root words which mean "abnormal tone." Dystonia refers to increased muscle tone, that is, the stiffening, pulling, drawing, cramping which can be associated with abnormal postures, particularly in the hands and feet. Other signs of dystonias may be such things as curling of the toes, a shoulder held too high, or torsion of one's neck. Dystonia is part of the disease process along with rigidity and bradykinesia.

Dystonia can occur as medication is wearing off or when the medication is not sufficiently effective, as might occur with absorption problems or a late or inadequate dose.

LOOKING BEYOND
THE GOLD STANDARD, L-DOPA

l-dopa is not a perfect diamond
but it has not yet been surpassed
it's failings have not been addressed

neither have the failings in thinking,
like, when the cascade of events in our brains happens
why do people think the lack of neuromelanin in our post mortem brains
is the most important sign of pd
when there are living specimens
ready and willing to be questioned, examined
at all stages of this condition
and show what PD
ACTUALLY IS
moreover
why do they have to prove it in creatures that cannot speak
when there are millions of creatures who can!

and again
all the non human models of pd
are not for us
not to prove what our condition IS
we are the proof of what our condition is . . .

our positions as stakeholders are different . . ." Lindy Ashford

DOPAMINE
· Dopamine is a small molecule, similar to an amino acid.
· Produced and stored in small vesicles within the neuronal cells of Substantia Nigra.
· Acts as a chemical messenger/neurotransmitter in the brain.
· Required for regulating parts of the brain that control our motor (movement) as well as non-motor (emotional, pleasure, pain and addictive) responses.

The Gold Standard.... L-dopa

Sooner or later if you are a PwP you are likely to come in contact with the drug that is called the 'gold standard' of treatments - levodopa/carbidopa - sometimes combined with a third drug, entacapone, to lengthen its period of effectiveness..

Once you start taking it you are likely to be on it for life, like insulin for diabetics. You are unlikely to be told this if it is the first treatment you've been offered. If you've hit a barrier with dopamine agonist treatment, you may approach l-dopa with some hesitation - it has a reputation of only being effective for around 5 years before disturbing side effects appear.

While this is true for some, patients have found a wide range of experience. Some go 20 years or more with no significant problems, others become sensitized within a year or two. Levodopa is highly effective in the treatment of PD, and has been around for over 40 years.

Since it was introduced, millions, probably billions, of research dollars have been poured into research for better treatments. Most do not get past trial stage. While there are promising treatments in the pipeline, there are currently few new medications that have been licensed for use in PD. Of those that are on their way, most are several years away from being approved for patients, who are weary of the ongoing 'five year' wait for new treatments. They are now busy lobbying for the most promising developments, in the hope that they will not come too late for the next generation of PwP.

Paula Wittekind

A major problem with current medications for Parkinson disease is that they do not control the symptoms all the time and do not address the non-motor problems of PD.

Seventy five percent of these patients experience an average of three hours a day in which the effects of their medications 'wear off' and symptoms of their disease returns.

Are All Generics Equal?
Linda Morgan, RPh.

Haven't we all wondered if our round yellow generic 'Sinemet' will work the same as the original yellow oval Sinemet? Are generics equal to the brand name medication? YES, according to the FDA. "When a generic drug product is approved, it has met rigorous standards established by the FDA with respect to identity, strength, quality, purity and potency." It must be therapeutically equivalent, meaning it must be the exact same active ingredient and act the same in the body - reach the same levels in the blood. A recent evaluation showed that the absorption rate of the generics studied varied 3.5% from the brands, some slightly less, some slightly more: an acceptable difference. What can vary from the brand name product and the generics are the inactive ingredients such as fillers and dyes.

Some medications have a low therapeutic index, meaning a very low increase in drug could produce toxic effects. These meds include digoxin, warfarin and phenytoin. It's best to stay with one brand or generic type for these medications.

With all this said, you and I, people with PD, know our bodies better than anyone. Do not use the information above as an excuse for not questioning why you have pink pills instead of white this month. Pharmacists make mistakes too; your prescription could have been filled incorrectly. In addition, a new generic may be causing headaches due to the inactive ingredients. If you have been given a generic and you truly feel like it doesn't work as well, talk to your pharmacist and/or physician. I've personally had one generic medication that did not seem to be producing the same results so I changed to another generic and have had good results.

In summary, generics are tested and are equivalent to brand name products. However, listen to your body and talk to your physician and/or pharmacist about any concerns that you may have.

I was diagnosed with Parkinson disease in October of 2005. The day before Thanksgiving of that same year I was enrolling into my first clinical trial at Duke. And ever since I have been involved in clinical trial advocacy. In July of 2008 I participated in the Parkinson's Disease Foundation's inaugural Clinical Research Learning Institute, a three day training that prepares people living with PD to serve as advocates within the clinical research process. I have presented to regional as well national groups about the clinical trial process. I currently serve on the Board of the Parkinson Association of the Carolinas. When not working with PD advocacy, I have a paid position as the director of a birth defects prevention program at Fullerton Genetics Center of Mission Hospital in Asheville, NC.

If you have been given a generic and you truly feel like it doesn't work as well, talk to your pharmacist and/or physician.

I've personally had one generic medication that did not seem to be producing the same results so changed to another generic and have had good results.

Linda Morgan, RPh

ONE LONG CLINICAL TRIAL?

Most people with Parkinson disease ultimately take medication to relieve some of the symptoms. Benefits and side effects vary in different people and can be successful for some and disastrous for another. This has led to speculation that there may be different causes and types of Parkinson.

Diagnosis itself can rely heavily on whether there is a response to medication. Once diagnosed and being treated, life with PD becomes one of symptom and medication management. Misdiagnosis is not uncommon as there are other conditions that have similar symptoms. A good Movement Disorder Specialist will know how to eliminate other illnesses and come to a diagnostic decision.

Finding the right medication can often be a matter of trial and error. Changing medications is not an easy process, but can become necessary if there is little or no therapeutic benefit, or side effects outweigh benefits. As a patient titrates down with one medication and up with another the condition itself can re-emerge with great force. Focus and care is needed to gain better symptomatic control without losing gains one has made.

As the range of symptoms that patients experience can be quite varied, many also search for alternative treatments and therapies and make lifestyle changes to help improve their condition. They have become aware of some of the shortfalls of current medications and of the difficulties of earlier generations of PwP who are now living with the result of longterm side effects of some medications, which are arguably as bad as the illness itself.

Until PwP find a medication balance that suits their needs it can indeed feel like one long clinical trial. Even if a balance has been achieved, the illness itself can progress, making further changes to medication necessary. **Paula Wittekind**

TALK ABOUT CATCH 22

Most patients taking carbidopa/levodopa experience an almost total reduction in symptoms in the beginning, the Paradise Period. Paradise will usually last for from two to five years, give or take, before the Paradise Lost Period. During the PP doses usually range from two to four per day often without a heavy price to pay for missing a dose. As Paradise is lost frequency of doses may rise to from four to six per day with fewer and fewer hours of symptom relief.

During the PP the effectiveness of each dose is almost immediately noticeable, but during the PLP it can take from thirty to ninety minutes for some without relief. These periods may be completely random and unexplained.

In addition to these "on" / "off" states continued increased use of carbidopa/levadopa in time nearly always causes the appearance of dyskinesias which can, in themselves, be incapacitating.

Occasionally in older patients the penalty for reducing motor symptoms is parkinsonian psychosis which may including hallucinations, paranoid delusions and/or confusion.

No wonder Parkinson disease is called the "gift that keeps on taking". Though medication does nothing to slow or decrease the progression of the disease, most patients, as they advance, become dependent upon it. Thus despite the difficulties caused by taking carbidopa/levodopa, without it a PwP may be unable to perform at all.

Girija Muralidhar

MOTOR FLUCTUATIONS TIMELINE: What Can I Expect with Levodopa?

Levodopa is the most effective substance for treating Parkinson symptoms. However, its dosage must be increased as time goes on, resulting in the appearance of side effects.

Melamed et.al., have divided its use into two time periods according to dosage and effectiveness and have mapped out an approximate timeline of what to expect for many people with Parkinson disease.

Note: Parkinson patients are so individual that there may not be a norm to response to medication.

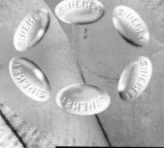

PARADISE PERIOD

Stable, smooth performance
Dose begins to works in 5 – 20 minutes
Dosage is 2 to 4 times per day
Period lasts 2 to 5 years approximately
Rarely lasts forever

PARADISE LOST PERIOD

Motor fluctuations less predictable
Begin to feel wearing off and getting on
Doses take longer to beome effective
Dosage increases to 6 to 8 doses
Unable to skip a dose
May need night time dose to avoid bradykinesia during sleep

AN INFORMAL OUTLINE OF DOPAMINE METABOLISM

Your brain needs dopamine. It might sound easy but it is a complicated process.

May Griebel MD

5. PROBLEM: As your brain decreases production of its own dopamine, the L-Dopa you swallow may seem less effective or may not last as long, because dopamine gets broken down in our brains by different enzyme systems called MAO and COMT

SOLUTION: Block those enzymes (MAO and COMT) with MAO and COMT inhibitors which as a result lengthen the lives of both exogenous and endogenous dopamine.

1. PROBLEM: Dopamine cannot get across the barrier that protects the brain called the Blood Brain Barrier (BBB) but L-Dopa can.

SOLUTION: If you can get L-Dopa into your brain, your own enzymes there can convert it to dopamine.

2. PROBLEM: To get L-Dopa into the body, it must be actively carried across the gut wall by carrier molecules. These same carrier molecules also transport amino acids. Protein breakdown results in lots of amino acids. That means too much competition for absorption, and L-Dopa can be wasted or too slowly absorbed.

SOLUTION: Limit eggs and Big Macs for breakfast and lunch. It is important to have a low protein diet until supper so the L-Dopa is absorbed completely.

Neurotransmitters

Neurotransmitters are chemicals that convey messages between neurons of the brain and along the nerve pathway connecting to a muscle or an organ. This chemical message induces a series of well-coordinated reactions in muscle cells leading to smooth movements.

4. PROBLEM: Vitamin B6 increases the efficiency of DDC and makes it harder to sneak the L-Dopa through the liver unchanged.

SOLUTION: Avoid excess B6 or B6 supplements unless otherwise necessary.

3. PROBLEM: The liver contains lots of an enzyme called dopa decarboxylase (DDC) which converts L-Dopa into dopamine. Dopamine, remember, cannot cross the BBB.

SOLUTION: DDC loves carbidopa more than L-Dopa. If the two are combined it will keep the DDC enzymes busy; then the L-Dopa part of the pill is free to go in the blood stream to the heart and then the brain where it can cross the BBB. Important point: Carbidopa does not treat PD. Its big role is to allow L-Dopa to pass through the liver without being changed to dopamine. .

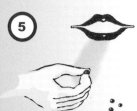

SIDE EFFECT CREEP

Is Levodopa Changing the Perceived Symptomatic Profile of Parkinson Disease?

The introduction of the drug levodopa in 1970 was a pivotal moment in the history of the treatment of Parkinson disease (PD). Since then, the impact of levodopa has been examined from many angles including its effect on life expectancy, quality of life and cost of treatment. I recently became interested in another angle—its possible impact on the perceived symptomatic profile of PD.

What follows is the outcome of research I did into that subject. I must preface it, however, by acknowledging that this was not done in a completely scientific manner. I was constrained by lack of both training and access to research papers as I am not (yet) a scientist. So, this should not be taken as a definitive work by any stretch; rather, it is a purely amateur investigation.

In my perusing of papers dating back to the mid-50s, I noticed that, in the last decade, at least, orthostatic hypotension is viewed variously as a symptom of PD by some[1], as a side effect of levodopa by others[2] and potentially as either by still others.[3, 4] However, it seemed to me that according to papers published immediately after the introduction of levodopa, orthostatic hypotension was considered a side effect, not a symptom. I decided to dig a little deeper and see whether my observation was valid. I reviewed 75 papers from three discrete time periods. The first time period was 1922 to 1968. I searched Pubmed for the terms Parkinson, Parkinson's, parkinsonian,

or parkinsonism. Within those parameters, papers in this time period were chosen solely on the basis of their being free. 1922 was the earliest paper that I could get for free and 1968 is two years before levodopa was put on the market. 17 of the 35 papers were deemed irrelevant as they did not contain any references to side effects of levodopa or symptoms of PD. That left 18 papers in the earliest time period.

The second time period was 1969 to 1975. 1969 was just prior to levodopa's entry onto the market and 1975 was chosen simply because I thought the five years post-introduction would be the most fertile for fresh impressions of the changes brought by levodopa. Papers in this time period were selected from among the 800 papers I have saved on the hard drive of my computer. I simply went through all the papers in that time period and culled the ones with references to symptoms and side effects. Since there were 18 papers in the previous time period, I limited the papers chosen for this time period to 20.

The third time period was 1996 to 2008, both of which years are arbitrary choices except that they are 25+ years post introduction and therefore might reveal the shift that I thought I had detected. The 20 papers in this time period were selected in the same manner as those in the previous time period.

A total of 40 phenomena were listed as either symptoms of PD or side effects of levodopa in the papers published in the latter two time periods. Of those 40, eight that were referred to almost exclusively as side effects in the papers published between 1969 and 1975 (Figure 1) were referred to more frequently as symptoms or potentially either symptoms or side effects in the papers published between 1996 and 2008 (Figure 2).

For these phenomena to be symptoms now, they would have to have been present before the introduction of levodopa. However,

Figure 1

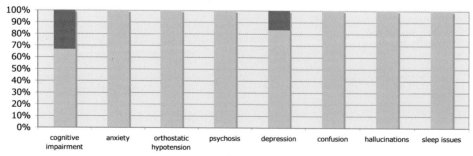

Percentage of References to Selected Phenomena Categorizing Them as either Symptoms or Side Effects Immediately Post-Introduction of Levodopa (Source: 20 research papers dated 1969-1975)

aside from one reference each to depression and cognitive impairment, these phenomena were not considered symptoms in the 18 relevant pre-levodopa papers I reviewed.

Possible explanations for this include:

1. The phenomena were present and noticed but not thought to be connected to the disease
2. The phenomena were present but not noticed

Regarding the former, since depression, anxiety and sleep issues occur frequently in non-disease-specific contexts in the general population and can also be reactions to having PD, it is possible that they were present and noticed pre-levodopa but were not considered symptoms.

However, cognitive impairment, orthostatic hypotension, psychosis, hallucinations and confusion neither occur frequently in non-disease-specific contexts in the general population nor do they manifest as reactions to the disease. Moreover, they are not phenomena that could be easily overlooked.

So, there is at least one other explanation.

Consider the fact that, having studied nothing but PD in the absence of levodopa for their entire careers, the researchers and clinicians writing in the 60s and 70s were uniquely positioned to observe the changes it brought.

Then consider the fact that levodopa has dominated the treatment of PD from the moment of its introduction, with the result that, unlike their peers three to four decades ago, researchers and clinicians today rarely see the disease progress to four years post-diagnosis before levodopa is introduced. Data presented in a 2005 study suggests that, on average, there was a 92% chance that a person with Parkinson (PWP) would be taking levodopa within four years of diagnosis.[5]

Indeed, the authors of a 2004 study found that 76% of PWP under 70 received a medication within one week of diagnosis, and that, prior to 1998, 63% of PwP under 70 and 80% of those over 70 were prescribed levodopa as an initial therapy.[6]

In view of all of the above, should the possibility be considered that these five phenomena are side effects of levodopa rather than symptoms of PD?

As I said earlier, this research should not be considered definitive by any stretch. Its weaknesses include a very small sample size, less than rigorous scientific method and limited access to research papers. And, though I did my best to select the papers from which this data was culled in a random fashion, because they were not selected via a formal literature review, the potential for bias exists.

Nonetheless, I think this subject bears further examination.

Kate Gendreau, MPH

[1] Hely M, Morris J, Reid WDJ, Trafficante R. Sydney Multicenter Study of Parkinson's Disease: Non-L-Dopa-Responsive Problems Dominate at 15 Years. Movement Disorders 2005; 20(2):190-99.
[2] Olanow CW. Levodopa/Dopamine Replacement Strategies in Parkinson's Disease – Future Directions. Movement Disorders 2008; 23(S3):S613-22.
[3] Rascol O, Goetz C, Koller W, Poewe W, Sampaio C. Treatment Interventions for Parkinson's Disease: An Evidence-based Assessment. Lancet 2002; 359:1589-98.
[4] Colcher A, Stern MB. Therapeutics in the Neurorehabilitaton of Parkinson's Disease. Neurorehabilitation and Neural Repair 1999; 13:205.
[5] Tan EK, Yeo AP, Tan V, Pavanni R, Wong MC. Prescribing pattern in Parkinson's disease: are cost and efficacy overriding factors? The International Journal of Clinical Practice 2005 May; 59(5):511-14.
[6] Zesiewicz T, Carter S, Sullivan K, Staffetti J, Dunne P, Hauser R. Initial Management of Parkinson's Disease in a Florida Community. The Journal of Applied Research 2004; 4(1):95-98.

Figure 2

Percentage of References to Selected Phenomena Categorizing Them as Symptoms, Side Effects, or Either 26-38 Years Post-Introduction of Levodopa (Source: 20 research papers dated 1996-2008)

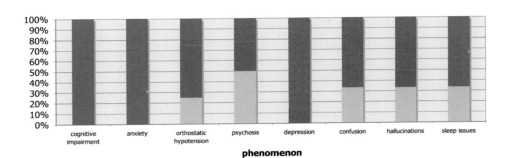

DOPAMINE AGONISTS:
"There are at least two sides to every story."

Very profound. Nowhere in medicine does that apply more accurately than in the controversy surrounding Dopamine Agonists.

The problem is, while we all want to know the "TRUTH", there is no single "TRUTH". What may be true for one is completely false for another. Without a standard to go by, how do we know what is best for us?

Unfortunately, informing yourself as thoroughly as possible followed by a process of trial and error, is still the only real way to find out. And sometimes even then……

The good...... Pam's story

When I was finally diagnosed with PD, I was prescribed Permax (Pergolide Mesylate) an ergot derivative dopamine receptor agonist at both D1 and D2 receptor sites. In plain English, it stimulates these two particular dopamine receptors to make them work.

For six years I was the poster child for Permax. I experienced near complete alleviation of symptoms, virtually no increase in un-medicated symptoms and no persistent or troublesome side effects after the initial period of titrating. In 2007, much to my dismay, it was taken off the market. I felt completely and utterly abandoned. After trying both Requip (ropinirole, a non-ergoline dopamine agonist acting on the D2 and D3 receptors) and Mirapex (pramipexole, another non-ergoline with an affinity for the D3 receptor), with totally unsatisfactory results (Requip made me sick and Mirapex simply didn't work), I was prescribed carbidopa/levodopa.

Still looking for the miracle relief that came from the Permax, I have had to accept the fact that I am no longer newly diagnosed and the freedom that I once experienced is not likely to be repeated.

The bad....... Girija's story

Are DA's my friend or foe? It is not an easy question to answer. I was on dopamine agonist (DA) treatment at the standard therapeutic doses for six years before I decided to quit. At first, treatment with DA was a blessing. It magically took away my PD symptoms and gave me the energy to live my life as I used to in my pre-PD days. In that DA-induced euphoria, what I failed to see was their effect on my non-motor symptoms, particularly behavioral changes. I was aware of my weight gain and hair loss, but did not realize that I was addicted to work, computer, shopping and that my actions were rather risky and impulsive.

Though I do not regret the decisions I made while I was on DA, they are not typical of me. As I look back, it feels like I am watching myself in a drama directed by a stranger. I am so thankful that this drama ended on more of a positive note for me. While my experiences with DA are mixed, it is not so for many others.

The ugly...... Fiona's story

I spent some years on a very high dosage of Mirapex. My behavior completely changed. I started staying up all night doing wacky stuff, lost my job and went into unbelievable debt. My life completely disintegrated to the point where I dislocated my hip and didn't know it and wound up in the hospital for over a month with pain so acute I couldn't move at all. I am amazed I'm still alive really. And it was worse than I'm telling it, too.

All of these behaviors COMPLETELY went away when I stopped taking the agonists. There is no way they are part of advancing disease, at least from my perspective. But see, that's how they use fear and a patient's self-doubt to corral us into not questioning the treatment…..

BUT beware, if one is going to stop the agonists, you have to do it glacially slowly . . . very, very, very gradually. And if you can get help, do so . . . I am so happy that the perils of the drug therapy itself are finally starting to be recognized. And for the record, now that I am off agonists, I have probably less off periods and dystonia. And I may be still struggling with the depression, but I was somewhat crazy and irrational while on Mirapex."

These diverse reactions to medication show how unique each one's PD is and how important it is to have a two-way communication between patients and doctors.

There should be more education about side-effects of drugs when a patient is offered the drug, in the interests of making a well-informed choice.

DOPAMINE-TRIGGERED CHANGES IN BEHAVIORS

Dopamine agonist treatment of PD carries a substantial risk of pathological behaviors. Compulsive behaviors provoked by dopamine agonists often go undetected in clinical series, especially when such behaviors are not specifically inquired about.

A recent study by the Mayo-Rochester Movement Disorder Clinic suggested that 22% of patients taking a dopamine agonist over a two year period experienced compulsive behaviors. Of 321 PD patients taking an agonist, 69 (22%) experienced compulsive behaviors, and 50/321 (16%) were pathologic. However, when the analysis was restricted to patients taking agonist doses that were at least minimally therapeutic, pathological behaviors were documented in 24%. The subtypes were: gambling (25; 36%), hypersexuality (24; 35%), compulsive spending/shopping (18; 26%), binge eating (12; 17%), compulsive hobbying (8; 12%) and compulsive computer use (6; 9%). The vast majority of affected cases (94%) were concurrently taking carbidopa/levodopa. Among those with adequate follow up, behaviors completely or partly resolved when the dopamine agonist dose was reduced or ceased.

Girija Muralidhar, PhD

From: Hassan A, Bower JH, Kumar N, Matsumoto JY, Fealey RD, Josephs KA, Ahlskog JE (2011). Dopamine agonist-triggered pathological behaviors: surveillance in the PD clinic reveals high frequencies. Parkinsonism Relat Disord.,17(4):260-4. Epub 2011 Feb 9.

The skeptic

"I have been on Mirapex at the max recommended dosage for about 6 years and I have engaged in compulsive behavior during that time – shopping. The onset of my behavior coincided not with any change to my DA, but to my mother being diagnosed with cancer. I was already depressed at that time and her struggle put me in a place I had never been before - and I found that shopping made me feel better, at least for a little while. The behavior resolved gradually, not with any change to my meds, but rather as I came out of the depression."

I would like to pose a question. If too much dopamine running around the brain is deemed responsible for such behavior, why would levodopa which turns into actual dopamine be less likely to cause these problems than dopamine agonists, which only mimic dopamine?

Another question I would pose pertains to the theory that it is the dopamine rush of an unexpected win that people with PD become addicted to. They suffer from a deficit of dopamine and are therefore more susceptible to the rush, shouldn't taking something that replenishes the ambient level of dopamine in the brain *reduce or eliminate* rather than exacerbate that problem?

Finally, I would point out that all of these behaviors are noted as beginning with the start or increase of a DA - maybe it is just me, but it seems to me self evident that a worsening of symptoms that requires the initiation of or an increase in meds is 'depressing!' and depression has long been correlated with gambling and - this is, of course, an extremely unrefined piece of information but there are over 600 hits if you search on the terms OCD and depression together in PubMed.

I remain unconvinced that DAs are any more likely than levodopa or buproprion (wellbutrin, a dopamine re-uptake inhibitor) to cause such behaviors and I have yet to see compelling evidence (excludes anecdote) that any of them cause such behavior.

My own advice would be to give close examination to the circumstances in one's life that could also be responsible for such behavior and to give serious consideration to the side effects of what one would probably take instead, i.e., levodopa - in addition to whatever your own personal priorities and symptom constellations are, and anything else that is relevant for you - and then make a decision. You could always just stop for a bit and see what happens - you can always go back on.

My 250,476 cents, Boann

IMPULSE ISSUES

I have been asked to write about the crazy stuff living with Parkinson disease can do to us.

After a year of trying to raise awareness through my fly on the wall documentary, "Sex, Lies and Parkinson's"* and the subsequent media interest and sensationalism which included a live TV interview where I was referred to as being "randy" and "fiddling in the corner" by the presenter, I am the perfect choice for this subject!

At one time an 'Impulse' issue would have been which body spray to choose!

Yes, I struggle with impulses, yes, I wear my heart on my sleeve. I don't mean to shock, I just tell it how it is, and that, my friends, is not pretty or funny.

Sometimes I'm asked, *"You got some of them tablets for my wife? Ha ha."* I feel like saying, *"In reality she'd be sick for months before her body adapted so don't get the impression we all turn into nymphomaniacs with no inhibitions."*

There might be an element of this but it can turn into a nightmare that people are desperate to escape. Unfortunately as a nation we are Victorian regarding our ability to discuss the 's' word. SEX. I'm not. It's not wicked not to find it a chore! What I find horrific and shocking is how condemning the reaction has been to my drawing attention to the side effects of some PD treatment, including hypersexuality. It isn't the only devil that can sit merrily on our shoulders either, nudging us, encouraging us, taking away our brakes. Gambling, exhibitionism, punding, shopping, overuse of the Internet. The list goes on, and on, and on.

There's no denying these drugs can be fantastic at treating the symptoms of PD. They have to an extent given me my life back, but they have also very nearly taken it away.

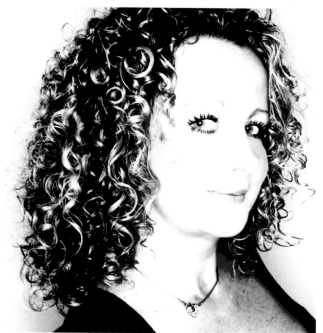

"How did they do this?", you may ask, "Aren't you using the drugs as an excuse for bad behaviour?"

I'll deal with both questions from my own personal experience, I repeat, MY own personal experience! I don't, speak for PD people as a whole, and never have. This is from me.

Quite simply the drugs removed my brakes, my inhibitions and to a certain extent my morals. Our secret thoughts and wildest fantasies can then easily become reality, but only, I think, if the seed of these thoughts were already there. I've always been a tad flirtatious and a keen shopper, so for me these have been the most noticeable areas where these tendencies have increased. It's not all bad though. I've discovered flirting with both sexes opens doors, i.e. a smile and a bit of banter can turn the sternest shop assistant into a pussy cat. It can get you served in a bar quickly while others are most upset that you are supping your gin & tonic within two minutes, while they've been waiting for ten! Flirting and I don't mean necessarily in a sexual way, can help people warm to you. It's amazing how most people become putty in your hands when you give them your undivided attention! Add a smile into the equation and interest in them as individuals, well.... let's just say it is not rocket science.

I may sound as If I'm making light of the impulse issues associated with our drugs. I certainly don't mean to. It's my flippant sense of humour, self preservation. In actual fact there have been times when my behaviour has been off the wall, causing my family, friends and myself considerable distress. My financial situation has near enough given my bank manager an ulcer!

I've come full circle now and I'm really trying to sort my head out. It's hard as you don't realise how much a drug can alter your personality until - well - until it is almost too late in some cases.

VICKI'S STORY

Non 'parkie' people may think "Why would you take them if that's what they do?"

Well, initially I had no concept of the effect they would have.

Yes, you are warned. Yes, I did read the list of side effects that came with the meds. But, "Nahhh! They won't affect me like that, I'm a strong feisty woman in charge of my life!"

Then, wham, before you know it you are out of control ....

The medication has been working on the pleasure seeking part of your malfunctioning brain, making you seek out adrenaline rushing little thrills. Or, as my other half puts it, they have turned me into an attention-seeking, shopaholic show off. Pre-PD I liked a night out, but probably liked a night in better. I was happy to wave my other half 'off t' pub' while I snuggled in with my boys and the latest chick lit. Now I've come full circle those days may soon be back, as quite frankly I'm bored with partying! It has kind of come to a crescendo, thank goodness! It has seen me get so drunk I couldn't pull my knickers up, or even at times walk. What kind of example Is that? Was it my way of blotting out the reality of my life? Or was it the meds? I'm not sure. I still drink, but to pleasant squiffiness now, not oblivion.

This impulsive lifestyle brought with it a need for new clothes, hairdressers, trips to beauticians, shoes, plus the drink money. I hate to think what I've spent....

Once I never would have dreamt of getting my hair blow dried for a night out, but that too became a necessity, as did acrylic nails and eyelash extensions. If I analyse things, it was a mask. I wanted people to see a foxy looking man-magnet, not someone with the degenerative neurological disease that was robbing me of my pride and self esteem.

I am no longer taking the medication that triggered the changes in my behaviour. Remember I was only 35 when diagnosed. It was one of the better treatment options for me.

I asked my GP to refer me to a psychiatrist as I felt I needed help. Did it help? No, but it did make me reflect and realise all my actions have consequences, drugs or no drugs and ultimately I have to be in charge of me. The other option of thinking "It was the drugs that MADE me" no longer washes with my inner self."

Vicki Dillon

DOPAMINE AGONISTS

Dopamine Agonists are small molecules that are "look-alikes" of dopamine and can bind to dopamine-receptors of a neuron. If you imagine a Dopamine receptor as a lock and dopamine as the key to open and send a message to the neuron, an agonist would be a duplicate key! A duplicate key is never the original and may open the lock with ease or after a bit of wiggling. Similarly, an agonist may not fit into the receptor with the same precision as dopamine - it may induce stronger and sustained signals, thereby altering the "message" to be delivered. To complicate this phenomenon further, there are at least 3-5 subtypes of dopamine receptors on neurons, (akin to opening different locks with the same key) some engaged in sending positive signals while other mediating negative signals, It is no wonder that responses to treatment with dopamine agonists are so varied among the patients with PD!
Girija Muralidhar, PhD

* Sex, Lies and Parkinson's was screened by the UK TV station Channel 4 in 2011, and is an honest and thought provoking look at Vicki's life with Parkinson disease. While most people felt it was a courageous attempt to 'out' the problems of some Parkinson medication, especially for Young Onset PwP, there were negative reactions from both the public and from within the PD community, some of whom wanted to distance themselves from the reality of impulsive behaviours. The unkind reality of Compulsive and Impulsive Disorders is that they may have a profound impact not just on the affected person, but on family members, friends and colleagues. PwP are not always warned that such side-effects can occur when they are prescribed, and it often someone they know well who notices that there is a problem. Vicki is not one of those people, she worked as a responsible paediatric nurse. Her article makes clear that she had kept herself informed. In spite of this she was unable to keep control of her life. There is a good case to be made for ensuring that all people who are prescribed such medications are informed of the possibility of impulsive behaviours so that they and their families are forwarned, and can avert some of the financial and personal damage that can occur.

THINGS WE HATE THE MOST ABOUT PD

1. FALLING
2. FALLING
3. FALLING
4. FALLING
5. FALLING
6. FALLING
7. FALLING
8. FALLING
9. FALLING
10. FALLING

dbiker2

1. I hate that it could take my capacity to think away
2. I hate the way it looks
3. I hate that it hurts
4. I hate that it causes me to not sleep
5. I hate that it makes people feel sorry for me
6. I hate that I am always looking for evidence that I don't have it
7. I hate that it has caused me to lose my ability to walk well
8. I hate that it has taken away my ability to sing
9. I hate that I have to take medicine every day
10. I hate that it is incurable

Pam Kell

1. I hate that it is degenerative.
2. I hate that it is viewed as an old person's disease.
3. I hate that I feel ashamed for having it and that I am somehow to blame.
4. I hate that I have to hide it.
5. I hate that it has made my life seem to center on taking pills.
6. I hate that doctors tell you that it progresses slowly when they really don't know how it will affect you at all.
7. I hate that it could rob me of valuable years with my young son.
8. I hate that it causes people to pity me.
9. I hate that people have extreme reactions to it.
10. I hate that the pharmacist now knows me by name.

Laura Brooks

1. Waking up off
2. Waking up off and needing a pee............
3. Picking up the phone and hearing myself weak and quavery instead of the person I know myself to be, and hearing the person on the other end of the line adopt a mildly patronising voice in response....
4. Being unable to make choices at the supermarket.
   This one drives me crazy!
5. People sometimes looking at me as though I am drunk, when I can't move out of the way fast enough, have a slurry voice, lose my balance, drop something, in fact I hadn't realized just how much was ascribed to alcohol abuse till I got PD!
6. Forgetting not to eat protein and going off, and not being able to do anything about it till I take my next lot of meds.........
7. Having to explain what PD is and why it is not the same as Alzheimer's, and why yes I am a bit young to have it...........
8. Dropping things
9. People thinking I am grumpy when I am off, and not understanding how I seem to be a different person when I am on...
10. Everything taking three times longer to do, and doing whatever it is with only half the efficiency!

Dr G

46

FALLING

SOCIAL ISOLATION, PEOPLE STARING INTERPRETED AS
BEING OLD AND/ OR DRUNK - WHEN AGE CAME UP, AND
MY GRANDSON DISCOVERED I WAS THE SAME AGE AS HIS
OTHER GRANDMOTHER, HE GOT A LOOK OF SURPRISE ON
HIS FACE. HE ASKED AGAIN, PUZZLED. OF COURSE FOR
AGE 6 I THOUGHT THAT WAS PRETTY GOOD THINKING...
LOL

BEING OFF WITH PERIPHERAL WEAKNESS IN LOWER LEGS
AND DYSTONIA

SINEMET COGNITIVE SIDE EFFECTS IMPULSE DYSCONTROL,
RAMBLING COMMUNICATION, DISTRACTION AND LACK
OF FOCUS AND CLARITY

FATIGUE, LACK OF ENERGY

APATHY, DETACHMENT, DULLNESS OF EMOTION

LAYING AWAKE AT NIGHT

NO APPETITE, WEIGHT LOSS, PROBLEMS MEETING
NUTRITIONAL REQUIREMENTS OR PHYSICAL PENALTIES
FOR EATING TOO MUCH TOO EARLY

ITS' TOLL ON THE FAMILY AND LIFE IN GENERAL....IT
CREATES A "CHAIN OF PAIN", DESTROYS FAMILIES, TURNS
MARRIAGE INTO A JOB FOR THE CARE PARTNER AND CAN
LOWER YOUR INCOME AND LIFESTYLE

Paula Wittekind

1. Lack of support and understanding from the
public and friends
2. A feeling of shame for being so "damaged" - like
I have to hide the disease
3. Lack of trust in my body
4. Loss of my job and all that went with that
5. Uncertainty about the future; lost feeling that
I can control my destiny, improve my condition
(well, maybe some shred left...)
6. Exhaustion: lack of stamina, insomnia
7. Anxiety
8. Dependency on a MDS whom I do not really trust
or like
9. Terrible loneliness
10. Never really comfortable in public but go stir-
crazy at home, miss activities that were such a part
of my life!

Sasha

We can't pretend it is fun having Parkinson
disease, so some of us said it like it is,
especially on a bad day. We even left a
space for your pet hates ! Grab a gold pen
or piece of chalk and fill yours in . . .

A PLACE FOR YOUR OWN PD GRIPE !

THE EVOLUTION OF A PSYCHE:
Adapting to Parkinson Disease

May Griebel, MD (Ret.)

"What could be happening to my body," I thought. My left hand was twisting in a dystonic posture as I dressed for work in the morning. I was a 45-year-old wife and mother, a pediatric neurologist with a happy family life and a burgeoning career. Given my training, I did a quick differential diagnosis on myself and was terribly frightened and worried by everything on the list.

So, I engaged in a very well-practiced skill: denial. Nothing was happening. After all, it seemed to go away as I moved around more. I was tired and stressed: certainly that had to be it. After six more months, I showed the hand I didn't even want to acknowledge as mine to my husband. "You are overworked and tired. You are entirely too paranoid about your body. Let it go."

Permission. The most important person in my life had just given me permission to continue my denial. This I did for another couple of years, then came the tremor, mild at first and then more pronounced. It really was more apparent with stress and effort and an element of it went away if I had a glass of wine. As I wrote notes when I rounded with our team of young doctors in the hospital, I found them staring – or felt them staring – at my left hand as it bounced up and down when I tried to hold a sheet of paper to write a note on a chart. A glass of wine would decrease the shaking, but I couldn't drink alcohol and work. I had to do something. I presented myself with my concerns to a wonderful neurologist at our medical center whom I deeply trusted, even though his specialty was multiple sclerosis and not movement disorders.

Even then, however, denial remained my mantle. I initially left out of my history the dystonia part, stressed the tremor and especially mentioned that it went away with alcohol: symptoms of benign essential tremor, except that it is not commonly unilateral. That part bothered the good doctor, but he listened to me as I urgently stressed the response to a glass of wine, a "diagnostic test" for benign essential tremor.

He prescribed propranolol, a beta blocker commonly used in essential tremor. My tremor did improve, for a while. I do truly have an element of essential tremor. There were a lot more symptoms, but I was practiced in hiding all of it as best I could. I scheduled follow-up visits early in the morning, after the dystonia had resolved but before I got too tired. Some part of me protectively recognized that the tremor and stiffness I was experiencing got worse throughout the day as I got more and more tired. I did not want him to see me then.

The symptoms, however, were relentless. The tremor and stiffness increased and increased. Finally, in what today would be a flagrant violation of medical privacy laws, my colleagues "told on me." It was hurting them to see me suffering so. They described to my doctor the full picture of what neither my husband nor I could really even see. I saw the neurologist for my standard morning visit and he asked me what else had been going on, had I experienced any other symptoms. He looked at me intently.

I guess at that point I wanted to end the charade. I WANTED help. I spilled out all my concern, but without diagnostic labels. Surely HE didn't really think that I had Parkinson disease. Then he said something, which gave me a huge chill: "I think we need to start you on Sinemet." He didn't even use the name Parkinson disease. He didn't need to. I started crying and he held me briefly and then wrote the prescription. Bawling so hard that he had trouble understanding my words, I called my husband to tell him that I had been given a prescription for Sinemet. Again, the name Parkinson disease remained unspoken. There was a long period of quiet and then he uttered, "Oh, my."

The diagnosis hit me between the eyes. Depression, as it often does, came on the heels of denial as the denial crumbled. I think it all hit me much harder because of my background. I could no longer intellectualize it all away. I couldn't even say the name Parkinson disease. I began to see a therapist to deal with my fears and anger: he suggested that to desensitize myself, I should shout "Parkinson disease" as loudly as possible and then say every curse word my brain could drag up as loudly as I could. That helped some, but I still could only say the words through sobs or while screaming expletives.

I needed to tell my family: both sets of parents, both brothers and their wives, most of all our bright and very sensitive fourteen-year-old daughter. I didn't want to sob and sob, so for all but our daughter, I sent explanatory letters. Somehow I managed to tell our daughter, who was furious not to have been told as all this was happening from the beginning.

I have thought proudly that I was "handling this well." My colleagues and friends all know that I have Parkinson disease and I have made myself widely available to talk to others with this diagnosis, newly made or long standing, who just want to talk about it, have questions about medications, or want to talk about side effects.

With all of this, I still have been scared. I have stayed away from contact with other people in the Parkinson disease groups. I have not gotten on a chat page to share my worries. I talk about them with my husband, but somehow that is not the same. With the people to whom I have spoken, I have been an information purveyor, a teacher, a guide. I haven't let my hair down and cried in a long time - and never with a fellow walker on this path.

If I had any recommendations to pass on to someone newly diagnosed, one would be that they need to get involved with a Parkinson disease support group as soon as they can, locally, by phone, on line, at national meetings, any or all of the above. Learn everything you absolutely can. You are the only thing that is guaranteed to go with you to all of your doctor visits.

Now I realize that in making some of my decisions, as scared as I was and still am to some degree, about what the future holds for me, that all along I was committing myself to life. To life as a healthy person who - yes, oh by the way - does have Parkinson disease.

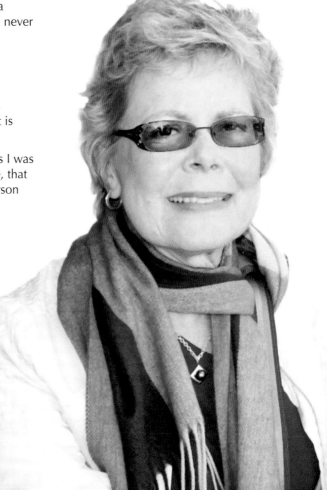

So my strongest recommendation is to deal with issues as you go along, but commit yourself to living and to living a full, involved and giving life. You don't want to wake up in ten years bitter about all the time wasted. Get with it.

DOCTORS . . .

Doctors; can't live with them, can't…. well, you know the old adage. After a diagnosis of Parkinson disease we all become more familiar with doctors (and with the medical community as a whole) than most of us could have ever imagined.

Because we require a closer than usual relationship with our doctors due to having a chronic illness, finding the right neurologist is no easy task. Each of us has unique issues and a unique personality. Some of us prefer the paternal type who takes charge; others prefer one who will act as a partner. Whatever your preference, know that you are entitled to a physician who fits your parameters.

If your neurologist does not spend enough time with you, is condescending or refuses to engage with you on issues that you feel are important, then find another one. Going to a doctor is not a contractual relationship. You are not married to your doctor and you don't have to divorce him or her. Your health will improve by seeing only doctors with whom you can establish, at the minimum, open and easy communication. You owe it to yourself to look until you find the physician you need. It is tempting to settle and in the beginning settling may cause no harm. However, the further into Wonderland we go, the more important it is to surround ourselves with competent people with whom we can be candid and forthright.

We should continually seek professional care from those of whom we can ask questions and feel assured the answers are well thought-out, informed and correct. We deserve it and nothing less will do.

However, the further into Wonderland we go, the more important it is to surround ourselves with competent people with whom we can be candid and forthright.

We should continuously seek professional care from those of whom we can ask questions and feel assured the answers are well thought out, informed and correct.

This, I think, is in no way, asking too much.

Pamela Kell

CHOICE OF DOCTORS

It is fair to say that not all patients with Parkinson disease will be able to choose where and who their neurologist or movement disorder specialist will be.

Depending on where you live, what health system you live under, or even your economic status, you may have fewer choices than you would wish for.

PD is such an individualized condition that it is important to be treated by someone who listens to your concerns and helps you obtain the best results from your treatment. If you have difficulty with this it is usually possible to get a second opinion.

If your choices are very limited there is something you can do for yourself and for others in the same situation. Ask your PD organization for any help and information they can offer and ask them to lobby for better healthcare options for people living with Parkinson disease. Many organizations are already doing this and need your support.

Lack of trust between patients and their doctors is a result of many things, lack of good communication, doctors' distrust and resentment of lawyers and insurance companies and patients who blindly accept inadequate medical care.

Patients deserve much better.

WHAT IS DEEP BRAIN STIMULATION (DBS) FOR PARKINSON DISEASE?

Deep brain stimulation (DBS) is a surgical procedure used to treat a variety of disabling neurological symptoms—most commonly the debilitating symptoms of Parkinson disease (PD), such as tremor, rigidity, stiffness, slowed movement, and walking problems. The procedure is also used to treat essential tremor, a common neurological movement disorder. At present, the procedure is used only for patients whose symptoms cannot be adequately controlled with medications.

DBS uses a surgically implanted, battery-operated medical device called a neurostimulator—similar to a heart pacemaker and approximately the size of a stopwatch—to deliver electrical stimulation to targeted areas in the brain that control movement, blocking the abnormal nerve signals that cause tremor and PD symptoms.

Before the procedure, a neurosurgeon uses magnetic resonance imaging (MRI) or computed tomography (CT) scanning to identify and locate the exact target within the brain where electrical nerve signals generate the PD symptoms. Some surgeons may use microelectrode recording - which involves a small wire that monitors the activity of nerve cells in the target area - to more specifically identify the precise brain target that will be stimulated. Generally, these targets are the thalamus, subthalamic nucleus, and globus pallidus.

The DBS system consists of three components: the lead, the extension, and the neurostimulator. The lead (also called an electrode) - a thin, insulated wire - is inserted through a small opening in the skull and implanted in the brain. The tip of the electrode is positioned within the targeted brain area.

The extension is an insulated wire that is passed under the skin of the head, neck, and shoulder, connectng the lead to the neurostimulator. The neurostimulator (the "battery pack") is the third component and is usually implanted under the skin near the collarbone. In some cases it may be implanted lower in the chest or under the skin over the abdomen.

Once the system is in place, electrical impulses are sent from the neurostimulator up along the extension wire and the lead and into the brain. These impulses interfere with and block the electrical signals that cause PD symptoms.

From the NINDS Information sheet at:
http://www.ninds.nih.gov/disorders/deep_brain_ stimulation/deep_brain_stimulation.htm

DBS is not for everyone...

Originally DBS was recommended as a last resort treatment. Recently it has been promoted as an earlier intervention. We begin with one PwP account of why he has not chosen DBS, then in the following pages a few PwP accounts of why they made this difficult choice and their results.

In the seventeen years since my diagnosis I have experienced a typical, gradual but relentless, increase in disability with a corresponding decrease in quality of life. So why have I and many other well-informed PwP chosen not to do DBS?

DBS is not for everyone. As I understand it, DBS mainly treats motor symptoms, but does not generally improve balance/gait and a range of non-motor symptoms that may have a bigger impact on quality of life than the dopamanergic functions.

PD has increasingly been shown to be much more than a movement disorder, affecting, mood, digestion, sexual function, speech /swallowing, and cognition. If a PwP is concerned about potential losses in these quality of life areas or is seeking to improve the non-motor symptoms, it is difficult to choose DBS.

There are no approved alternatives for advanced patients like me. Many of the more promising new therapies involve brain surgery as the way to get the medicine into the brain. You can only receive these new therapies through a clinical trial. If you have already had DBS or another brain surgery you usually will be excluded from participating in a trial.

In my case, I have been waiting since 2009 when I first learned about the resurrection of GDNF - using gene therapy to deliver it to appropriate locations in the brain. (see Chapter 7 for details). Having worked on GDNF advocacy since 2005, I am well aware of the issues and promise of GDNF.

I see other promising therapies moving too slowly to be helpful to me any time soon, so I have decided to use my one token on the experimental highway. to not just relieve symptoms and feel better but to take a chance at getting back part of whats left of my life before I am too old.

If I do not qualify for gene therapy, I will most likely have DBS as a last option for some immediate relief.
Perry Cohen, PhD

Note: Perry participated in the GDNF trials in May 2013 averting the need to choose DBS for the time being.

DEEP BRAIN STIMULATION

"What if" questions are usually difficult to answer. This time it isn't. If I hadn't had deep brain stimulation surgery, I wouldn't be able to sit at this desk and type out this account on a computer. I think I would have led an increasingly isolated life in my Washington house and ultimately in a nursing home (if you can call that a life). My wife thinks I'd be dead.

Instead, I'm an almost fully functioning member of society. I retired as an editor and reporter with the Washington bureau of the Los Angeles Times about three years ago at age 64, but only partly because of my health. More important, the journalism profession was collapsing all around me, under pressure from a young generation that preferred cable television and Internet blogs to newspapers as information sources. Within a year or two of my retirement, the LA Times Washington bureau was no more.

Several years before, I had staked my future on DBS. Diagnosed with Parkinson disease in 1990, I had adjusted comfortably to the disease once I had got over the initial shock. Within six months, the Times sent me, with my wife and three children, to Europe to open a bureau on Brussels, the capital of what was then the European Community. In Brussels I enjoyed the three best years of my professional—and personal—lives. To this day I thank the Times for having the guts to send a potential cripple overseas.

As it happened, the two pioneers of DBS could be found in Grenoble, at the foot of the French Alps. I spent most of an afternoon talking with one if them, Dr. Pierre Pollak. He described the pros and cons of the procedure, which was still very much in the experimental stage. To see if I would qualify, he tried to hook me up to a harness to measure my tremor. I was shaking so hard that he couldn't get the harness on. "You qualify," he said. My tremor wasn't usually so violent, and for my three years in the Brussels bureau I held up pretty well. But as my regular tour was drawing to a close, my condition had deteriorated sufficiently that I wasn't sure I could make it for another three, particularly if I were sent somewhere that lacked Belgium's quality of medical care. So the

Washington bureau took me back in an editing job, in which I wouldn't have to explain to interview-subjects that I was shaking not because I was afraid of them but because my Sinemet, the anti-tremor medicine, was wearing off. I filled the writing void by starting work on a book ultimately entitled, **A Life Shaken: My Encounter with Parkinson Disease**.

In late 2004, as I was finishing the paperback version of the book, I wasn't quite ready to let surgeons go poking around in my brain. Shortly thereafter, I was. I consulted with three surgeons, two local as well as Dr. Ali Rezai of the Cleveland Clinic (he's since moved to Ohio State), said by two neurologists I knew and trusted to be the best in the business. Despite the inconvenience of regularly schlepping to Cleveland, I signed up with Dr. Rezai. Not a bad choice.

Before I could undergo the operation, I had to pass a series of psychological as well as physical tests. My Cleveland neurologist, Dr. Thyagarajan Subramanian (the only person I ever knew with 10-syllable name) was alarmed by my tremor and thought it might indicate not Parkinson but essential tremor run amok. To find out, he wanted to see how I looked first thing in the morning. Trouble was, he was usually asleep first thing in my morning; I couldn't sleep past 4 or 5 a.m. So he sent me home with instructions to use a camcorder (insurance didn't cover it) to tape myself tying my shoes. It may not have been an award winner, but the film persuaded him that I really did have Parkinson. So one spring morning in 2004, Dr. Rezai implanted two electrodes in a part of the brain on the circuits of many Parkinson movement disorders. The operation was a success.

End of story?

Hardly. First, the operation itself. It's no fun having all the paraphernalia of brain surgery screwed into your skull. But for that part of the procedure they knocked me out, and I hardly felt a thing. You have to be awake when they experiment with various electrode placements so that, as in an eye doctor's office, you can tell them which location feels better, A or B. That's no fun, but it's only a few hours of discomfort—about five in my case. I'd gladly take that over a lifetime of tremor. (Speaking of tremor, mine was so bad—you can't take any medicine during the operation—that a 220-pound orderly had to be recruited to lean in my shoulders and try to hold me still.)

Then there are the psychological considerations of having a surgeon fooling around with your brain. There are people I know who won't have DBS for this reason. I can't blame them. I'm lucky to have the ability, possibly from a career as a journalist, to step outside myself and be a mere onlooker at things that are happening to me. So it was in the operating room. I was even taking mental notes for stories I might write one day.

That was only a middle chapter in the DBS saga. I had to return to Cleveland in about two weeks to have batteries implanted in my chest and wired up to the electrodes. Then Dr. Subramanian, with almost an infinite number of combinations to choose from, decided how much juice to send pulsing to the electrodes. Finally, I could feel DBS's full effects. The hated tremor was gone. My care at the Cleveland Clinic was then turned over to a full-time programmer, Sierra Farris. At least initially, it would be her job to adjust the electricity as the underlying disease progressed. Because I trusted her, I commuted to Cleveland about every six months for a couple of years. I stopped only when Sierra moved to Seattle. Traveling through three time zones seemed a little excessive for a medical appointment. It was then that I learned of the shortage of programmers in Washington and probably a lot of other places. The number of Parkinson patients with DBS is growing fast as more neurosurgeons do more operations. The number of programmers is not growing nearly as fast. It's not as if I didn't need some mid-course corrections. Most seriously, the electrodes interfered with my gait; one morning on my way to the bus stop I fell head-first three times, breaking my wrist. Finding someone to deal with this kind of situation has been no cinch.

Would I recommend deep brain stimulation for other Parkinson patients? No, but I wouldn't recommend against it either. Every Parkinson patient is different. Some (like me) benefit from the operation, some don't. I'll leave it to the doctors to decide who's in which category.

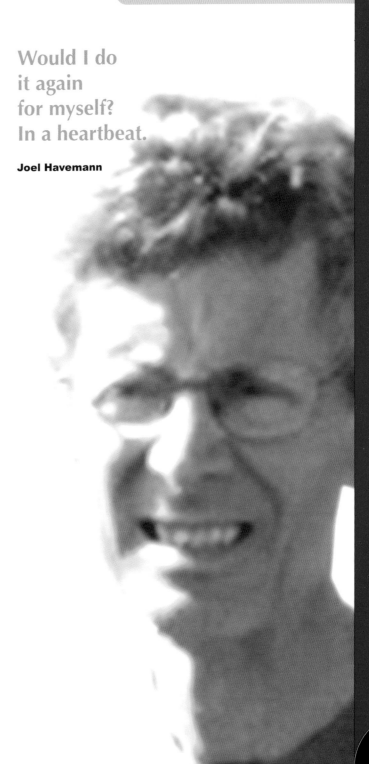

Would I do
it again
for myself?
In a heartbeat.

Joel Havemann

DBS was the best option for me with my Parkinson symptoms to give me a better future, even though I knew it would be a very complex and long operation, for me and my family.

Clifford Williams

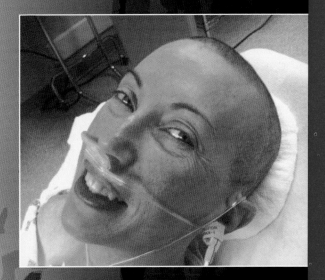

MICHELLE & HER DOCTOR ON DBS

DR. RAO'S STATEMENT:
After nearly 10 years of PD Michelle had developed severe L-dopa induced dyskinesia and off periods. She had more severe dyskinesia of the left-sided limbs than the right side. We chose to do a DBS of the right subthalamic nucleus. Since surgery her peak and end of dyskinesia of the left-sided limbs have completely disappeared; her resting tremor of the left-sided limbs, arm more than leg, has also been under excellent control. She sleeps much better and requires very little anti-PD drugs to control resting tremor of the right hand and leg. We are planning to do a left STN surgery sometime during November of this year. Hopefully after the second surgery her quality of life will improve even more.

MICHELLE'S STATEMENT:
After a two year sudden progression of my Parkinson and numerous intolerable side effects from long-term use of the medication, I rarely left the house in the last 12 months. I finally decided it was time for DBS as it could only offer improvement of my current situation. I am in shock at the amount of improvement and return of quality of life I have received. I am able to leave my home and drive short distances unassisted. Never would I have imagined that I would have benefited this much from one side of the DBS surgery. I am actually looking forward to the second surgery and praying for the same results! Less medication and regaining quality of life is a wonderful feeling!
Michelle Lane

MIRACLES DO HAPPEN

I had no energy. My doctor laughed and said I was no doubt pre-menopausal and I should make another appointment to discuss hormone replacement therapy. She then examined me physically. Noting some tenderness in my lower right abdomen, my doctor stated that she suspected appendicitis.

After a battery of tests she returned with an inscrutable smile and said, "Well, I know it's impossible, but you are pregnant, my dear." I immediately burst into tears.

I was 47 years old and had never been pregnant. I had been diagnosed with Parkinson and took an elaborate cocktail of very powerful drugs several times a day to control the symptoms.

Afraid to believe the news, I explained to her that obviously the test had resulted in a false positive. For the briefest moment she seemed to entertain the notion as she acknowledged the possibility. More likely, she said, I had an ectopic pregnancy that, if proven, would require immediate termination.

From joyous, albeit incredible notions of pregnancy one moment to contemplating the prospect of an abortion, what an enormous swing in life's pendulum....

I dialed my husband's office. I heard him ask, "Are you calling me from your doctor's office?" I meekly replied, "Yes."

"You're pregnant, aren't you?" he simply asked without betraying any emotion.

"That's what they think," I remember stuttering, before a jumble of words and emotions spilled out of me. "They've scheduled an ultrasound later this afternoon. If it's an ectopic pregnancy, my doctor said it will have to be terminated."

"It's okay. I'll be there with you, honey," he reassured me.

Later that afternoon the technician efficiently conducted an ultrasound of my uterus. Miraculously, an image resembling a pinto bean in size appeared before our eyes, unremarkable except for the distinctive rhythmic pulsing that was to be Abigail.

It is now around ten years since the birth of our miracle baby. Within the first year my Parkinson disease began to rapidly accelerate, resulting in gastroparesis due to the Parkinson meds I was taking. The situation culminated in a 3 week hospital stay, liquid feedings and crushed meds through a j-tube every two hours around the clock. I was forced to face the reality that I could no longer pursue my chosen profession and ultimately resigned from the law firm where I worked and applied for social security disability benefits.

In one fell swoop, my role as a gainfully employed professional career woman ended, and my roles as wife, mother of a toddler and stepmother to two teenagers changed forever. I had planned to care for my aging mother, who had endured quadruple bypass surgery mere months before Abigail was born and to care for my younger sister, who had become permanently physically disabled a few years previously from a head-on car collision. Instead, I was transformed into a person who not only was unable to look after the significant others in my life, but now required nearly round-the-clock care myself.

Following gastro surgery, I was deemed to be a candidate for Deep Brain Stimulation surgery, a treatment that had just been approved by the FDA. On August 30, 2002, I had my first brain surgery.

In retrospect, mine has been a journey filled with good and not-so-good days, as is true of everyone, even those not directly affected by Parkinson. Among the worst moments for me was the day when, after observing me writhing in pain on the floor from a dystonic spasm, then four-year old Abigail plaintively inquired, "Mommy, am I going to get Parkinson disease?"

Rivaling this painful memory is the time when, during parent's day at her preschool, I flipped expectantly in her family notebook to the page prepared especially for the mommies where she had reported in a matter of fact fashion that she wanted to be just like me when she grew up and "laze (sic) around in bed all day," then had drawn a stick figure of me laying in a bed! The fact that this was during my recuperation from many surgeries had apparently escaped my young daughter's consciousness.

I realized at that point that Abigail would never know me as the physically active person who once climbed 14,000 foot peaks, ran 5k races, backpacked into the wilderness and rode and showed horses, or as a career woman who enjoyed an intellectually challenging and busy professional life.

Such moments have, however, been offset by those more frequent and compelling moments during which I have observed my daughter growing into a much more compassionate and understanding person than she might otherwise have been, a person who takes adversity in her stride, hopefully having learned from my example that it is possible to live life with grace and dignity, no matter what may come your way.

As a direct consequence of DBS surgery and the reduction in meds that it has allowed me, I have also been able to have the gastro tubes removed, another momentous occasion in my life. Since DBS, I have been able to accompany my husband and daughter bowling, horseback riding, roller skating, and even downhill skiing - activities that I had erroneously concluded I would never be able to enjoy again!

In hindsight, the gifts that this chronic, progressive, currently incurable illness have revealed to me have far outweighed the burdens, not the least of which includes the satisfaction that comes from having stumbled into a new calling that is much more fulfilling than my prior career in law. Though it may not be the life I had originally envisioned for myself, it is a rich and worthwhile life and one in which I believe my daughter can also take great pride!

Valerie Graham (Copyright © 2007)

See Postscript section for an update on Valerie's story.

PREGNANCY & PARKINSON

.... a cautionary tale

Despite the fair weather forecast from my neurologist that I might enjoy a med free pregnancy, it never came to pass. I remember her saying that at 13 weeks I would start to feel noticeably better and might even enjoy a med holiday. I never made it to 13 weeks. Following a fairly rapid downward titration (from three levadopa a day, an agonist and a Klonopin) I thought the worst was behind me. Off medication, I felt for the first time noticeably Parkinsonian, but besides an amped up tremor and a little lean to the right, I was not bad.

Over the course of six weeks, I saw myself glide right on through the Hahn & Yoehr staging for PD. I am still wondering where being akinetic from the neck down only while sleeping, falls on the scale. My mother and I, still in denial over my diagnosis, experienced a rather brusque awakening. I was alarmed that I now sensed a tremor in my left hand, categorizing me as bilateral. I shared my fears with the neurologist who thought I had come off medication too suddenly. All I heard was that I could slowly re-inroduce Sinemet at 12 weeks. We prayed it would work and only talked about that time in hushed and hallowed tones reserved for sharing family secrets, adult ones. Have I remained that bad in the off state? No, but I now have to take much more medication than I ever did. Would I have another child? Not likely.

I don't wish to scare or deter other Young Onset women wanting children, but make them aware that case studies show pregnancy and PD are not always a good mix. This is odd because estrogen is considered neuro-protective. Parkinson does nothing to help our systems maintain homeostasis.

With the hormonal upheaval going on during pregnancy it is no wonder our brain is speaking up! Now, if only someone else could hear what it is trying to say....

There are answers here - and clues. Dr Lisa Shulman is the only researcher even broaching what pregnancy may tell us. When I have suggested that more research on us is needed (I keep meeting other PD moms who also worsened) I was told that it is a too ethically delicate a research area. It is vexing because there is a window of time for us that seems exponentially smaller. We need to move closer to a model of Patient Driven Research to address these important issues. **Laura Brooks**

W ith the hormonal upheaval going on during pregnancy, it is no wonder our brain is speaking up! Now, if only someone else could hear what it is trying to say . . . . .

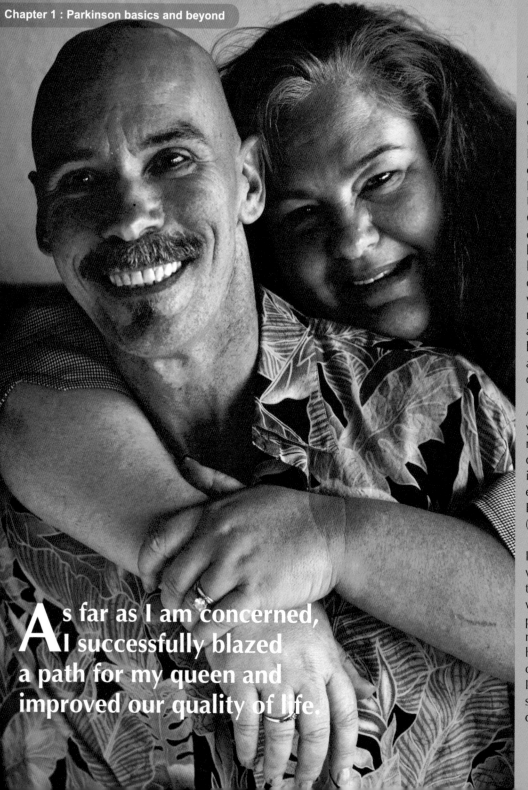

GRETCHEN, MICHAEL & DBS

As far as I am concerned, I successfully blazed a path for my queen and improved our quality of life.

After living with Parkinson Disease for over 13 years, you would think I could catch a break, right? That is what I asked myself as I sat in my neurologist's office at the Movement Disorder Clinic at the University of Florida, Gainesville, in February of 2007. Although, I must have been thinking out loud because my wife and care partner, Gretchen, who also has PD said to me, "quit complaining and sit still!" I would have given my last nickel at that point to be able to do just that.

A lot of things go through your mind when you make the conscience decision to go forward in the process of being evaluated to have Deep Brain Stimulation surgery (DBS).

I recall my first thought was, "Why do I have to go first?" My wife was real clear on this point: "Because a real man blazes a path for his queen." Not very comforting but what could I do, my manhood was at stake, not to mention my quality of life.

THE WORLD'S FIRST DBS COUPLE....

My PD had progressed to an unhealthy and debilitating state. I could not dress myself, buttons were a challenge, shoe laces bothersome and forget about wearing a tie. It's funny how you can justify something as serious as brain surgery when the quality of your life is a series of comedic errors – dropping food in your lap, struggling with the phone and hoping you dialed information correctly and not 911.

Gretchen's turn for DBS came in November of 2008 with similar results. Her gait and balance, although improved, are still a problem and make her susceptible to falls, but there are little to no symptoms of dyskinesia and we have eliminated frequent trips to the emergency room for Ativan injections to release her muscles from their curled up state of dystonia, and only a slight tremor which signals time for meds. Together, we daily celebrate the new and improved Michael and Gretchen.

Has DBS surgery changed our lives? Absolutely! Would I ever reconsider having brain surgery knowing what I know now? Not in the least, I would have it done again tomorrow if necessary. DBS surgery, although the procedure is being constantly improved, will not cure you of PD and there is no guarantee you can stop taking medication. Gretchen never fails to say that having brain surgery was never a walk in the park, but it is a blessing in disguise. It has far exceeded our expectations and restored to us a quality of life that we continuously celebrate. Every Thanksgiving we always remember to say a special prayer of thanks for the technology that has given us our lives back.

I would be remiss if I didn't say there are some trade-offs associated with DBS. DBS surgery creates a certain heightened sense of awareness of your surroundings. It changed the way we travel, the way we shop, even the way that we feel emotionally. There is a euphoric period after DBS that when you feel invincible but it usually does not last. Ultimately, we rely on each other to gauge the appropriate emotional responses to certain situations that are related to DBS. One such example: Gretchen likes to point out to people is how sensitive I've become because I will tear up over beer commercials! These and other "side effects" should be brought to the attention of your doctor and can usually be programmed out if these feelings continue. Uncontrolled crying, laughing, depression, apathy are all common with DBS surgery. DBS surgery has changed the way that we travel. No longer can we zip through the magnetic field generating security systems used by the TSA at airports. Instead we must submit to the very thorough hands of airport security personnel. Additionally, I've found that even hunting for a snack in the refrigerator can be hazardous. The magnetic strip around the door can shut the stimulator off. The return of symptoms is usually a clue.

Both Gretchen and I are grateful for the commitment and dedication of our doctors, nurses and medical students pursuing this career choice. It has truly changed our lives for the better and we live each day with more purpose. We give thanks to our creator and have found a renewed sense of living. Walks on the beach, holding hands, playing with our children, eating out; these are some of the things PD had taken from us and we missed them.

Because of DBS we can now plan for the future. We set goals that are attainable and we pursue new ones. We are able to travel and attend more PD events where we readily share our experiences with our new "battery-operated brains" (borrowed from Jackie Hunt Christensen's book).

As far as I am concerned, I successfully blazed a path for my queen and improved our quality of life.

Michael Church

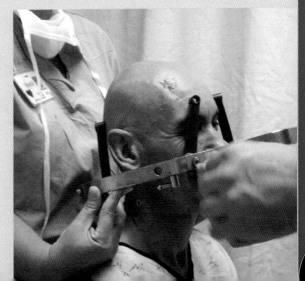

BE AWARE,
DBS IS NOT A PANACEA

I was 38 when I heard the military neurologist say those dreaded words, "I'm pretty sure you have Parkinson's."

Having completed my Ph.D. in clinical psychology and working on active duty in the U.S. Air Force as a military psychologist, I had some knowledge of what those words meant for me and my wife Sandra's future. Still, I was relieved, in a way, that it wasn't what I had been fearing.

At least I hadn't had a stroke, or worse yet, a brain tumor. I had been turning these over in my mind as explanations for the foot-dragging that hampered my running ability and the annoying twitching in my little finger. Being diagnosed with a chronic disease, especially an old person's disease, seemed particularly unfair and annoying - other than the occasional seasonal allergy, I was seldom ill.

Despite the relief of finally getting a firm diagnosis, I was skeptical. Before I saw the neurologist, my physicians had dismissed my complaint of 'forgetting how to run' as a sign of stress, or advancing age, or being over-worked. I knew something was wrong, my body wasn't acting right. But Parkinson? At my age? After a positive response to Sinemet, the diagnosis was almost certain. We researched the symptoms and saw that PD explained the nightly cramps, and food didn't taste or smell as good as it used to. Even my constant dandruff seemed associated.

Our lives went on. In the early stage of PD the Air Force deemed me healthy enough to be transferred to Okinawa, Japan. For the first two years, Sinemet worked well and I was able to function as chief of Kadena air base's mental health clinic. When tremors spread to both hands, making my handwriting nearly illegible, I compensated by typing everything. I learned how to time my medications to best hide the symptoms.

During my third year overseas I started having severe dyskinetic movements brought on by the Sinemet. Soon, I was no longer able to hide my symptoms from my co-workers and patients. My commander initiated a quick medical retirement and before I knew it, I was a civilian again. Unwilling to let PD win, I landed a job teaching at one of the universities on Okinawa. The decrease in stress due to the slower paced lifestyle allowed us to stay an additional two years--some of the best years of our lives.

Finally PD caught up again, and I had to stop teaching face-to-face classes. After Okinawa the symptoms started to progress more rapidly. I went from being able to type forty words-per-minute to five. Dyskinesias started interfering with my ability to walk and I started having freezing episodes. At times my tremors would be so violent there

was concern I might fracture the bones in my hands. Sandra had read about deep brain stimulation surgery and, after much thought, we applied for it. With Sandra navigating the red tape of the VA system after two years on the waiting list I had the surgery.

Immediately after the surgery I was ecstatic. Nearly all tremors were eradicated along with all the dyskinesias. Freezing was eliminated. I went from 36 pills per day to eight. We had been cautioned that DBS tended to give a 'honeymoon period' right after surgery where long-term difficulties hadn't yet arisen. For eight months I was nearly back to my early PD functioning. I even went back to work, part-time, working with another psychologist.

Eight months and about ten reprogramming trips to the neurological clinic later, a 90 miles trip from our home, the programming specialist finally conceded there was little else she could do...my speech was, for all practical purposes, gone. The left DBS lead was leaking electricity into the speech area of my brain, causing muscle rigidity in my jaw, tongue, lips and throat. We knew it was a side-effect of the DBS stimulator - if we turned the DBS lead's electricity off my voice returned to normal, but the tremors also returned on my right side. Without the stimulator the tremors were so violent my whole body shook so hard I opted to go without speaking as the best of choices.

For the past two years Sandra and I have learned, to some extent, to compensate for the loss of my speaking ability, but, no bones about it, it has been difficult. I had to quit working entirely. Unable to speak, I found that the slowness of my typing made working unfeasible. Just typing this 1,000-word article took the better part of four days. Still, we are getting by.

I use a (supposedly) portable touchscreen speaking device, primarily designed for wheelchair-bound patients to say complicated sentences, but the general slowness of the PD (not substantially improved by DBS) makes two-way conversation halting and frustrating. At times, when it mispronounces words, I can sound like a drunken Stephen Hawking. For shorter communications I use a small whiteboard with a dry erase marker, but my cramped PD-sized, nearly illegible handwriting (also not DBS improved) can be hard to read.

All in all, would I recommend DBS? Most certainly. But, be aware, it is not a panacea. Tremors, balance and freezing are definitely improved but nearly 70% of DBS patients experienced some degradation in speech, although complete loss of speech is rare. For some patients DBS also requires frequent follow-up visits to a DBS-trained neurologist, which can be hard to find in some rural areas. Finally, I would recommend not giving up. Accept help when needed, keep active and, above all, keep a sense of humor and perspective.

Christopher Herron PhD

WHY DEEP BRAIN STIMULATION?

I'm definitely in favor of the DBS-STN. I would do it again. In fact, I have done it again, with no regrets.

I had a thalamotomy in June 1996, for tremors on my left side. This is an invasive and non-reversible surgery that permanently damages cells in the brain. When tremors showed up on my right side I couldn't have another thalamotomy because of a high risk of side effects due to excessive stress on the thalamic region.

My first stimulator implant (the forerunner of DBS) was done October 1998. Due to a rare infection, my stimulator was removed in January 2001. My last surgery was August 2001, when I had a a bilateral DBS-STN. Those seven months were the longest of my life. For all practical purposes, if you have Parkinson disease and qualify by need, the DBS is truly a life support system. With it, you have a life. Without it, you are alive - BUT have no life. For seven months my only reason to go on living was the promise that my DBS was coming.

The difference between the surgeries was amazing. In the first surgery, I was fully awake and aware through the halo, MRI, drilling, implanting and testing. The last surgery, they phased me in and out of lala land as needed. There was not near as much stress or pain during the later surgery, and it was bilateral. I had DBS for tremors and they are GONE.

NEGATIVES:

- Once you've had surgery, you no longer qualify for most med studies.

- I believe the stress from surgery awakens dormant symptoms. After DBS, I had balance and rigidity problems.

- Others have mentioned "side effects" but most agree that quality of life is better, overall, with DBS.

- It is normal to have a euphoric "honeymoon" phase, where the patient feels "cured" of PD. Then when reality hits deep post-op depression can occur.

- DBS is an effective symptom reliever, but NOT A CURE.

- It may take from months to years to find your "magic" calibration. There are literally thousands of combinations.

- There are trade-offs. Your best calibration for tremors may give you balance problems and/or slurred speech, etc.

Having Medicare coverage is essential because many with Parkinson disease cannot work and thus have no opportunity to attain insurance through employment and private insurance is not affordable.

In many cases, if not most, the need for PD meds is reduced with the DBS.

From a medical standpoint, the advantages of DBS have been documented. However, the reality of regaining functions of the body, once thought lost forever, is nothing short of an amazing miracle. Try tying your hands to a short cord attached to a ceiling fan blade & you'll have an idea what it's like living with severe tremors: you're rendered helpless. Trapped in your own body as if it were remote controlled and the controls had an erratic short circuit.

Is it a cure-all end-all? NO! Does it give back your life? In most cases, NO! But for me and countless others, it gives a life worth living, and when a cure for PD is found, it can be reversed.

If you don't have a ceiling fan, or are afraid to be connected to it 24/7, I could take you on a verbal journey through Hell and then you'll know why Medicare should approve DBS!

In closing I must say that even though I'm a DBS-STN advocate, I do NOT believe that it's for everyone. With any surgery, a positive attitude is paramount for optimum success and a negative attitude is like wearing an anchor to a pool party.

Jimmie 'Toad' Turner

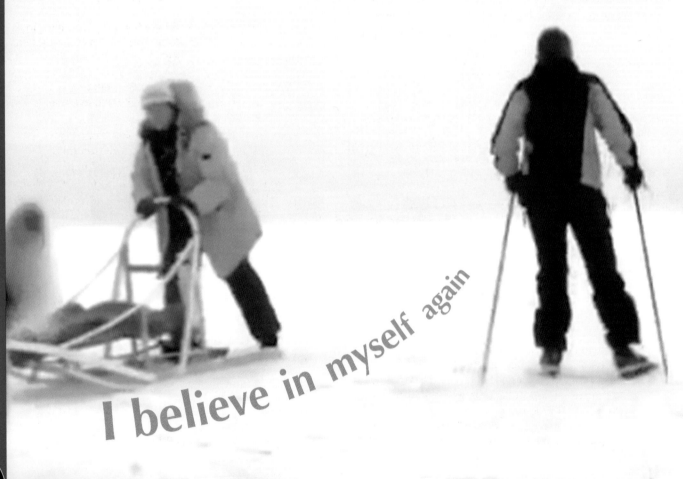

Duodopa is licensed for use in some countries in the European Union and elsewhere. Patients in the USA have been watching its progress through the regulatory process for years. It is hoped that it will be available there soon.

I believe in myself again

PÄR'S DUODOPA STORY

Back to life with Duodopa

This a short summary of my experiences using Duodopa.

Duodopa has changed my life as a Parkinson disease patient. I have literally got my life back.

My name is Pär Ohrberg and I was with diagnosed Parkinson disease early in 2000. I am married to Mia and we have two youngsters, Lovisa aged 17, and Marcus who is 19. We live in Stockholm. I work in the IT business in sales and management. Until the end of 2008 I worked full-time and then for six months I only worked for 75% of my usual hours. We have a rich social life individually as well as a family. We like to travel, ski, cook, watch films and enjoy outdoors activities.

My Parkinson diagnosis was made in early February 2000. During 2000 to 2004 I lived a rather normal life, taking oral medication only. Work and career mean a lot to me and I have always been very focused, an overachiever with definite targets and time limits. I have had goals since early on which have followed me all the way through my life - until the diagnosis of Parkinson disease.

In 2007 my symptoms became more problematic and it felt as if function after function of mind and body were being lost step by step. Chores and jobs that used to be done with little effort suddenly became very challenging and took a lot of time to do.

Before Duodopa

A normal day in October 2008: My morning started, often very early, around 5 o´clock. Most of the time I had a hard time moving myself and I was very stiff, so one Madopar dissolved in water gave me a good start. Most mornings my feet were severely cramped and the pain was terrible. I got a maximum of 5 hours sleep a night - almost never in one go. I would go to bed around midnight and take a sleeping pill to help me sleep. Often I would wake up during night very hungry. Mornings would start at around 5-5.30 am.

All the usual symptoms of PD were there: Tremor, slowness (bradykinesia), rigid muscles, impaired posture and balance, loss of automatic movements and:

- Speech changes, dementia.
- Feeling very down, even depressed, for several days of the week.
- I sometimes had suicidal thoughts.
- It was getting much harder to type and write by hand.
- During off periods it became difficult for me to express my thoughts, ideas etc.
- As a result of this I tended more and more to keep away from social happenings, events, parties, etc.
- I couldn't smell anything, apart from odours produced by my brain, ghost smells.
- I frequently needed the men's room.
- I needed Viagra to improve my sex life.
- I had an increasing need for sweets.
- My memory was getting worse every day.

Worst of all, my personality had changed. I went from being reliable, sociable, strong-minded, decisive, engaged, quick, and a high achiever, to something rather different and less attractive.

After Duodopa

In April 2009 my DuoDopa pump was "installed". I had a team of three nurses from Solvay and a team from the hospital who supported me during the pre-op phase, the operation and during the initial phase managing the treatment. I didn't feel nervous - the team was extremely professional.

The effects were immediate and extremely positive. If we look at the situation now, 15 months after I started on the treatment, following effects are noticeable:

- I have no tremor and no on-off effects.
- I am only rigid in the morning and evening.
- I can think clearly all day long.
- I am performing much better at work.
- My enjoyment of a social life has returned.
- I am not nervous any more when doing. presentations, meeting large groups of people,etc.
- My speech is normal - I have a strong clear voice.
- I can remember things again.
- I believe in myself again.

Pär Ohrberg

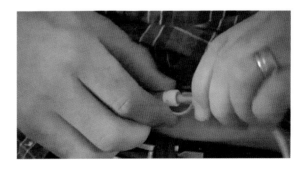

LIFE LESSONS, ENOUGH!

I was diagnosed in 2001 after a string of misdiagnoses. I was fifty-four, not young, but not old either. Being diagnosed was as difficult a moment as I have ever had but only for a while and then everything, more or less, went back to normal. Coping with Parkinson disease has been demanding, but I am fortunate to have progressed slowly. I am fortunate to have an attentive and supportive family. I am fortunate to be tremor dominate. I am fortunate to have Parkinson disease instead of one of the other brain maladies. I am fortunate, I am fortunate, I am fortunate.......I know that, however, if I'm so damn fortunate how come I don't really feel fortunate? I am fortunate that I know that answer. Today my meds aren't working largely because I got up late and the timing has been thrown off all day, I am tired from preparing for week-end house guests, a fact which delights and destroys me and finally I don't sleep.

The last decade has changed my life, but the last year has changed me. I used to be physically strong, now I am not. I used to sing, now I cannot. I used to be athletic, now I am not. I used to work, now I do not. These are only a few of the ways in which Parkinson disease has changed my life. These changes happened over time and I have learned , fairly successfully, to adapt my new life to the demands of the changes. My life is slower now, more contemplative, more self-aware. I have reduced the number of things that I consider really important, I have prioritized the things that I value and I have let go of old slights and perceived offences. For better and for worse my life has changed.

Seldom, when things are going well, do we examine the reasons. It is only when something bad happens that we really take the time to consider all the "whats" "whens" and "whys".

Good things make us happy, bad things make us smart. I have learned a great many things in the last decade, I have committed to memory a great many life lessons and if it's ok, I would just as soon not learn any more. My life is just fine right now, just the way it is.

Life change is inevitable, without it we would still be living in caves and hunting our dinner with sticks. Personal change is desirable but not a real requirement. Until this past year I had spent my time managing the changes in my life, coping with an unpleasant disease, reordering my spending habits and in lieu of a job, organizing all the drawers in my house. Then, after a rather lengthy absence I discovered NeuroTalk. At the time I thought I had rediscovered the MGH forum BrainTalk, a place that had been instrumental in sharing with me the skills I needed, at that time, to keep moving forward. The names were unfamiliar and the subjects seemed less about emotions and more about science, but the feeling was the same. It was a place of sharing and comparing, exchanging and informing. I began reading about a proposed project that entailed writing a book about the value of the experience of communicating virtually with strangers. I had met one of the parties once or twice and asked if I could join in.

That's when I began to change. For the first time in many years my days were filled with "occupation", genuine, meaningful, productive work. I began to see myself in a new light, a light that included being a contributor to a cause that I cared about. The writing was difficult in the beginning, requiring draft after draft, edit after edit. Many of the early pieces found their way to the trash can. The time passed, the barricades came down and the truth began to spill out. I have become a new person. I still have Parkinson and I still have to cope with the disease, but the terms of our arrangement have changed. There are times that I know I must acquiesce but now there are more times that I overrule my condition and do what I want. By participating, I have become powerful, not in the way I once was, but in a new and profound way. I have learned to demand and not be still, to insist and not be silent. I still cannot sing but I can be heard.

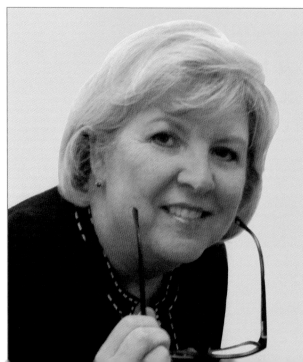

I can join my voice with others and together we can make a real difference.

Now that's power . . .

Pamela Kell

A FEW QUESTIONS FOR MY NEUROLOGIST

Pamela Kell talks to her neurologist Dr Samer Tabbal

Why did you become a Movement Disorders Specialist?

Did you have a personal connection with movement disorders, or a particular intellectual connection?

My interest in movement disorders grew steadily during my first year of medical training when I started learning about a mysterious collections of brain cells (neurons) that are located in the base of the brain, called the basal ganglia. Aside from their beautiful unusual shape, the electrophysiological function of the basal ganglia fascinated me enough to light up my whole brain! They receive connections from the entire brain and contribute to the generation of movements as well as to thinking and behavior through intricate little circuits that cross purposefully numerous surrounding structures. By my second year of neurology residency training, I witnessed first-hand the clinical manifestations of the injuries of the basal ganglia when I listened to and examined patients with parkinsonian syndromes, various forms of tremor, gait problems and unusual involuntary movements (such as tics and dyskinesia). I was genuinely amazed by how a tiny lesion in a strategic location of the basal ganglia caused widespread symptoms and signs that can be picked up on exam (even without brain imaging). Parkinsonian syndromes were particularly special in their wide spectrum of unique clinical manifestations and their response to treatment.

By then, when I gave a lecture to medical students, I consistently started it with my standard statement: "I can't imagine how someone who studies medicine can choose any specialty other than neurology. After all, what is more interesting in this universe than the brain? Once you become a neurology resident, I can't imagine how you can choose any neurology sub-specialty other than movement disorders. What is more interesting in the brain than the basal ganglia?"

In your practice what has been your biggest surprise or disappointment?

When a disease, such as Parkinson disease, or a structure, such as the basal ganglia, is so mysterious, any little new discovery brings a surprise. There have been many little discoveries in the 13 years since I became a movement disorder specialist. The biggest surprise was probably how well deep brain stimulation therapy improved the symptoms of Parkinson disease and tremor. I was still a movement disorder fellow when this was presented in the late 1990s as a "miracle treatment" for such patients in France. Since there had been many "pretended miracle treatments" that did not stand the test of time, the movement disorder community (including me) was quite skeptical of DBS's effectiveness. When examining patients before and after DBS therapy, it became obvious to me that this tool is quite valuable in conquering Parkinson disease and essential tremor. Indeed, Parkinson patients do reasonably well in the first 10-15 years on medications, but motor fluctuations and dyskinesias become difficult to control satisfactorily thereafter on medications alone. DBS therapy can patch this disease for another 10-15 years. DBS therapy is a major breakthrough in the treatment of Parkinson disease. What is not surprising is that DBS therapy is obviously not a cure and it has some adverse effects that are fortunately tolerable in most patients.

My biggest disappointment in 13 years of practice was leaving my patients at the University of Arkansas for Medical Sciences in Little Rock, when I moved to Washington University in St Louis. When I see patients in the clinic for several months, they become in a way family… each one with his unique personality, his unique family and unique stories as well as unique disease … It is never easy to leave family, even for good reason. What made my move to St Louis even harder was that the people of Arkansas were particularly appreciative of my services.

How optimistic are you about the future of those with Parkinson disease?

We have learned more about Parkinson disease through research over the last 30 years than we have over the last 100 years. When I started my movement disorder fellowship training in 1997, we had six medications for the treatment of Parkinson disease. Ten years later, this number doubled and DBS has become an established therapy. We now have technology to study the brain and its diseases. We are quite close to identifying the cause of Parkinson disease and I have no doubt that we will discover how to slow down the progression and/or prevent the disease, probably within the next 10 or 15 years. However, I doubt that we will be able to re-grow brain cells to cure advanced Parkinson disease.

What area of the current research do you believe is the most/least promising?

By far the most promising area of research in Parkinson disease is that of identifying drugs to slow down the progression of the illness. I believe so because we know that the degenerating brain cells and their connections are extremely difficult, if not impossible, to regenerate (say with drugs or tissue transplant). I doubt that tissue transplant will ever be the cure of Parkinson disease, but I hope I am just as wrong as the person who did not believe a hundred year ago that humans would be able to fly. For now, it is best to keep the brain cells and their connections from degenerating in the first place.

Studying combinations of drugs that could slow down the progression of the illness will be the next step in drug therapy. It is unlikely that the progression of Parkinson disease will be halted with one "magic" drug. Just as in the treatment of cancer, it is more likely that a combination will be needed for this end, especially because Parkinson disease is not one disease.

Identifying the cause of the degeneration of brain cells in Parkinson disease is also key for beating the disease, especially in light of growing evidence that the cause of idiopathic Parkinson is genetic as well as environmental. In other words, patients with Parkinson disease (especially those with no family history) probably developed it because they have a genetic predisposition superimposed on exposure to an environmental toxin. Identifying such toxins is key to preventing the disease.

What is your definition of a good movement disorder specialist?

A good movement disorder specialist is a "good doctor" who has been trained in a good movement disorders program. The definition of a "good doctor" varies with the needs of each patient. Some patients prefer authoritative doctors to draw confidence from, while others patients prefer a more give-and-take attitude. The attributes of a "good doctor" however remain the same: one who listens well, who is patient, compassionate, understanding, knowledgeable, experienced and passionate about his/her mission.

I usually recommend doctors involved in research (such as those at reputable universities) because their knowledge tends to be more up-to-date and deeper than that of busy private practitioners. However, I am not sure this is necessarily a requirement since there are also excellent movement disorder specialists in private practice who are not involved in research.

What characteristics make a good patient?

A good patient is the one who exercises regularly, who has reasonable expectations and the "right attitude", who is educated about Parkinson disease and who provides accurate information to his/her neurologist.

There is growing evidence, in animal and human studies, that regular exercise improves symptoms and may even prevent developing Parkinson disease. Even walking and dancing count!

The right attitude consists of a whole-hearted attempt to make the most out of the situation despite the physical and psychological limitations imposed by the illness. A social support system of family and friends is most useful. Antidepressants may also often be useful since more than a third of Parkinson disease patients have clinical depression due to chemical imbalance in their brains resulting from degenerating brain cells.

Learning about Parkinson disease helps a patient fight it. A good patient therefore should ask his/her neurologist questions in clinic and should seek information from every reliable source. When choosing a source, keep in mind that not all of what is on the internet is accurate. Some patients and caregivers find support groups useful, others find them depressing (it is sometimes not a good idea to compare notes because there are no two Parkinson disease patients who are alike).

I am sorry to say that to date, there are no drugs or food supplements that slow down the progression of the illness. This does not mean that you should not adhere to a healthy diet that keeps you from having heart attacks, strokes and cancer.

Knowing about the manifestations of the disease makes it less unpredictable and leads to reasonable expectations. Knowing the adverse effects of medications helps in recognizing them and learning about treatment modalities makes the patient seek them at the appropriate time.

Accurate medical history allows the neurologist to make the best decision in the plan of care. In my experience, compliance in taking medications (as instructed and on time) is usually not an issue in Parkinson disease patients because non-compliance leads to immediate worsening of symptoms.

How have the roles of the patients and doctors changed since you began practicing and how have those changes, if any, been beneficial?

The role of patient has not changed much since I began my practice (see "characteristics make a good patient") except that patients have more access to more (good and bad) information through the Internet.

The role of doctors has grown to encompass a much larger body of medical information that is growing at a tremendous rate, thus the imperative need for sub-specialists.

Unfortunately, for many reasons related to malicious regulators/lawyers as well as inappropriate doctors' behavior, physicians have had to assume the role of businessmen. They are now required to increase their efficiency at evaluating patients and change their documentations of patient encounters to shield themselves from medico-legal problems. These changes unfortunately are at the expense of patients as doctors have had to cut the time they spend with each one.

What is the single most important piece of advice/ warning you would give to a young doctor entering your profession?

My advice is to treat your patients like you would like to be treated if you were the patient. (Isn't it interesting that all religions give this same advice to humans about dealing with their neighbors?) This sounds like one advice, but it actually encompasses several requirements, such as integrity, motivation patience, compassion, understanding, knowledge and experience. In other words: be a "good doctor."

My warning to a young doctor is to watch out for arrogance, hypocrisy and greed.

What is the greatest impediment to the success of future research?

The greatest impediment to the success of future research is conformism of researchers and under-funding of research (usually brought about by shortsighted and/or ignorant politicians).

Is there anything you would like to see implemented universally to improve the general standard of care?

I would improve young doctors' education in every respect.

Namely, instilling in them the attributes of the "good doctor", providing for them free access to information and relieving them of debt related to medical school tuition fees in return for some medical care service that they provide to their community.

In what area, if any, do you see input from patients being necessary or beneficial to determining the direction of research?

Research starts with listening to patients. Patients already know what they want and have set the direction of research. The direction is straight forward: The cure of Parkinson disease.

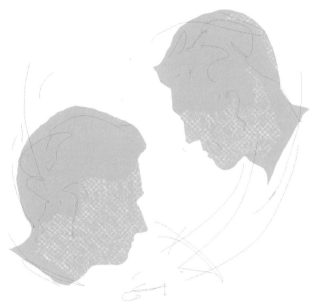

Dr. Samer Tabbal, recipient of the Sven Eliasson Award for Teaching Excellence, joined Washington University at Saint Louis in June 2003 as Assistant Professor of Neurology and Director of the Deep Brain Stimulation Program for Parkinson Disease and Other Movement Disorders. In January 2013, he returned to his native Lebanon.

Research starts with listening to patients. Patients already know what they want and have set the direction of research.

The direction is straight forward: The cure of Parkinson disease.

BRAAK'S HYPOTHESIS

Girija Muralidhar, PhD

The first detailed report of Parkinson disease was published by James Parkinson in 1817, as a monograph titled "An Essay on the Shaking Palsy." Parkinson described tremor or trembling movements, particularly while at rest; stiffness or rigidity of muscles; slowness of movement; and difficulty with walking and maintaining balance as major symptoms of the disease which we call PD.

Interestingly, Parkinson's monograph was based on his analysis of just six patients, yet his portrayal of PD has been used as a standard for diagnosis for over 150 years. The standard mode of treatment for PD has been to revive motor responses via dopamine-mediated mechanisms while the non-motor symptoms were neither acknowledged nor treated.

What are the non-motor symptoms? Many non-motor symptoms such as hyposmia (decreased sense of smell), gastrointestinal dysfunctions (constipation), sleep disorders (trouble falling asleep, REM disorders), pain and/or depression, anxiety and panic attacks, dementia and psychosis have long been a part of Parkinson disease from the patients' perspective. In the last decade, these non-motor manifestations of PD have been accepted as components of Parkinson disease mostly due to Braak's hypothesis of PD, as well as voices of patient activists who believed that PD is more than a movement disorder.

What is Braak's hypothesis?

In 2003, Heiko Braak proposed a novel hypothesis of development of PD, based on the distribution of Lewy bodies and Lewy neuritis in the brains of elderly people during postmortem examinations. He proposed that the pathological changes in brains of patients with Parkinson disease begin in the olfactory regions and the lower brain stem (two non-dopaminergic areas), then spread to the midbrain, i.e., substantia nigra (dopaminergic areas) and in the final stage, pathologic changes spread diffusely throughout the cerebral cortex. He believed that non-dopaminergic regions are affected long before dopaminergic ones and non-motor dysfunctions precede motor difficulties.

According to Braak, Parkinson disease has six stages.

Stage 1&2 are considered preclinical. Lewy bodies are seen in medulla oblongata and olfactory bulb. Hyposmia and dysregulation of autonomic nervous system initiated. The symptoms include constipation, orthostatic hypotension, urogenital disturbances, sialorrhea, excessive sweating and temperature dysregulation.

Stage 3 & 4: Lewy bodies appear in substantia nigra and forebrain. Pontine cholinergic functions are affected. Neural degradation seen and dopaminergic function deteriorates. Patients may have akinesia, fluctuating attention, REM sleep disorder, day time sleepiness, mild deficits in executive function and depression. Patients will start to manifest classical Parkinsonism.

Stage 5: Lewy bodies progress to the amygdala. Emotional and motivational disorders become more common

Stage 6: Lewy bodies may progress to cortex, fibrillary tangles and sporadic senile plaques are common. Parkinson disease dementia may develop.

While Braaks' staging of PD appears to validate many of the observations of patients who are "experts" in their disease, it is not a perfect one and may not explain every feature of PD. However, the impact of Braak's hypothesis is big and is already visible. Treatments targeting non-motor dysfunctions are available, early diagnostic tools as well as disease-modifying therapies based on non-dopaminergic pathways are being developed. It is an exciting time in PD research and drug development. Time to hope for a cure!

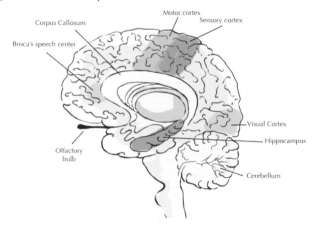

Ref:
• Braak H, Del Tredici K, Bratzke H, Hamm-Clement J, Sandmann-Keil D, Rub U. Staging of the intracerebral inclusion body pathology associated with idiopathic Parkinson's disease (preclinical and clinical stages). J Neurol. 2002; 249 Suppl 3:III/1-5
• Braak H, Bohl JR, Müller CM, Rüb U, de Vos RA, Del Tredici K. Stanley Fahn Lecture 2005: The staging procedure for the inclusion body pathology associated with sporadic Parkinson's disease reconsidered. Mov Disord. 2006 Dec;21(12):2042-51. Review.1.

THE GENETIC BASIS FOR PARKINSON DISEASE

Most cases of Parkinson disease are classified as sporadic and occur in people with no apparent history of the disorder in their family. Until 15 years ago, idiopathic Parkinson disease was thought to have no genetic basis. However, approximately 15 percent of people with Parkinson disease do have a family history of this disorder. This suggested that certain genes may be involved in developing PD.

What are genes and how are they responsible for causing PD?

At the simplest, a gene is a unit of genetic information carried on a chromosome which we inherit from our parents. Genes code for proteins and proteins are the building blocks of our cells and body. Genes are arranged along these chromosomes in a linear order with each gene located at a specific spot called a locus (plural: loci).

The discovery of SNCA locus, coding for alpha-synuclein protein being linked with PD, and further observations that mutations in SNCA result in a faulty alpha-synuclein protein (a component of Lewy bodies), supported the idea of genetic basis for PD. Furthermore, mutations in genes such as LRRK2, PARK2, PARK7, PINK1 are shown to be linked to the development of familial PD. Now the race is on to find other genetic sites which are connected with PD, and discoveries are being made all the time.

Going hand in hand with defining loci, the opportunity to relate that information to understand PD and its clinical course is emerging. For example, mutations in PARK2 locus (coding for Parkin) affect mitochondrial

function and seem to contribute to PD development. This form of PD is characterized by slow and relatively benign course and a marked sensitivity to dopamine unlike with typical late onset IPD.

The scientific community is also beginning to define the risk for genetic disease in the Parkinson population, based on race and ethnicity. For example, in East Asian populations there are a number of LRRK2 gene variants that considerably alter the risk for Parkinson disease. Genetic variability at this locus explains about 10% of risk in the East Asia populations. PARKIN and to a lesser degree PINK1 mutations are common, yet most often seen in early-onset disease. They actually may explain about 50% of the disease that is young onset. Overall, the loci identified explain about 10 to 40% of the risk in most populations. That is to say, about half the risk of getting Parkinson disease has now been identified on a genetic basis. As more loci are discovered, the proportion of identified risk will increase significantly. The interaction of these gene products (proteins) with environmental factors is another challenge.

While genetic testing to predict the onset of PD is certainly possible, it still remains in the realm of research studies. Moreover, there also are ethical issues in relation to genetic testing. Specifically, if one is found to be prone to develop PD, how would that affect such things as job availability or the possibility of getting insurance? If people become "rated" for insurance policies based on genetic risk for Parkinson disease, genetic testing certainly will be much more problematic.

Another issue is the emotional basis of knowing that one is highly prone to developing Parkinson disease. As of now (2013), there are no known medications or other treatments to prevent Parkinson disease. How would it affect the life of a 30-year-old to realize that he was prone much more than an average person to get the disease, as he watches his parent suffer from PD?

All of these ethical issues remain unanswered.

Girija Muralidhar, PhD & May Griebel, MD
Ref: Hardy John. Genetic analysis of pathways to Parkinson disease. Neuron 2010 October 21; 68 (2): 201-206.

THE GENETICS OF PARKINSON DISEASE

Mutations in 6 genes (SNCA, LRRK2, PRKN, DJ1, PINK1, and ATP13A2) have conclusively been shown to cause familial parkinsonism. In addition, common variation in 3 genes (MAPT, LRRK2, and SNCA) and loss-of-function mutations in GBA have been well-validated as susceptibility factors for PD.

Bekris LM, Mata IF, Zabetian CP 2010 The genetics of Parkinson disease.J Geriatr Psychiatry Neurol. 2010 Dec;23(4):228-42. Epub 2010 Oct 11.

ONE MORE GENE MUTATION:
Protein Mutation in VPS35 is associated with late-onset PD

Dr. Carles Vilariño-Güell and colleagues have discovered a mutation in vacuolar protein-sorting associated protein 35 (VPS35) that may signal a higher risk for Parkinson disease. VPS35 is a central component of a protein complex, is critical for endosome-trans-golgi trafficking and membrane-protein recycling. One specific mutation (VPS35 c.1858G>A) was found in all affected members of the Swiss kindred and in three more families and one patient with sporadic PD, but it was not observed in 3,309 controls.

Zimpric, A et al., (2011) The American Journal of Human Genetics, Volume 89, Issue 1, 168-175, 15 July 2011 online publication

What we learned in 1998

- **Parkinson is a movement disorder caused by a lack of dopamine.**
- **If you had to have a neurological disorder, this was the one to get.**
- **Researchers were closer to curing Parkinson than any other neurological illness.**
- **They predicted a cure in 5 years.**
- **Neurologists felt conflicted about when to start patients on Sinemet.**
- **Parkinson was only rarely genetic and this was mainly in younger onset patients.**
- **Pesticides were suspected as causal.**
- **Parkinson was not painful.**
- **It could take 20 to 30 years to become disabled.**
- **If Sinemet worked, you had Parkinson.**
- **Parkinson doesn't kill you.**
- **But there are no survivors.**

What we are learning now.....

The Parkinson community has blossomed online, though it is still fragmented across national and international borders in its offline activity. During more than a decade, (1998–2012) PwP online have become informed and involved in their own medical care and have learned about the role of economics in the treatment development process. Though some stakeholders are now reaching out and communicating with them, patient activists feel PwP should play a larger part in decision making. Some PD organizations and foundations now have patient advisory councils.

Scientists are less inclined to make predictions about a cure, or even a treatment. Parkinson is no longer viewed as simply a movement disorder; rather it is now viewed as a more extensive Central Nervous System disorder, with many non-motor symptoms and an emerging pattern of pre-motor symptoms that might begin in the gut, or in the olfactory system. (Braak)

Genetic analysis is set to play a much larger role in diagnosis and in the search for bio-markers and treatment targets. Genetic factors alone do not predict or diagnose Parkinson. It is still believed environmental triggers, possibly in combination with gene mutations, may cause the condition, but genetic susceptibility alone may increase the chances of developing the condition.

Parkinson presents in highly individual ways and generally speaking, it is more often recommended that patients are prescribed dopamine agonist therapy before l-dopa. There are sophisticated, more revealing scans, such as the PET scan, that are able to pinpoint the damage or progress in clinical trials. Scans are expensive and not yet widely used as the norm in the course of most PD patients' diagnoses or treatment.

Young onset patients, disturbingly, are increasing in number, as are the aging 'baby boomers', who are plentiful and at a more typical age for the development of PD. There is still no accurate accounting of numbers of PwP. The often used figure of 1.5 million in the USA and 120,000 in the UK may be an underestimate, especially considering the many early onset patients misdiagnosed or not openly sharing their diagnoses.

People with Parkinson would like to argue the assertion that PD is not painful. Accompanying effects such as dystonia can be crushing. Malfunctioning nerves and muscles can lead to a spectrum of painful conditions resulting in disk replacements and other surgeries. The addition of painkillers to medication protocols complicates matters. L-dopa, used for more than 40 years as the gold standard for symptom relief, is proving to have troubling side effects with long term use. It is, however, heartening that along with the knowledge gained in the search for treatments, there appears to be a shift toward exploration of newly discovered non-dopaminergic pathways and non-dopaminergic therapies.

There are still no survivors.

Paula Wittekind & Robert Cummings

PD THEN AND NOW • A PATIENT PERSPECTIVE

Not That You Asked

Kathleen Cochran

Previously published in
the Yale Journal of the
Humanities in Medicine
in October 2010

Walk…
slow—
shake…
so—
want
to know?
Let me
explain…
about my
brain —
how it
constrains.

Muscles don't move
right.
Can't walk loose, stride
light,
can't make my pen
write
or hold a knife
tight.

I tend to drop
stuff
and if I chop
stuff
it's very
carefully,
don't want to be
an amputee.

My clothes put up
a fight;
gotta dress with
foresight.
Silky-loose works
just right.
Stretchy, clingy really
bite.

Nightmare
scenarios?
Consider
pantyhose…
or icy
intersections,
city drivers'
predilections:
a mini-
marathon
for this would-be
carrion.

Well, it
could be
worse.
Hell, I've got
words.
Though it's hard to find
ones
that rhyme with
Parkinson's.

HOURLY TRANSFORMATIONS

Like the big-hearted Tin Man in the Wizard of Oz, before and after Dorothy finds his oil can, we spend our days at the whim of our own oil cans, i.e. our levodopa treatment. In the later stages of our disease, we may need our Parkinson medications as frequently as every two hours. When they fail, we're stuck in the body of a feeble elderly person, but when the meds kick in, we may recover our real selves, transformed to an exuberant, limber 57 or 85-year old scampering up a hill after a child. These fluctuations may leave us feeling extremely fragmented.

In the course of any given day, a PwP (unlike someone without Parkinson) essentially has no fixed physical identity. When our meds work, we say we are 'on', and when they fail, we say we're 'off'. Our good 'ons' make us forget we have PD. We prefer to skip our bad 'ons' (caused by our meds over-working), which can cause writhing, embarrassing, unwanted movements called dyskinesias. The casual observer may misinterpret our appearance with dyskinesia as drunkenness and our 'offs' may make us appear 'stoned'. Our best 'ons' lead observers to believe that we must be getting better, and then cheerfully congratulate us!

The truth is far more complex, unique to every individual and difficult to digest. Until there is a cure our disease inexorably progresses. No one actually gets better or cured, nor has the equivalent remission of some cancer survivors. If PwP intermittently feel and appear better throughout the day it is because of a combination of meds kicking in, consistent mental and physical exercise, adequate sleep, good friends and support systems, creative pursuits, eating well and limiting major stressors. Unfortunately, even if we do all those things, it doesn't eliminate the daily, extreme pendulum-swings between Rusted Tin Man and Skittering Scarecrow.

During my own demoralizing 'offs' I try to remember that like the rise and fall of the tides, my 'on' state will always return. Try as we may to manage interfering factors sometimes our meds kick in and sometimes they don't. We live with these ephemeral realities, as do our loved ones. For friends, co-workers or family members who spend many hours in our presence, the dramatic "shape-shifts" between our many selves can feel bewildering and scary. Like us, they wonder if our 'offs' will become a permanent state.

The good news for all is that PD does not decrease our basic intelligence or creativity. Through the daily yoyo swings between identities, we remain, in our cores, the people we have always been. So, rather than exclaiming, "You've gotten better!" when our meds kick in, we ask those around us to join us as we ride the choppy tides, cheering when the temporary good 'ons', like friendly waves, lift us up high!

Leonore Gordon, LCSW

BE YOUR OWN PARKINSON INVESTIGATOR

You may wonder why we end this chapter with an article on how to do medical research. We couldn't possibly include everything there is to know about PD, besides things are always changing. It's important to double check information you receive, from any source. We urge you to do so - your health may depend on it.

For those of us who like to check information, it's a treasure hunt. But, if you don't like to research, perhaps there's someone in your extended family or support group that could help you with it. There is power in knowledge.

Advanced medical research for e-patients

If you are one of the 61% of adults who go online to search for health related information you are most definitely an e-patient according to Pew Charitable Trust researchers. Not surprisingly, over 90% of e-patients consult Wikipedia for medical information. While it is reasonable that patients use Wikipedia to gain an overview of a disorder; the librarian in me trusts that it is common knowledge entries there can be written by nearly anyone. Too often, we must try and convince our health care providers that we may need more diagnostic testing, or we may want to try an anti-oxidant like Curcumin, etc. This means you need evidence to make your case and Wikipedia, though great to get the basics, is not very persuasive. Where do you start when you need more substantive health information?

On your mark...

Instead of homing in on Wikipedia every time, try looking at some of the major consumer health-related database websites that show up in your search results, keeping in mind that Google makes money off the top five in your list. In other words...

1. Don't be afraid to look beyond the first page of your search results. The results are weighted to give you quality information but you overlook hidden gems when you limit yourself.
2. Think like a computer. Always be thinking of your keywords or search terms. Google will not even search for superfluous words like "the" and "and". Focus on being as specific or descriptive as you can. Keying in "Parkinson" and "exercise" will be okay but if you want results focusing on a specific activity like "PD" and " running" just go for it.
3. Learn how to truncate. Instead of "Parkinson's disease" type in "Parkinson" if you are looking for anything beyond Idiopathic PD.
4. Spelling usually does not matter but logic does. All keyword searches scan text for exact occurences of what you type. If you type in an acronym like LID it does not know you mean "Levodopa Induced Dyskinesia" unless you give it a context to go with it like "Parkinson".
5. Know why quotation marks makes a world of difference. Use them when you are seeking info on an exact phrase.
6. Become more intimate with the advanced search features of Google. Scholar and Translate are potent weapons in your research arsenal.

Get Set...

1. Try tips 1-6 on Google. Have a stiff drink whether it be a shot of bourbon or wheat grass to prepare yourself for Boolean searching.

2. Boole was a mathemetician who used some circles to show algebraic relations between words or something like that (I am merely a mathphobic librarian). On paper it is hard to see the practical benefit, but try it to search a computer and you will see how it works (hint: mind your search results). It involves using operators or computer commands to relate words within a context. The commands are AND, OR and NOT. The first one AND is implicit in any keyword search, so you do not need to type it. Definitely must type the others. An example is "Parkinson NOT plus" means the computer will eliminate all results that would have any mention of Parkinson Plus Syndromes like MSA. Use NOT to narrow your topic and OR to expand.

3. This is really the only algebra that ever made any sense to me. Test it out on Google Advanced or go straight for the gold at PubMed. Note: Boolean searches must be done on a separate advanced search feature page on most web database sites and in quality search engines.

4. Impress your doctor or frighten him with your expert research skills and he is more likely to either elevate your status to partner in your care or eliminate you because he feels threatened (the defensive response). In fact, this is a great litmus test for the doctor-patient relationship we all hope to have in living with this cursed disorder. Your quality of life is only as good as your doctor, so make sure that you are on the same page.

5. Do not unleash these new skills on your family all at once. They already worry that you spend too much time researching PD anyway (ie. They have no clue what "incurable" feels like).

6. Do remind yourself how fabulous you are for learning something new. Please tell everyone how wonderful librarians are. Shameless plug, what can I say?

Go!

Before you take any of this seriously, check out the tips provided by years of experienced Medical Librarians:

A User's Guide to Finding and Evaluating Health Information on the Web

Bypass Wikipedia and go straight for the sunken treasure known in the Deep Web:

Medline Plus

Healthfinder

PubMed

Laura Brooks, MLS

Living with the non-motor effects of PD

She studied the basics of this new condition. Now that she had a name for her problem, she read everything she could find out about Parkinson disease. There were many other changes in her body.

She was having trouble organizing her day, getting things done, was tired and even constipated! Could this be part of PD? So she kept looking and discovered many more unexpected symptoms.

Some PwP talked about "clognition." What did that mean? It's not in any dictionary. So she did what she had to do. She continued to look for information online and asked new friends who also had PD.

In this chapter you will find information on how PD can affect your mind, organizational skills, and almost every part of your body.

If you're as strong as those living with PD, read on.

CHAPTER TWO
PD is More Than a Movement Disorder

The condition our condition is in is heavily
influenced by the spirit our spirit is in.

Which also influences the production of
chemicals in the brain.

Bob Dawson

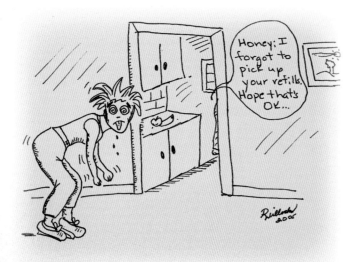

Honey: I forgot to pick up your refills. Hope that's OK...

The longer I live with PD, the more I think that to term it a "movement disorder" is limiting and misleading.

PDaffects everything, including cognition and mood. The sooner we all admit that, the sooner we can break out of the box our fragmented, competitive system of health care and medical specialties has put us in.

Kathleen Cochran - 2009

A Movement Disorder ?

Many people with Parkinson feel that the initial symptoms that led to their diagnosis are not their biggest concerns. Often the symptoms that cause the greatest difficulty are not treated by their neurologist; they are dealt with by specialists that deal with other areas of the body than the brain, such as urologists, gastroenterologist, cardiologists, dieticians, physiotherapists . . .

Some people require treatment by psychologists or psychiatrists for depression, obsessive compulsive disorders or sleep disorders. The doctors who treat these conditions may have a limited understanding of PD and the way PD medications can be affected by other medication, or may even be the cause of the problem.

At times, the patient's non-motor symptoms are misdiagnosed. Before and after a PD diagnosis, people may be treated for many years with drug or surgical therapies, sometimes inappropriately.

The wide range and variety of symptoms in each patient may result in PD not being diagnosed at all. Patients wonder why PD is categorized as a movement disorder. First symptoms may not be motor-related. Unfortunately, this may lead to delays in initial diagnosis, confusion in confirming the presence of PD and treatment that is not necessary.

Communication between patients is helpful in filling in some of these information gaps and empowering them to manage their own condition.

Although the non-motor symptoms of PD are now being recognized and written about, not all physicians are aware of this and do not ask their patients about the broader range of PD symptoms. Better communication between patients and doctors could help improve outcomes.

More education for the medical community and the general public is still needed. **NeuroWriters**

A CASCADE OF CHEMICAL EVENTS?

For many, the cardinal signs of PD are the least of their worries, even though they are more visible. Forum discussions among PwP made it clear that 'non-motor symptoms' (NMS) and the side effects of Parkinson medications were causing problems.

New research points to a cascade of chemical events in the brain and body that may cause non-motor symptoms. While medication addresses the lack of dopamine, this cascade is not yet fully understood or treated.

Researchers have discovered that non-motor symptoms may fluctuate as motor symptoms do. Dr. K. Ray Chaudhuri MD FRCP DSc and others are developing NMS assessment tools. Because doctors and patients don't talk about these NMS, many patients do not receive treatment which is available to relieve many of these symtoms. Check the article noted below for more information.

NeuroWriters

Note: Anne Marie Bonnet, Marie France Jutras, Virginie Czernecki, Jean Christophe Corvol, and Marie Vidailhet, "Nonmotor Symptoms in Parkinson's Disease in 2012: Relevant Clinical Aspects," Parkinson's Disease, vol. 2012, Article ID 198316, 15 pages, 2012. doi:10.1155/2012/198316
This article is also the source of the list (developed from Dr. Chaudhuri's work) to the right, reprinted under a Creative Commons Attribution License.

PD affects every part of my life; therefore I vote for calling it a "life disorder".

(I would call it several other things but that type of language would not be tolerated on a public listserv!)

Joan Blessington Snyder

NON- MOTOR SYMPTOMS

It is extremely important to recognize the complexity of PD, and for both patients and physicians to be aware that it is far more than just the symptoms described by James Parkinson. The following is a fairly comprehensive list of the Non-Motor Symptoms (NMS) of Parkinson Disease:

(A)Neuropsychiatric Symptoms:
(1) Depression
(2) Anxiety
(3) Apathy
(4) Hallucinations, delusions, illusions
(5) Delirium (may be drug induced)
(6) Cognitive impairment (dementia, MCI)
(7) Dopaminergic dysregulation syndrome (usually related to levodopa
(8) Impulse control disorders (related to dopaminergic drugs)

(B) Sleep Disorders:
(1) REM sleep behaviour disorder (possible premotor symptoms)
(2) excessive daytime somnolence, narcolepsy type "sleep attack"
(3) restless legs syndrome, periodic leg movements
(4) insomnia
(5) sleep disordered breathing
(6) non-REM parasomnias (confusional wandering)

(C) Fatigue:
(1) central fatigue (may be related to dysautonomia)
(2) peripheral fatigue.

(D) Sensory Symptoms:
(1) pain
(2) olfactory disturbance
(3) hyposmia
(4) functional anosmia
(5) visual disturbance (blurred vision, diplopia; impaired contrast-sensitivity)

(E) Autonomic Dysfunction:
(1) bladder dysfunction (urgency, frequency, nocturia)
(2) sexual dysfunction (may be drug-induced)
(3) sweating abnormalities (hyperhydrosis)
(4) orthostatic hypotension

(F) Gastrointestinal Symptoms:
(1) dribbling of saliva
(2) dysphagia - swallowing issues
(3) agueusia - loss of taste
(4) constipation
(5) nausea
(6) vomiting

(G) Dopaminergic Drug-Induced Behaviour NMS:
(1) hallucinations, psychosis, delusions
(2) dopamine dysregulation syndrome
(3) impulse control disorders.

(H) Dopaminergic Drug-Induced Other NMS:
(1) ankle swelling
(2) dyspnea - breathlessness
(3) skin reactions
(4) subcutaneous nodules
(5) erythematous skin problems

(I) Nonmotor Fluctuations:
(1) dysautonomia
(2) cognitive/psychiatric
(3) sensory/pain
(4) visual blurring

(J) Other Symptoms:
(1) weight loss
(2) weight gain

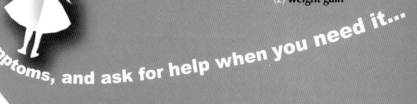
Keep on top of your symptoms, and ask for help when you need it...

EXECUTIVE FUNCTION

Executive function refers to a set of mental processes that help connect past experience with present action. It includes initiating and stopping actions, planning, organizing, strategizing, paying attention to and remembering details.

We use our executive functions when we monitor, anticipate outcomes and adapt our behavior to changing situations. All of these abilities are used when we set and meet goals.

As a PwP gradually loses the ability to perform executive functions, it may affect many areas of life such as being unable to plan your day or a special event to altering your normal speech. It also may be confused with dementia, by PwP or people they interact with. The reality is that it is not dementia but a failure of executive function!

COMMUNICATION BREAKDOWN

The issue of speech processing was discussed on the NeuroTalk forum in January 2010. An excerpt follows:

Happy talking, talking .... not.....

• I am having a problem communicating....... well with spoken communication and I don't know what to do to make things any better.

I've had a little difficulty with words and getting them out at the right time before.

When I do manage to speak, I often think that I am not finding the right words, or to formulate sentences easily - my lips and tongue that won't do the right thing, instead of tripping over my feet, right now it seems to be my tongue.....

Does anyone know what to do, how to get that easy flow back again - or it this something that I am going to have to live with, and get used to? Lindy

• I have had similar things happen. It's like my mouth is running faster than my brain and the result is gibberish. I have no advice other than I practice what I'm going to say in my head first and count the words on my fingers then when I say it out loud I speak slowly and count on my fingers again. It doesn't make for spontaneous scintillating conversation but at least I can make the occasional comment or response. Not much help. Pam

• Do you mean that you know the words you want, but can't articulate them fast enough - they're kind of lost or stuck somewhere in your head sort of feeling? Or is it a fluency in your speech itself? I tend to experience the former. I feel your pain!

I think it is an executive function malfunction we're experiencing... I suspect that conversing does not flow like it used to for us because our brains are working overtime compensating and it takes longer for us to find words.

I have read that the word being 'on the tip of our tongues' but not making it out is fairly common in PD- we know the word(s) we want but they just don't pop into our heads and out of our mouths like they used to do. We have a loss of fluency to add to the list of what is taken away from us. :(

Laughing to keep from crying, Laura

• What I am hearing from you all is that this is something that does impact your life, it certainly does mine!

From all over I am also hearing messages that say we have to keep devising strategies just to be 'normal'. This is a big part of the problem for me, and I suppose a reason for why I like writing. It can be done in my time, and if I get it right, the communication is good.

But I can't use this device in normal life. You cannot pass notes around, and besides, unless I'm at a screen my writing is too awful to read..... :eek:

So this impact of communication must be a major one. And implies major personal losses over time......... and it changes not only our perception of ourselves, but other peoples perceptions about us. But intellectually on the inside we are mostly the same people...... Thanks. Lindy

LANGUAGE PROCESSING & PWP
A Dutch researcher, Katrien Colman showed that problems with executive functions affect language processing in PwP. She found that it affects understanding complicated sentences, makes it difficult for the person to change the subject of the conversation and to use grammatically correct sentences.

She believes that this deserves serious attention and says:
'If communication is difficult, this does not necessarily mean that the patient is tired or depressed, or that there's something wrong with his intelligence.... We could spare patients a lot of suffering if we learnt to better understand their language impairments and developed suitable ways to communicate with them.'

Study: Parkinson's disease undermines language processing ability in Dutch native speaker patients. The Medical News, 9. February 2011

KEEPING IT SIMPLE

Nowadays any kind of complexity sends me in a spin, and it doesn't take much. Take the dishwasher, my kitchen monster.

I open it, and stare at the contents, knives, plates, dishes, pans, a whisk, a wooden spoon ... I sigh, where does it all go. Looking around my kitchen, all those cupboards and homes for things, I look back at the dishwasher and it overwhelms me. I shut it. If we washed only cups, I could cope, one cupboard, one shelf.

Simple.

Then I turn to my to do list; it is rammed. I don't miss deadlines, but my 'to do' list stays in my head. If I attempt to write it down I would implode. Did I really commit to so much? do I really have to do all that this week, and how will I get through today?!

I would curl up under the duvet if I faced it in its entirety. So I keep it floating in my head and hope that I keep enough wits about me to avoid failure. I only pull forward one thing at once, do it, 'cross it off' and then pull the next activity forward.

Simple has to be my operating code.

I am finding more and more that busyness also stops me functioning such as a supermarket aisle filled with stuff I go 'product blind'. I see everything but can focus on nothing.

A clothes shop, my favourite, I will select something, then another, then another put back the first, select 3 more, swap the second for a different colour, put back the last, pick up the first again..... and then buy nothing! Exhausting? Yes it is.

What is most frustrating about all of this is ..... I never used to be like it. I was always clear, direct, decisive. To be reduced to a quivering jelly by the thought of a dishwasher would seem preposterous to the old me. The new me accepts it albeit with some reflective sadness, and ultimately I have to smile, who wants to be clearing up pots anyway!

Colleen Henderson-Heywood

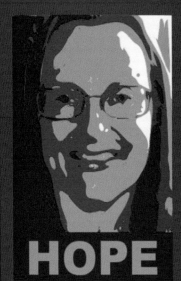

Almost anyone who has heard of Parkinson disease knows about the physical symptoms of PD, including tremors, generalized slowness of movement, stiffness of limbs and gait or balance problems.

What is less well known about PD is that it is not the motor symptoms that tend to do the most harm to quality of life.

Clognition coupled with stress is more often than not the culprit that precipitates job loss and family discord.

There is not much information available about the effects of Clognition or strategies to cope. Talking with other PwP reveals the problems to be similar and ubiquitous, including unpaid bills due to inattention and habitual all-night computer use. Although the behavior is "normal" it is far from healthy.

The discovery that Clognition was normal for PD sufferers gave me the strength to take steps towards managing my life and alleviating stress. It's not easy, and I can't do it alone. Counseling sessions with a neuro-psychologist plus conversations with PD compatriots give me strategies to maintain and the motivation to follow through.

Drug therapies are available as long as you take the time to find the right one. PD is an extremely individualistic disease. Loss of motor control, mental changes, drug treatments, surgical treatments, diet, exercise – the menu is long, the choices and combinations infinite.

Young Onset PwP present a new public health challenge: keeping healthy, active and productive in order to raise families, go to work, survive for many years as medical science continues to make our bodies stronger so that we live longer. But our brains have to keep up with our bodies and clognition remains a huge but elusive challenge to leading full and healthy lives. Education and "brain re-training" are necessary, along with more funding for research in this area.

Access to information is essential to good health and a well-balanced life. PD is tough to live with, balance is difficult to achieve. Information enables; education gives hope; advocacy increases strength; and knowledge is power.
Carey Christensen

Take control of your life!

PD is a tough disease to live with. My words are brave; the reality of my life is much different.

The struggle is daily; hope not always evident. I am working hard to find the right path.

Ahhh, PD cognition - they should call it CLOGNITION

**Greg Wasson 2002
MGH Forum**

CLOGNITION

CLOGNITION

A few years ago I started losing my mind . . .

I thought I might have Alzheimer and feared that diagnosis. I felt as if little pieces of my mind were falling away. It was terrifying. My memory, once precise and quick, was now deteriorating beyond my ability to recover.

I can't say it's gotten any better since I was diagnosed in 1997. I've had some harrowing experiences, but I've learned to deal with them. It took a while to get used to the short spells of forgetting who and where I was. It's disconcerting to find yourself driving along, suddenly realizing you don't recognize anything around you.

When I say I've learned to deal with it, I mean that I just stopped getting upset about it. I keep driving, knowing that soon I'll remember where I am. So far I've found that I'm near home when I do regain my memory.

People who know me are aware of just how bad my memory problems are. There's a difference in how someone with Parkinson will perceive my forgetfulness and how a non-Parkie will see it. That's interesting to me because I find this true about other Parkinsonian behaviors as well.

Usually a non-Parkie will say something like "I have the same problem with my memory that you do". When a person with Parkinson says that to me I know it's true, but when a non-Parkie says it, I know they don't get it. They don't realize that people with Parkinson worry about more than memory, we worry about our sanity. Losing the ability to hold a thought, to focus, is more onerous than just forgetting where you left your car keys. In a naturally aging person who notices that they are becoming more forgetful it may be frustrating, but that's probably all they'll have to face.

My deteriorating memory is my enemy and I do battle with it daily. It's a problem that you can't really quantify. All I can do is repeat (often) "I have a bad memory" and hope for the best. Most of my friends know this to be true and so they remind me of things I need to attend. Occasionally I offend someone who thinks it is an excuse.

I go to great lengths to keep the collection of facts, promises and responsibilities necessary for the maintenance of my daily life in order. I feel that if I fail, if I lose control, it could be the start of a long slide downward. This is why when I have too many episodes of 'forgetfulness' it is so disturbing.
Idiopathic PWP

Clognition is not dementia. It is not mental retardation. It is distractibility, focusing and concentration lags, time and space misperception, loss of ability to plan accurately, loss of ability to complete tasks, as well as a slew of social/emotional baggage that either accompanies or results from these losses.

Paula Wittekind

The term CLOGNITION, coined by Greg, was quickly taken up by the PD community, who knew a good word when they saw it. Carey took this one step further. Her pioneering Clognition website was a milestone in opening up the cognitive issues of people with Parkinson. This helped pave the way to accessing some recognition of the obstacles that we face in our ordinary lives, and to professional help that would allow a better quality of life. Nevertheless there is still much to be done in raising awareness of clognition, and ensuring that people suffering from it are able to access the help they need, at home and in the workplace.

Pain In Parkinson Disease

Many People with Parkinson were told at diagnosis that there is no pain involvement; some of us would beg to differ. The cardinal signs of PD do not seem to indicate pain in themselves, however, those who present with shoulder and neck problems and difficulties associated with rigidity may have had pain prior to diagnosis. Medication sometimes alleviates this, at least for a while.

As their condition progresses PwP often speak about the presence of pain and while we believe more doctors now have a better awareness that it can be a problem, there may still be a perception that it is not a 'real' issue, or that it is not a major problem.

Dystonia and dyskinesia can be painful, especially during 'wearing off' and 'wearing on' times. Some people experience 'moving pain' - where there does not seem to be a specific location, such as a joint or limb that is solely affected. PwP have also reported having operations for shoulder, neck and back problems that have not resulted in expected relief from pain, only to be told later that the culprit could be dystonia. Dystonic pain is sometimes used as an indicator of whether medication needs to be increased or decreased, depending on whether it occurs at 'off' times or at peak dose times. It has to be said that, from a patient perspective, this is a difficult place, where medication both resolves the pain and is the cause of it. This is especially true for those on levodopa for some years whose treatment options have become limited. If their medication regime is a close schedule, say every two hours, it can mean frequently recurring pain. Often ordinary pain relief is ineffective, leaving patient and doctors with fewer choices.

Rigidity related problems can be a source of pain. Some wake with pain and stiffness due to immobility during sleep (nocturnal akinesia). Some have facial pain related to jaw (temporo-mandibular joint) problems; clenched jaw and grinding teeth during sleep (bruxism) seem to be fairly common. Some experience abdominal pain related to their medication cycle, with less pain when medications are working well. This and pain in the chest and pelvic areas are thought to be related to receptors being activated in the viscera. A type of disregulation of blood pressure called postural hypotension can be the cause of 'coat-hanger' pain in the shoulder area. People also relate how they have pain from 'curly' (dystonic) toes and in their hands and wrists. Postural problems cause pain on the more affected side, through poor gait or 'leaning' when seated. 'Poverty of movement' - not moving enough - can cause peripheral edema leading to painful legs. Pain can also be caused by central nervous system (CNS) lesions.

The experience of PD differs widely and these are just a few of the ways pain manifests. Many of us would like a wider recognition of the role of pain and its impact on our lives. This is especially important in the later stages of PD, when PwP are more fragile and less responsive to medication.

If you have a problem with pain, discuss it with your neurologist and your general practitioner.
Paula Wittekind

Ref: Non-motor symptoms of Parkinson's disease: dopaminergic pathophysiology and treatment. Chaudhuri KR, Schapira AH. Lancet Neurol. 2009 May;8(5):464-74.

PAIN & PD

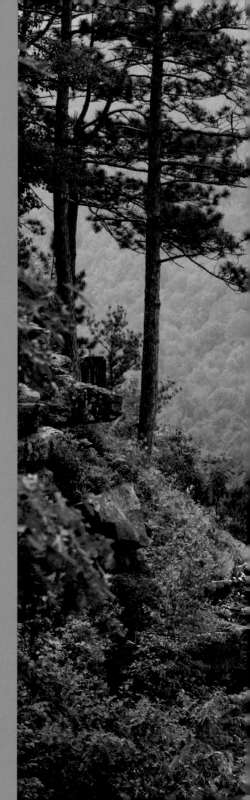

Stress vs Distress

We all experience new symptoms from time to time because we have a progressive disease. In fact, a lot of us have been through some really rough times lately with such changes. Some of us seem to be able to handle those changes without distressing ourselves, while others feel devastated by them.

Having PD is like being shot with an arrow called Disease. We all felt the hurt when we were first diagnosed with PD, and we feel the hurt with each new symptom. Ranting to myself about how terrible and unfair it is that I have yet another symptom would be like grabbing hold of that PD arrow with my hand and twisting it, making the wound bigger as I lapse into worry and "awful-izing." ("Isn't it AWFUL that I have this disease!") Instead of dealing with PD, I would be fighting it and getting more stressed and worried. I'm learning to not make the injury worse by twisting the arrow.

REDUCING DIS-EASE

There's a big difference between disease and dis-ease. I'm learning some ways to reduce my dis-ease (dis-comfort, dis-stress) over Parkinson. I'm learning to focus on today, on what I **can** do rather than on the things I can't do that I used to do. Focusing on what I can't do just stresses/distresses me, so I'm learning to work **with** rather than against my PD.

Some people believe that we should never accept PD, but instead, we should fight it. But "accepting" PD does not mean giving up and giving in to it in a weak, wimpy way.

On the contrary, real acceptance is:

- **Going with what IS rather that what should be**
- **Looking for ways to counter new symptoms, to reduce them, and to live better with them**
- **Being pro-active by tackling a problem and resolving it as well and thoroughly as possible**
- **Acting out of practical adaptive thinking about what will help you most, rather than out of anger or embarrassment. The focus is on thinking, not on upset feelings, because the latter tear you up.**
- **Changing what you can change, and letting go of the need to change what you can't (Serenity Prayer)**

It is true that I **strongly** dislike PD, but I don't HATE it because that level of anger makes me twist the PD arrow and adds dis-ease to the disease. And I don't need that!!! When I am angry enough to cause dis-ease and dis-stress, my PD symptoms get worse.

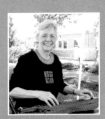

The issue isn't so much "don't fight." It's "use your head, not your emotions." In "western" cowboy movies, the "hot heads" always end up getting killed or hurt badly when they fight. It's the ones who stay cool, though determined, who draw quickest, shoot straightest and hit their target. So in this sense, acceptance doesn't mean to take off your guns. It has to do with fighting cool and not dis-easing yourself. Yes, PD is stressful. But if you dis-stress yourself over it, you will shoot yourself in the foot, for sure!

Judith Giddings, PhD

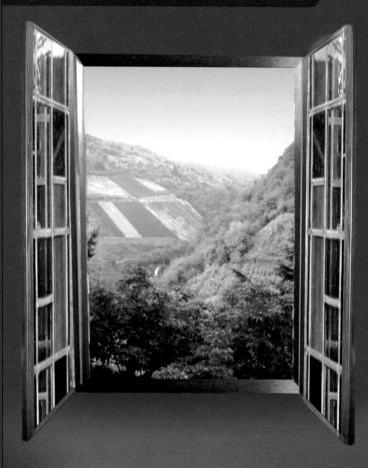

APATHY

OUT FROM UNDER THE COVERS

Deep inside most of us lurks a child, who, when he is afraid, feels an overwhelming desire to crawl into bed and pull the covers over his head. As we age we learn to face those things we fear without resorting to the cocoon of our childhood. We learn through experience that by tackling problems head-on we are often able to avert the worst of them and then someone says to us, "You have Parkinson disease." I am sure the statement could end with a number of other debilitating incurable diseases and the result would be the same, a desire to find the warm safety of our hiding place under the covers.

By the time we hear those dreaded words we are too old to really believe in the refuge of quilts and pillows, but our eagerness to escape our surroundings remains. The experience of hearing our diagnosis, the gathering clouds of apathy, detachment, depression, the loss of grace and the ultimate decline of confidence, make the urge to seek asylum seem reasonable to us, even desirable. The questions "Where is this haven?" and "How do we get there?" hang in the air. They are not questions asked aloud, but they are implicit in the kinds of action we take. Rather than confront the issues of life, friendships and abilities inexorably changing and then cope with them, we prefer to avoid it all and allow the dread and fear accompanying the change to grow unfettered in our mind. When this kind of thinking is compounded by apathy the problem grows exponentially. Apathy may cause the pain of these losses to fade simply due to lack of interest, while at the same time increase our preference for our own company. The addition of detachment and/or depression completes our submergence into the sanctuary of solitude.

Solitude, in and of itself, is not a bad thing, but for the chronically ill, it may be catastrophic. The solitude we crave is not that of the contemplative life but that of the recluse or the hermit. It is a life in hiding, a life turned inward. Fighting the allure of social separation is a perpetual battle in which we are often disinclined to engage. But without the battle we become concerned with only what is happening to us, our bodies and our minds; an existence that is the antithesis of living, that is entirely composed of separation and loneliness. An existence that is the beginning of dying, for once the isolation is complete there is no further use for anything, not friends, not family, not joy and is that not the definition of death, nothing left to lose?

Pam Kell

BLACK HOLE

At some point in the course of this disease many of us find our way to depression, a dark and ugly place. It is very individual, experienced differently by each person. Winston Churchill, who was a fellow sufferer, called it his "black dog".

Depression is an inky, thick, restricting, place where direction is not possible to divine and hope is absent. When at the bottom of this black all-consuming hole no light can penetrate. The weight and mass of depression does not preclude cognitive awareness of its depth but can rob us of the ability or motivation to alter the circumstances.

The origin of depression is not yet completely understood nor is its apparent connection with Parkinson disease. It is not the same as sadness caused by external events such as our diagnosis, loss of a loved one or other events we all experience. It may be caused by faulty chemical transmissions for which we bear no guilt and yet the guilt can be overwhelming even given that knowledge.

Sometimes depression resolves itself spontaneously, in other cases it requires serious medical intervention.

The one characteristic of depression that is crucial to remember is that it is no different from any other illness. There is no separation between physical illness and mental illness, regardless of the less than progressive attitude shown by some health insurance companies, among others.

When depression strikes, seek the help of a medical professional in order to achieve a resolution as quickly as possible.

The stigma of mental illness, though not yet eradicated, is dimming and will continue to do so with the open acceptance of those of us who experience it.

Pam Kell

The stigma of mental illness, though not yet eradicated, is dimming and will continue to do so with the open acceptance of those of us who experience it.

"...it is so bad, you are so glad you have it and it is not your wife, or other family. It is so bad, you would not wish it on your worst enemy. It is so bad, that the sheer unpredictability of when an off period will occur makes normal life impossible. It is so bad, that if you dose up to go out for a meal, to avoid a freeze, dyskinesia will cause you to throw your food in all directions. It is so bad, that you are totally amazed at your ability to cope and to accept that in the 21st century there is no cure...."

Ron Hutton

Having PD is like having 1-2 six packs of beer in you, listening to Hank Williams singing YOUR CHEATING HEART and you're all alone on Saturday night. PD is a slow insidious disease. That word insidious, means PD comes over you slowly in a not easily apparent manner, more dangerous than seems evident. When I was first diagnosed I said to myself, look at me I can run, lift weights and have all the energy to do most anything, I'll beat PD because I have a strong body and mind. 16 and 1/2 years later, I'm crawling to the rest room, barely able to lift myself up off the floor.
BUT I'll make it to the other side. I will survive. **John Gillespie, Jr.**

for me
it's a gift
a tough slap-upside-the-head kind of gift

but a gift nonetheless
it forced me to look hard at my life

and at my priorities
I had to make some changes
what I had thought was important

suddenly wasn't

what I had thought was cornball
sentimentality

suddenly wasn't

I grew to learn that I had not received

a sentence to a living hell
I grew to learn that any 'hell' was

of my own making and my own thinking
I grew to learn that this is a tough test

is all

I am in competition with no one
I am not being punished
I am being challenged
I will rise to it
and thus find the gift in it

janet313313

"You become a prisoner trapped in your own body.
You lose your dignity when someone has to help you do a task as simple as going to the bathroom." **Peg**

...I have this new kind of loneliness sometimes, unlike any I've ever experienced before. It's not a people loneliness, because I have plenty of friends - some of the best ones I've ever had as a matter of fact, and many of them happen to be you people. I miss the part of me that's gone forever kind of loneliness. It's like you get up in the morning and think, I'd like to do this n' that today, but first I have to check with the board of directors and Mr Parkinson is the Chairman of the Board.... **stevem53**

PWP ON PD

It takes all your concentration to get across a room **Sparky**

My voice will be silenced.
My hands wili not respond.
My legs will not move.
My face will no longer register emotion.
Rigid and frozen my body will become
While my mind, ever aware, constantly thinking, processing, understanding
Will become desperate to communicate, connect, be understood
But unable to be heard.
We MUST talk while we can!

indigogo (Carey)

My symptoms are still mild, but I can best explain what it is like through examples.

Parkinson is all encompassing, things like a pervasive fear of the future. It is simple things, like giving up on necklaces because you can't work the clasp. It is carrying tea to your guests across the room as your hand rattles the cup, drawing attention when you don't want it. It makes you count out your money into your hand long before you get to the cashier, so that you don't hold up the line. It is fearing the sales person at Macy's will think you are using a stolen card when it takes you so long to write your name. It is the shame you feel while speaking in front of a group while your hand flutters and others assume you are nervous. It is the guilt of knowing your children are worrying about your decline, and, unlike when they were little, you cannot reassure them. It is looking with envy and even anger at others who walk, dance, write, gesture and count change with ease as you once did but no longer can. Finally, it is knowing it can only get worse. **AnnT**

OUR BODY LANGUAGE DOES NOT TELL THE WHOLE STORY

In the beginning, we may feel like our nerve endings have been exposed, and complain about the raw deal we've been handed. These are the good times. PD can also bring apathy and detachment.

These differences in the way we are used to feeling, possibly never experienced before diagnosis, can become unwelcome companions as we journey with Parkinson disease. Though not identical, they can overlap. Apathy is marked by aloofness, disinterest and a lack of involvement, a condition that leaves us without enthusiasm or energy for the things we were once engaged in and loved doing. Detachment is the feeling of being separated from our surroundings and the people and the activity associated with them. Detachment leaves us aware of what is happening, but disinterested in the outcome.

Both can result in intensifying the isolation so often associated with this illness. Without a stake in the results of the events occurring around us, we become less interested in things that we previously enjoyed and as interest diminishes so does involvement.

It is not unknown for these two intertwined states of mind to cause even long term relationships to collapse under their weight. For one partner to carry the entire emotional burden of a relationship is unrealistic, yet nevertheless it is sometimes necessary, if the relationship is to survive.

Apathy and detachment can be mistaken for boredom with family and friends, or disinterest in the things they share with us; then they may feel rejected or no longer welcomed, or needed. Combined with a sense of personal distance that comes with apathy and detachment and the unexpressive masque of a Parkinson face - and it is no wonder that friends and even family often feel rejected, or misunderstood.

Apathy and detachment can result in a deepening of the isolation often associated with this illness. For many this sense of disconnection is catastrophic and makes successful social contact seem an impossibility.

It is very important that we take a positive stand against these aspects of PD, because they do not represent the people we really are. Both PD and the medication used to help our symptoms can cause these two problems. Simply knowing that apathy and detachment are frequently encountered by PwP and are treatable, can make all the difference.

Discuss this with your neurologist because skilled counseling or adjusting medications could help.

Pam Kell

Apathy and detachment can be viewed by others as boredom with them, or disinterest in the things they share with us, consequently they may feel rejected or no longer welcomed, or needed.

Combine the aloofness and distance that comes with apathy and detachment with the stony masque of a Parkinson face - and it is no wonder that friends and even family often feel rejected.

MANAGING APATHY & DETACHMENT

THE FENCE IN MY BRAIN

Movement disorders create disturbances in movement and that is what movement disorder specialists are trained to look at. They may tell you not to tell them about your despondency and your difficulties getting through the day, because what they're interested in is "your mobility".

Movement is their thing. That's all they want to deal with.

There is a fence in my brain between the psychiatric and neurological symptoms and there is a kind of closet for gastrointestinal functions and there are all these different doctors that work on opposite sides of the fence in my brain.

If I go into the psychiatric part, there's a nice voice coming over the speaker system in the office saying, "Come in! Sit down. Be calm. We'll be with you in a moment and we can help you with your difficulties." In that office I even find out that if my Parkinson is treated it will have no effect on my depression, but if my depression is treated, however, it will improve my Parkinson symptoms.

So it's all quite pleasant and cordial. The only problem I have with that is all my ancestors are standing outside the window and peering in and saying, "Hi! Hi, Crazy head. Crazy head, we always knew it!" and everyone I went to school with is saying, "Did you hear about her, what happened to her brain? She's crazy, she's got Parkinson, definitely demented."

- Which is not true.

And if only those people would go away I could be very happy in the psychiatry department, because they're helping me with things like my cognitive losses and my difficulty with thinking of words and stuff like that . . . What were we talking about? . . .

However, if I go into the narrow-ish side of my mind, on the other side of the fence - and I don't know where that fence is because all of these look mixed up together on the chart on the wall of the brain - but anyway . . .

Movement disorders create disturbances in movement and that is what movement disorder specialists are trained to look at. They may tell you not to tell them about your despondency and your difficulties getting through the day, because what they're interested in is "your mobility". Movement is their thing. That's all they want to deal with.

Now, the fun part is that other neurologists, general neurologists, are not trained sufficiently in movement disorders to be able to diagnose and treat movement disorders very well. Now, you and I picked it up after a couple of years of taking the meds, but they didn't have our advantage and they have trouble even comprehending that there are other symptoms to Parkinson disease than those which they have been trained to care for.

That makes it kind of complicated to be a patient, see, because you've got the fence in your brain and that's your biggest problem. The doctors don't want to admit it and you have to co-ordinate conflicting orders from different kinds of doctors who can only see one part of the fence inside your brain . . .

J.L Wheeler

WILTING WITH FATIGUE?

Many months before learning I had PD, I began having periods of wilting fatigue. I was forty-nine when it began and put it down to my job, which was high pressured and very stressful. Not long after it started I had that birthday with a zero in it, always a big deal for some reason and entertained the thought that I was simply growing older - this sort of thing was to be expected. It bothered me that the fatigue coincided so perfectly with my fiftieth year as though zero years really are more significant than all the others.

When I say fatigue, I don't mean "boo-hoo I'm tired", or "I never get enough sleep and I'm worn out", or "I've worked so hard today that I'm whipped". I mean bone-weary, debilitating, crying tiredness. Tiredness without limits or explanation. Nothing remarkable had changed in my normal routine and yet the feeling of not having the requisite energy to lift my arm up to comb my hair often engulfed me and it was getting worse.

Some days, still, every action, every movement, regardless how small, can feel as though I am doing it in a vat of Jello with weights tied to my limbs. Walking up a flight of stairs can leave me breathless and aching. Vacuuming a single room can put me down for an hour.

Any time I mentioned fatigue to a physician I was told I should get more exercise, eat less and lose weight. (Thank you very much, I never would have thought of that!)

The only other explanation ever offered is depression. I understand depression and have dealt with it on occasion, but for me, there has never been any correlation with depression and the fatigue I experience. When I was younger and more willing to accept stock answers to my questions, I even began to believe I must be depressed - though I thought I was happy. My perceived happiness must be another form of denial. I'm older now and smarter and better informed.

I have been fortunate enough to have met others with PD, to have talked to them and compared notes on our individual journeys. I have come to understand that while fatigue is not universal, it is fairly common.

I am no longer willing to accept what I am told when it makes no sense to me. I am unwilling to believe I am depressed because I am excessively tired and I am unwilling to accept that no one else experiences the same kind of apparently unwarranted fatigue, because now I know better.

To this day none of the neurologists I have gone to take me seriously when I tell them fatigue threatens my quality of life; that fatigue is the main reason I stopped working early; that fatigue is the reason I tend to withdraw from social interaction; and that fatigue is the one thing I believe my family and friends do not understand. Then again, why would my family and friends understand when neither I nor my doctors do?

It wasn't so long ago that the cognitive issues connected with Parkinson were not given serious consideration. Without the efforts of a small number of determined individuals who had learned from their own experience, cognitive issues might still be dismissed as unrelated to PD.

Knowing that others experience the fatigue that I contend with gives me hope that it will be recognized by the medical community. When we stand together and speak with one voice we are heard.

We can help ourselves if we are honest when discussing the things that are obstacles to our quality of life and steadfast in refusing to accept a dismissal of fatigue as unrelated or insignificant when we know better. It takes a measure of confidence to disagree with a physician on medical matters. By being well-informed about this and similar issues and remembering that we know our own bodies better than anyone, we can help the medical community recognise fatigue as a facet of Parkinson.

What is the answer if you are struggling with this kind of fatigue?

Inform yourself, talk to others, pay attention to your body and don't relent when you know something is not right. Don't back down if you are told the cause of your fatigue must be unrelated to PD, or that it is a symptom of depression. It might be, but equally it might not be. Finally, do not let anyone tell you that what you are feeling is not real. The very fact that you are experiencing it makes it real by definition.
Pam Kell

FATIGUE

My apathy emerged separately from depression. I was missing deadlines, which I never would have done in my life pre-PD. But the strange thing was that I wasn't upset about it; I was neutral or even slightly bemused. I still cared about the people I worked with and for the people we served but not about the work itself. Nothing about it moved or impassioned me anymore. I thought it might be career burnout and began to consider other options. Yet nothing appealed.

Now I consider a dash of apathy one small mercy among a sea of trials. How merciful to have the loss of one's abilities mitigated by a reduced attachment to them. Still, if apathy is problematic, it is no gift. Though I don't think there is any medicine that successfully treats it, there may be other strategies.

Rose of his heart

WE ARE NOT ALONE . . .

In some ways PD resembles such conditions as Autism. Dyslexia, Dyspraxia and Aspergers - also cognitive and problematic as well as very misunderstood and sometimes denied by 'experts'.

Such denial can lead to all sorts of misinterpretation of behaviour and intent, and to potentially serious and difficult issues relating to work, communication, relationships and social status. If these things, which are on the edge of general understanding, are to be truly aired with a view to enabling people who suffer from them, then it is exactly those people who need to be advocates to both medical & social science communities, as well as the general public.

After many years of working with disabled people, from those with most difficult and disabling physical and mental conditions, to those with relatively slight impairment, it became extraordinarily obvious that what effectively disabled them AS MUCH AS their own condition were the misperceptions about what they were suffering from and the prejudice that arose from the misperceptions.

Education is the key to breaking down these misperceptions. It brings a whole new level of meaning to 'life-long learning'.

Linda Ashford

COGNITIVE DIFFERENCE

I am naturally an early riser. Sleeping late has never had any real appeal, but even if it had it would not have been possible. I come from a long line of early risers who view anything past 8:00 am as positively decadent. I never had any difficulty going to sleep either.

Then suddenly, without warning or explanation, I stopped sleeping. Nothing of any consequence had changed except I could not go to sleep. When I did, in less than four hours I was completely, irrevocably wide awake. For weeks I fought it. I did relaxing exercises, drank warm milk, fantasized about spending lottery winnings and ultimately took pills, all to no avail.

I was one of those lucky people for whom wakefulness was a binary state, either asleep or awake, with no middle ground, no rising slowly out of sleep into a fully awake person. Those of us, the binary ones, secretly considered ourselves slightly superior to the Others, those who can't be spoken to until they have a cup of coffee and an hour or two has elapsed, who cannot shut off the day without routines and rituals meant specifically for slowly finding unconsciousness.

That was then, but when the sleep switch was turned off I became one of the Others. Sleep became as elusive for me as flight.

I would go to bed and I could hardly blink - my eyes were so wide open. I would toss and turn and fidget. Eventually I would creep out of bed and move into the computer room, where I could connect with other PwP who also could not sleep. I soon made fast friends with others who had stayed up late communicating in the dark. It was private, personal, intimate and anonymous. The night-time quiet made it almost addictive.

Over a few months, I became friends with these denizens of cyberspace, confessing, listening to confessions, confiding in them and learning from their experience, while being reassured that everything that was happening to me had also happened to more than one of them.

I was spending more time online with my distant empathetic friends than I was with my loved ones. This social contact allowed me to accept my insomnia and gradually enabled my family to accept it.

Embracing insomnia was a great relief. Thinking about it no longer occupied most of my waking hours. I was able to relax knowing that I had somewhere to go late at night, where I was welcomed.

I have had two periods of extended insomnia since my diagnosis. I am in one now. This time I have been lucky enough to find a new group of people to share time with. Some of them are collaborators in this book, one is a friend rediscovered after many years and one a relative who is invariably up and always amusing.

I expect this time will be like the last, just as suddenly as it began the insomnia will stop. No explanation, no lifestyle or medication changes, it will just stop. I will begin sleeping a reasonable number of hours, stop waking up at night and struggling to go to sleep.

It will be a great relief as I have let many things go because of the fatigue that comes with getting only four or five hours of sleep. I will feel better, I will probably even look better. With days and nights back in their proper order, I will be more engaged, less apathetic and detached, more focused and more accomplished. My family will be thrilled, as will I. On the other hand, I will miss my nocturnal friends and the warm cozy feeling that came from our sharing our lives without guard rails or speed bumps in the anonymous late dark night.

Pam Kell

Embracing the insomnia was a great relief.

I CRY . . .

I don't mean just when someone dies, or when I have injured myself, or when some foreign tragedy occurs, or even when I am faced with grave disappointment. In fact, at those times and all the other real life times when crying is appropriate, I am more likely than not to be found completely dry-eyed. I don't consider myself a particularly emotional person and I have always been very guarded with my feelings, but the longer I have Parkinson the more crying triggers I seem to develop.

I am not depressed, nor do I cry exclusively in response to things that are sad or sentimental. Mostly I cry at the sight of anyone else crying. I cry at the sight of anyone being sweet to an elderly person or the winners of foot races, at presentations of awards and groups of children singing. Sometimes it is spontaneous and without any obvious cause. It is not emotional crying and it does not come from a sense of loss, pain, disappointment or failure. It nearly always surprises me, always embarrasses me and I am completely powerless to control it.

I have been told by other PwP with similar experiences of inappropriate emotional responses that it is a Parkinson symptom. That means just possibly it isn't the beginning of mental demise but just another bump in the road.

Whether it is caused by Parkinson, or medication, or is unrelated to PD entirely is less important to me than whether or not my problem is taken seriously by the medical community. In any case I always know there are fellow travelers who have walked in my shoes and are willing to share what they know and how they feel. When they don't have an answer or a similar experience, they are ready to support me, acknowledge my frustration, endure my venting and see me through until someone shows up who does have an answer, or the directions to one.

Pam Kell

Sometimes it is spontaneous and without any obvious cause.

EMOTIONAL LABILITY

Pseudobulbar effect is a secondary symptom to neurological disorders or brain injury. It is also sometimes called emotional lability, or involuntary emotional expression and can occur as episodes of crying, and sometimes laughter, that are exaggerated or contradictory to the triggering event. Those who experience it are aware of what is happening but have no control over it at the time. It can be unpredictable and at its worst can occur several times a day. It can coexist with depression, but often occurs in contrast to mood.

Being proactive in maintaining health

She was finished with research for now. She needed to do something to improve the situation. If she couldn't fix the PD, maybe she would feel better if she took some control.

There were many possibilities that went well beyond doctors' prescriptions. She could join a choir, start going to the gym regularly or begin to write a blog.

Tango lessons or mountain climbing - maybe not yet- but tomorrow she could start a walking program using ski poles....

In this chapter you will find ways to improve your body and mind through exercise, meditation, nutrition and the arts.

If you're as strong as those living with PD, read on.

CHAPTER THREE
Helping Ourselves

keeping moving is probably the BEST
single thing that you can do to help yourself

YOU MAY NOT WANT TO CLIMB MOUNTAINS -
BUT DON'T RULE OUT THE POSSIBILITY

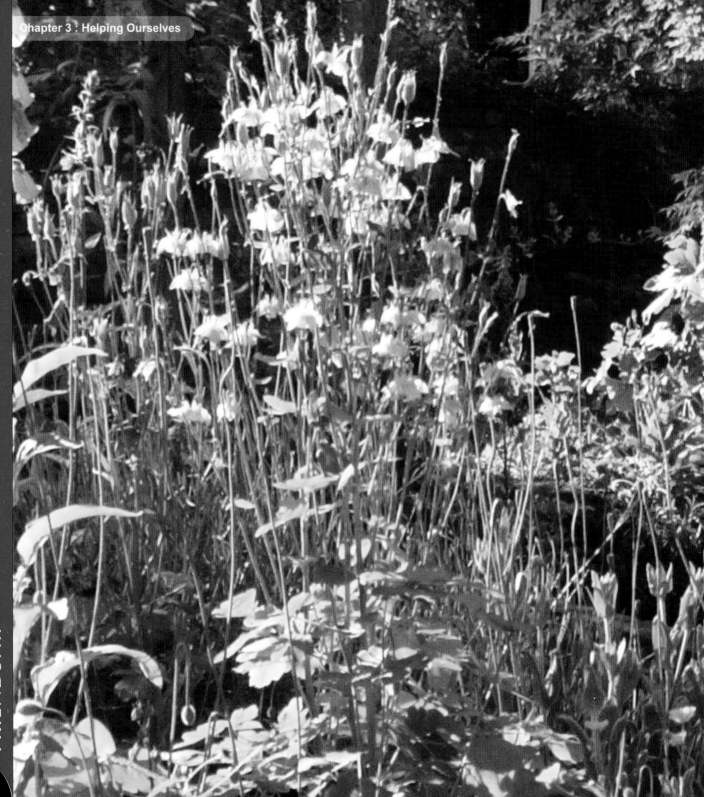

FRIENDSHIP

Make New Friends....

A song I remember fondly from day camp had the refrain "make new friends but don't forget the old, one is silver the other is gold…"

When I think of my life since being diagnosed with Parkinson three years ago, that refrain has significance. I live where I grew up which means I have maintained friendships for the better part of 70 years.

I have friends from elementary, junior high and high school. I have met people professionally and socially over the years and thus have expanded my circle of acquaintances.

However, since my diagnosis and involvement in the PD community, I have met incredible people and made significant new friends.

These are accomplished folks professionally and artistically. They are empathic, witty and engaged and engaging. There is certainly concern about being a PwP. Most important there is concern about one another. They add the gold to my life.

Judith Kapustin Katz, Ed.D.

SO HOW DO WE IMPROVE OUR LIVES TODAY?

For better living, a key element is to revisit, rekindle, or create a PASSION in your life! Find a cause or activity that you want to devote energy to. For those of us who produced this book, the challenges and opportunities have given us purpose and pleasure far beyond any contributions to society and the PD community.

You might express your passion in creative outlets like crafts, the arts, advocacy or anything else that speaks to you. Many PwP have reported that they can reduce or ignore their PD symptoms when they're totally involved.

A corollary passion or mission is to help others. Many people agree that when we do things for others we get back much more than we give. When my mother was in her 90s and totally forgetful, she still wanted to be useful. Given her limitations, it was hard to find a suitable task but we did - rolling wool into balls from the original skeins. Very simple work but she felt better knowing that others relied on her "work".

Then there's exercise - as they say, "use it or lose it". Also, recent studies show you may be able to build new pathways in your brain.

Another concept is "slippery." If you get stuck, i.e. turning in bed or putting your arm into a coat sleeve, think "SLIPPERY" - a silky type bottom sheet or a smooth polyester shirt might help "grease " the non-cooperative body part. And sing when you freeze while walking -- did you ever think a song might work like anti-freeze or oil with no mess? And "LOOSE" - your clothing may act as a straitjacket if it is too tight but if it's too loose, it may trip you. Beware of extremes!

Finally, laugh as often as you can. In the 1970s Norman Cousins wrote **An Anatomy of an Illness**. His self-prescribed cure consisted of watching Marx Brothers movies for pain relief. Genuine belly laughter worked for him! Today researchers study laughter and humor; back then it was a frontier subject.

Remember, laughter:

- has no side effects except aerobic breathing (and that's good for you)
- feels great
- boosts endorphins
- and even if it works only as a placebo (and as we know, PwP are more sensitive to placebos) do you care why?

Because we all react differently, keep track of what improves your life and when something does, share it with your PD community. You never know - what helps you, might lead to the next real breakthrough in PD research. **Katherine Huseman**

Neuroplasticity and the PD brain

While recently watching a programme about disabled athletes, about how their brains adapt to their losses and start to expand activity into areas that are not usually used for that purpose, I wondered whether this is what is happening in some of the exceptional results that active PwP are having in two areas. One, when active PwP learn new skills and their PD symptoms improve; and two, when PwP who have lost mobility due to PD, can cycle or dance, or do fine motor work like drawing when their signature is illegible. Is this a way to overcome the limitations of PD?

As a practitioner of Tai Chi Chuan for many years, I was aware that I could do things involving turns and balance within the practice of the art that were at odds with my everyday abilities. I was also aware that some of the Tai Chi skills spilled into my routine activities. The years of practice had in someway embedded certain skills that I was using unconsciously to good advantage.

One of the most obvious of these was the 180 degree turn from my kitchen worktop to my sink, which I mainly manage, medicated or not, with no problem, due to a fundamental heel turn specific to Tai Chi. Another is the heel-toe movement in walking that every practitioner of the form that I am familiar with is drilled in.

I knew that we can learn to move differently and that the new learning, when added to the original movement skills we learned in infancy, gets embedded elsewhere in the brain. They do not even 'feel' as though they are coming from the same place.

Watching the remarkable footage of a young man with serious debilitating Parkinson going from crutches to bicycle to participate in a long distance challenge that would floor many able people, or hearing of the studies on tandem or forced pace cycling and its effect on PD - these inexplicable stories of people feeling symptom-free while doing an enjoyable activity made me very curious.

The questions that I found coming up again and again were these:

- **Why is targeted physical therapy not offered as standard to people with PD?**
- **Why is there a common medical expectation for many patients that they will physically decline?**
- **Is the thinking about Parkinson and movement fundamentally flawed?**

Again, I had to go back to the last question and ask myself: Is this a fair question? Surely among medical professionals there must be some who do go counter to the general flow and actively encourage patients to do more, to think outside the box about their own mobility. From where I stand these things fall into a medical bracket that shouts NEUROPLASTICITY! And that surely is the province of neurology......

This led to another thought: perhaps the view of Parkinson is also linked to its historical stereotype, that of the elderly person in late slow decline. In fact, within my own family circle, there are people now in their late 70's with tremor, shuffling and poor balance who do not complain to their doctors and insist they are just 'getting old'. This may be the case - an inevitable late life loss of neurons. I also see people of the same age who are spry, flexible and very functional.

I know many people who are, or were once, Young Onset, and started losing mobility in their 20s, 30s or 40s. The older of these, like myself, had no medical encouragement at all to be more active, rather than less active and there is little evidence of targeted provision. In fact, nearly all of the provision of this type, outside of general physiotherapy, seems to have come about by accident, through the efforts of interested and engaged individuals with a special interest in PD. Their efforts have resulted in walking, cycling, dance and singing groups, specialized Tai Chi classes. In my own home town I found a programme of Conductive Education, run by people trained at the famed Peto Institute which has had notable success with children who have cerebral palsy.

- **Has this notion that we have to accept these losses been derived from a view of old age that itself might be flawed?**
- **How are Young Onset patients changing this perception?**
- **How is the medical profession in general adapting to these changes, and neurology in particular?**
- **Given research that highlights the benefit of exercise for PwP, are the majority of neurologists and MDS doctors prescribing exercise?**

Lindy Ashford

So my big question is:
"How best can we harness the gift of neuroplasticity and use it to our benefit?"

If patient anecdotes reflect the reality on the ground, then awareness that there are strategies for wellness that involve being actively engaged in creative movement and processes are not yet being medically promoted to patients.

On the other hand, we feel that there is a growing awareness that the medical view of PD is far from complete; patients are saying that more doctors are curious about what we are doing and are prepared to discuss it!

TAI CHI CHUAN AND QI GONG

Tai Chi is a slow graceful martial art which was traditionally practiced in China by people over the age of 50. The dance-like 'form', which one should learn slowly, taking years rather than weeks, is beneficial for PwP. This is because it involves slowly repeating each move until perfected. If you are interested in exploring what Tai Chi has to offer, you will need a good teacher who views Tai Chi as a health art, plenty of patience, a commitment to practicing daily for a while, some loose clothing and soft shoes.

Tai Chi will help exercise the small muscles of the body that usually do not get exercised well with faster activities. These muscles are the ones that get affected early in PD, so it can help you maintain flexibility. It is useful for breathing, balance and, if you are adventurous, for learning how to fall well! Once you know the basics, you may also want to explore energy exercises known as Chi Kung or Qi Gong. Anecdotally, these have a profound effect on PD when practiced daily, though they do require nearly as much commitment as you would need to run a marathon to achieve a lasting result.

Exercise is something that everyone can do, even when your mobility is limited. You may not climb mountains or run marathons, but out there, or even in your home, there are ways for you to keep mobile. Everything you do to keep your body moving will ensure that you have more energy and a better quality of life.

EXERCISE

Exercise vigorously.....

People with Parkinson may not know they are entitled to physical therapy and often get discounts at health clubs. The importance of exercise cannot be overstated, especially the older we get when the lines between PD and aging become blurred and aches and pains are numerous. Each person has a preference for types of exercise. Here are a few recommendations: recumbent exercise bicycle (this is a stationery bike with a back to the seat), tandem bicycling, regular bicycling, treadmill or brisk walks.

Aqua Therapy

There are many locations at which one can find exercise classes, but those in the water lessen the impact on painful muscles, joints and bones; at the same time, the water provides resistance that strengthens the body. Classes improve strength, balance, and cardiovascular function and build muscle. Many classes on the floor have been adapted to water exercise, such as aqua zumba and aqua chi. Treadmills have also gone aquatic with the AquaCiser available at some physical therapy centers. This is basically a hot tub with a treadmill floor. It fills up around you and has several therapy jets. The water drains quickly when you are finished. As a twenty year plus PD veteran, I strongly recommend aqua therapies. They alleviate some of the pain and increase stamina, providing some of the energy that PD has left us incapable of producing.

Paula Wittekind

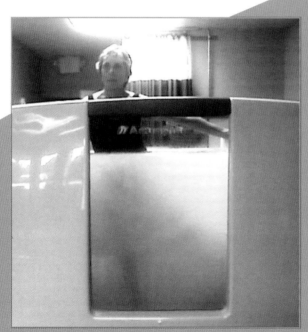

Paula exercises in the AquaCiser

The importance of keeping moving cannot be over estimated

EXERCISE

An exciting finding about the value of exercise was reported at the 2010 meeting of the Radiological Society of North America.

A group from the University of Pittsburgh showed that in patients with minimal cognitive impairment or Alzheimer disease, those who walked just 5 miles a week had more than 50% less cognitive decline and memory loss, coupled with significantly less loss of brain volume on a 3-dimensional volumetric MRI, than did those persons with cognitive decline who were sedentary.

Even more exciting, the preservation of brain volume was maximal in those regions which often affect people with aging and cognitive decline: that is, in the cortices of the temporal and pre-frontal regions. These effects of preservation of both structure and function were actually greater in affected individuals than in those without any cognitive problems. They seemed to hold up over a ten-year period. Those PwP for whom cognitive decline is a major fear will find hope in this study for the cognitive rewards of getting on our feet and moving around a walking track or our neighborhoods. Get off your duff and go!!!!

From Raji CA et al.
Abstract from Radiological Society
of North American, 2010.

HANDY TIPS FOR EXERCISE

1   START SMALL Do something you know you can accomplish. Maybe it's just walking to the mailbox once a day; maybe it's going on a treadmill for two minutes! Don't feel that you have to start five times a week with a half hour per session. When I'm at a conference about exercise and participants are being told to do x, y and z, I feel this collective internal sigh that if expressed out loud would say, "Sure...I'm really going to get up tomorrow and walk for a half hour and then I'm going to do it all week long! And after that, I'm going to train for the marathon!" Start small. Choose an activity that will give you pleasure - do it to your favorite music and make sure it's something that you can accomplish. We all build on success and success gives us energy; failure brings us down.

2   MAKE A COMMITMENT TO SOMEONE TO EXERCISE WITH You will not honor a commitment you make to yourself, but you will to another person. Involve a friend, a grandchild, a trainer, even a pet. You will even honor a commitment to your dog over yourself! So don't do it alone; involve others if you can.

3   DO AN EXERCISE THAT YOU DID AS A KID The neuromuscular pattern is there. Have you seen Michael J. Fox on hockey skates? We all have physical memories which we can draw on to help us move. Something as simple as bicycling can be good. Even playing catch has something to offer. It's not a cardiovascular workout, but quick shifts of weight involved in catching the ball work your balance. You are more likely to do something if you enjoy it and enjoy it if you can do it!

4   EXERCISE AT A REGULAR TIME Do you watch the news or a show that you could see while you're on a stationary bike? Or do you like mysteries? You can make a rule that you will only listen to a book on tape when you're exercising on a treadmill or a stationary bike.

5   GO TO A MOVEMENT OR EXERCISE CLASS WITH OTHER PWP You will make friends: you will go to the class to see them, to have fun together, to exchange ideas and to move and enjoy one another. Social contact is very important for a disease that affects how we're perceived by others and tends to isolate us at home. Getting out and seeing friends and moving together in a non-judgmental environment is a very good thing.

Also, beware of very high intensity workouts. A study by Lisa Shulman from the University of Baltimore shows that moderate activity done for a longer period of time is more beneficial to PwP than intense activity done for a shorter period of time.

Use music you like, it will help you move.

Find a way to make it work for you. When do your meds kick in? What climate do you live in? How often can your schedule manage? If you have balance problems, how can you be supervised? You need to know who you are, what your particular needs are and what you like to do. Remember, "A dream without a plan is only a wish."

Pamela Quinn, professional dancer for 20 years, was diagnosed with PD at 42. She uses her training and experience to develop movement therapy programs for PwP.

A SET OF EASY GENTLE WARMUP EXERCISES.....

 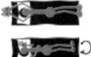

SIMPLE WARMUPS TO GET YOU MOVING

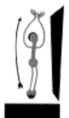

before you get up . . .   then . . .

1. Mindfully stretch your arms and legs, then wriggle your fingers and toes - gently - then stretch your arms over your head . . .

2. Really scrunch up your face muscles as hard as you can - then relax. Repeat, and imitate a goldfish - open and close your mouth!

3. Still lying down - rotate your feet slowly to the right, then to the left, dipping your feet make little circles with your toes . . .

4. once you are up, meds taken, and you are having coffee .... you can exercise your hands and feet. First circle your hands, then . . .

5. ... place your hands flat on your table, feet flat on the floor, and lift up your fingers and toes - 10-15 times . . .

6. When you are done with coffee try standing at a table or counter, swing one leg back and forward, then the other, a few times . . .

7. Lift your shoulders up as high as you can, then circle them back and round, then forward and round, they will feel looser . .

8. . . . then rotate your head, dropping it to one shoulder, circle your head round and back, then repeat the other way. . . .

9. Use a chair or wall if your balance is poor, and stretch yourself upwards as far as you can, raising your heels and making yourself really tall.

10. With your feet apart, and body well balanced, gently shake your body all over, from your head to your toes, gently loosening up.

11. A little more energetic; Stand with feet apart, hands on your hips - rotate those hips in small circles, then as large as you can.

12. You can circle your knees in the same way, then make 'windmills' with your arms, small circles first, then grow them, and shrink them back . . .

13. Now swing your whole body from side to side, let your arms hang loosely, making the movement first bigger, then small again . . .

14. Standing with feet apart, hands by sides, gently slide one hand down your leg as far as it will go, bending your torso, and back again. Repeat on other side . . .

15. Raise arms shoulder high and wide apart. Turn to your left and touch the left fingers with your right hand, then your right fingers with your left hand . . .

16. Finish with a big conscious yawn, and stretching everything you can - gently!

You should by now be ready for the day!

even if we are stiff and find exercise hard . . .

I think John was amazing on the ride.

Of all the Parkinson people in the world with mobility problems, he has achieved more that anyone I have heard of.

His 1000 miles Land's End to John O'Groats cycle ride was a unique, single-minded demonstration of determination and effort in overcoming extreme difficulties.

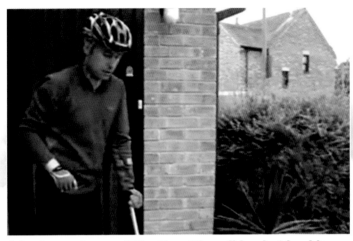

John has extreme difficulty with walking but is able to cycle. With help he completed this amazing journey from the northern most point of mainland Britain to its furthest southern point.

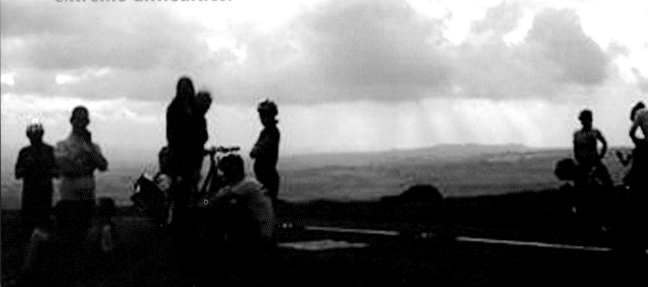

"When I cycle, I don't feel like I have P.D. MAGIC!"

I have found that people newly diagnosed with Parkinson fall into two camps; those who were relieved, because they thought they had something worse, or those like me who were completely devastated. My diagnosis was brutal. "You've got Parkinson. You won't need any medication just yet. I'll see you in six months time and you'll need to tell the DVLA*." Then out on the street. I immediately plunged into a black hole. I couldn't say the word 'P..........' without bursting into tears. I had been a sportsman all my life, who, through exercise and a healthy diet, planned to outlive my 95 year old Dad by at least ten years. "It's just not fair, I kept repeating". This for me was the worst possible scenario. I'd lost control.

It took me two years to climb out of that black hole. I went through all the stages of bereavement for my old life, mourning its passing but at the same time, deep down a smouldering ember of determination not to let this thing beat me, ignited into a life plan to do everything I could to help fund a cure for Parkinson. This was perhaps the ultimate denial. This thing wasn't going to beat me. I was back in control.

In the early stages, I just didn't want to meet anyone with Parkinson. I was not like them. Eventually my wife persuaded me to go on a Parkinson fund-raising trek to Corsica and it was there that I discovered other 'Parkies' with interesting pasts, like me, struggling with their new lives, trying to make the most of a bad hand. A fellow trekker, Bruce Lorimer, inspired by the determination of Tom Isaacs, suggested we pedal from Lands End to John O'Groats to help fund research into a cure. It was during that journey North that the third member of our Parkie trio, Neil Manning, pointed out to me that I was a man on a mission. "You're being driven," he said. He'd watched me surviving on four hours sleep a night, planning how I would involve every Parkinson Branch in Britain in funding a cure, through cycling.

Two years on, two End to End trips completed and £45,000 in the kitty, Pedal for Parkinson is going from strength to strength. With a growing band of Patrons, including the Arch Bishop of York and Graham Norton, our profile has soared. There are plans afoot for an even more ambitious ride in 2011 and Pedal for Parkinson is to become an annual feature of Parkinson UK events.

The bonus has been that I have discovered that regular exercise is half the treatment for PD and cycling in particular is being recognized as a sport which seems to improve symptoms.

My life now is so busy and exciting, I can't fit everything in. When we emerge at the end of this journey to find a cure, I will be able to say, hand on heart, that having Parkinson has been a valuable experience.

David Greaves, Pedal for Parkinsons
http://pedalforparkinsons.co.uk
* UK newly diagnosed PwP may need to inform the DVLA (licensing authority) if they are deemed unfit to drive.

SERENDIPITY AND OUT-OF-THE-BOX DISCOVERIES

One day Jay Alberts, PhD, was riding a tandem bicycle with a person who had PD. When they stopped for a break, the PwP realized that her symptoms were greatly reduced. This led Professor Alberts to investigate whether forced exercise improves Parkinson symptoms. His initial research says yes.

There is another theory of exercise that finds that it is the learning of new, intense physical skills that creates the improvement.

From a practical point of view, while those 2 theories battle it out, the best thing for PwP is to just get moving. Aerobic exercise is probably best but aim for a balanced exercise program. (E-patient Dave quoting Peter Schmidt, CIO and Program Director at the National Parkinson Foundation.)

http://epatientdave.com/2012/01/16/e-patient-resources-for-parkinsons-disease/#.UGEwdhjD57

DANCE TO RAISE A QUESTION

It seems so long ago.

2003, The Tennessee Waltz Lady, Edith.

Her husband, Clive, wheeled her in.

In a wheelchair for 3 years, except for a few hours a day shuffling painfully with a walker. The Tennessee Waltz was the first song she and Clive had danced to, decades ago.

We put on her song, loud.

She got out of the wheelchair, into Clive's arms and they danced. At times when Clive was not there, she danced alone, with her arms embracing air; you could see love as it moved her gracefully. We had to keep people away if they disturbed her with their weeping. You could start at the beginning of time and go to the end of time and never see anything more beautiful than that.

It seems so long ago.

2004 I started dancing in my living room, to alleviate the symptoms. I started writing my acceptance speech for the Nobel Prize, but then noticed on the Internet that there were hundreds of Parkies who were dancing against the pain.

2005 We fancied ourselves to be the Parkinson Underground. We launched chain-letter CDs; exchanging our favorite dance music.

2006 I realized I could improve my walking by singing in my head and pretending to dance down the street, pretend I was floating, my feet 6 inches above the ground. Part of my brain died, but dance and music are controlled by a different part of the brain. Its is my contention that Parkinson is a cowardly disease, and it is too chicken to attack the re-inforced primitive areas of the brain; the parts where 50,000 years ago, we banged on sticks and chanted and danced to scare off predators such as sabre-tooth tigers. Parkinson, the killer of brains, does not dare attack the place where the drums are playing.

2007 We e-mailed 6,000 people the following question: Dance as therapy, Dance for flexibility, strength, endurance. Dance for joy. Dance in defiance of the disease. I agree with all of that, and all of that has been accepted and approved. It is clear that dance, like exercise, combined with meditation, like physical and spiritual movement joined together, is benefical to PwP - or to anybody.

But here is what it is really about: Dance for a cure. Dance to bother the scientists. Dance to raise a question. The question is: if you cannot walk without falling down, if you cannot hold a spoon to feed yourself, if you choke when you swallow, if your mind is losing its ability to give instructions to your muscles, then how come you can get up and dance? Eh?

How come? What's up with that?

The next day, I got 400 e-mails.

From Parkies, caregivers, dancers, dance teachers, dance choreographers, an orchestra conductor, drummers who teach drumming as therapy, Blues artists, visual artists teaching the handicapped, some nurses on the night shift in a hospice for terminal cases… they were all dancing in defiance of the disease.

Dancers all around but not a scientist in sight, I put on earphones all day, plus music playing at night. I attended business meetings with music playing in my ears. Sometimes I would take them off just to give myself a break, but mostly I listened to music 24 hours a day for three years.

It was excellent but excessive; after a year I was talking in song lyrics. John Lee Hooker pointed the way, (in his song "The Healer") His words do it for me. Buddy Guy or Mozart cannot do it for me. I was selecting the playlists to match the occasion, or the place, or the visitors, or some abstract impression. I was changing the way other people appeared by changing the sound track. The movie would change, of course.

Things got complicated.

Dance for flexibility and happiness: that is underway, massively, thanks to the dancers.

Olie Westheimer and the Mark Morris Dancers spreading the miracle to so many cities;

Royal Ballet in London offered themselves up for medical experiments to find out what parts of the brain are dancing.

Many local PD groups promoting dance:
Parkinson's Disease Foundation
London Arts for Health
Arts4Life
the PD association in Greece
the Dana Alliance
Nurse Jeanine Young-Mason,

Jill Bunce
American Dance Therapy
American Music Therapy
The Mysterious Anuket singing to her computer at 3 a.m.,
Fiona (Dolenga) McCarty at Hidden Arena Dance…
thousands more…

Parkies dance is a huge grass roots movement, growing at startling speed. Because it works. You can debate an idea; but when your body does not function and it hurts and later your body functions and no longer hurts…. Yeah, I'll try that.

The human race had music and dance tens of thousands of years before we knew how to build shelter, before civilization; dance is pre-verbal, deep in the sensations; we danced before we had language, before we had names for each other.

Then Margie Gillis, dancer, said this:

"**M**y approach is based on listening to the connection between thought, emotion, spirit and body. This is the natural kinetic process whereby our inner landscape translates into electrical impulses that transmit to the muscles the message as to how, and with what quality, to move.

I explore the physical manifestation of this pure experience of being; the neuromuscular interrelationship."

Dancers know about neurology; the neurologists do not know about dancing.

That's where you will find me these days. Following the Continuum movement; training by Linda Rabin; not for dancing as such; going below intellect, below concept, below argument, below opinion, below words - and here's the startling part: below emotions. To get to the sensations inside; pre-verbal and with a solid anchor. There are many schools of thought about this, free innovation dance or pre-planned movement dance? Solo dance or social dance? Hey, baby, whatever rings your bell!! Go for it!

The dancers answered the call; the scientists did not. So, I repeat the question from 2007: how come some people cannot walk, but they can dance? Eh? Doc? Scientist? What's up with that?
Bob Dawson

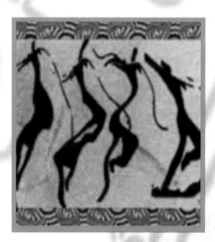

DANCE FOR MOBILITY

DANCE, PARKINSON AND HEALING

Actually, it seems I have had to go deeper into the world of illness in order to find a way out. A spinal infection compounded medical maladies in the 13th year of my life with Parkinson. The subsequent six years of rehab have been difficult ; a confusing time emotionally as well as physically. I barely have had the energy to get out of my bed; the feeling of trapped fluid in my body - so heavy and making my gait so tentative. When I told each doctor about these sensations, I was always dismissed as delusional and offered drugs and/ or surgery. However, proprioceptive intuition (developed through a decade of dance training, three decades of yoga studies, a lifetime immersion into the ways music motivates movement) would at intervals provide a clue as to the direction to go and the will to stay this unmarked course.

One of these clues was provided a few years ago when a cousin stopped by with an invitation to a theater fund raiser. I balked. She persisted. I went. The food, the people watching, the change in venue from my bedroom were all therapeutic. But it was when the DJ started with the dance tunes that this therapeutic outing took on the joyous expression of body.

Alas, the next day the heavy feeling of being immobilized by trapped fluid returned, but the memory of freedom through dance remains in me still. Four years later, I heard about a professional dance studio in Chicago, where the teacher was offering dance for Parkinson. She refused to teach in the space of the local hospital. She did not believe that it was a therapy for sick people, but a vital outlet, as well as exploration, for people suffering Parkinson.

Our group of dancers are about to begin our second year next weekend; I look forward to physical and emotional freedom that those Saturday afternoon classes give me. Doctors still do not know what I am talking about. My family and friends still think I am delusional, but I know that it has something to do with the fluid in my body.

I was just discussing with my care-giver this afternoon, that illness is as much physical as it is emotional. I see both avenues being addressed at these classes. Erect spinal posture feels like being released from a prison of forward flexion. Arms reaching out, up and over head, seem to allow the fluid to move more easily through out my body.

Lastly, as for those Parkinsonian masks: they seem to slip away with the music, laughter and movement, and emotional expression.

My visit with the new neurologist last week, who pronounced my Parkinson to be mild. I still have other maladies to work through, including finding shoes, but next Saturday I am ready to hit the dance floor for another year.

Maureen Stricker

Hubbard Street Dance Chicago's Parkinson's Project

MUSICAL CHALLENGES

I purchased my piano in 2005 after I had a diagnosis of focal dystonia (FD). This came after not playing, or hardly playing for nearly a year, as I found I was more and more stiff and had more and more coordination and hesitation problems. The neurologist said that things would get worse and I had already started down the path of no return. Deep down inside I knew he was wrong, but I was not a doctor and others kept telling me he knew better and I was crazy. I then went to another doctor a year later and that proved to be the best thing in my life. It was with neuro two that my diagnosis was more affirmed and confirmed as not being FD, but more of an atypical PD. I then blew more cash on my clavichord.

Anyway, the piano turned out to be my godsend. As frustrated as I was then and I remain, I kept at it, and after 6 month, I was back playing again. I played well enough before to not lose the technique completely but I've lost enough never to have the real facile playing I had.

I practiced piano exercises every day. I did the Schmitt finger independence exercises a few at a time, slowly and with as relaxed hands as I could. If I fatigued or tensed up, I'd stop. At first I got in probably no more than 10 minutes maximum. This was a far cry from my 2-plus hours every day plus 4-6 hours on a weekend. Eventually I was up to one half hour and then an hour or two a day. Now, 4 years later, I'm back to about 2-3 hours per day on a consistent basis.

The thing is, you are going to suffer from 100 steps backward. You will want to toss the piano out of the window, sell the guitar and anything else to move as far away from your passion as possible. Even today I get very frustrated particularly when I want to play some of the more demanding keyboard literature such as piano sonatas by Beethoven (even his easiest aren't so easy for me now), or some Chopin Etudes, which I could hardly play before, let alone now.

The other thing I learned is to know your own limits. I believe I've said this before. I can't play the fast ferocious Etudes anymore or other really demanding concert pieces I was working on. I now have to play the slower, less challenging technically, but more lyrical pieces. These alone have proven to be plenty to do and in some cases just as difficult. Not in the technical sense, but in the musical challenges they present. It really takes a whole lot of work to play slowly and to play with emotion that comes of being sincere and true to the music and not in a contrived way, as some playing comes across.

John Citron

Anyway, don't give up on your passions.

I learned the hard way that no matter what you try to do to divorce yourself from them, they will come back at you, and drive you back to them no matter what.

My advice is to play a little of whatever you can every day. I find that the more I play, the more I can play. If you play a little every day, you might be able to increase what you can play.

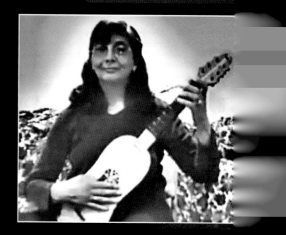

I wonder if this phenomenon of transient reversal of PD when your mind is focused on something you are passionate about is common among PwP or just in some cases.

The opposite effect is from stress. Most of us know and have experienced the negative effect of stress, with PD symptoms getting worse.

This mind-body connection and the neuro-psychology is another piece of the PD puzzle.

Have any of you talked to your doctor about it? How many of you had such experiences - both feeling great when you are doing something you love and the opposite when stressed?

It could be one of those things the doctor doesn't know and only a PwP knows !!

PARKINSON & CREATIVITY

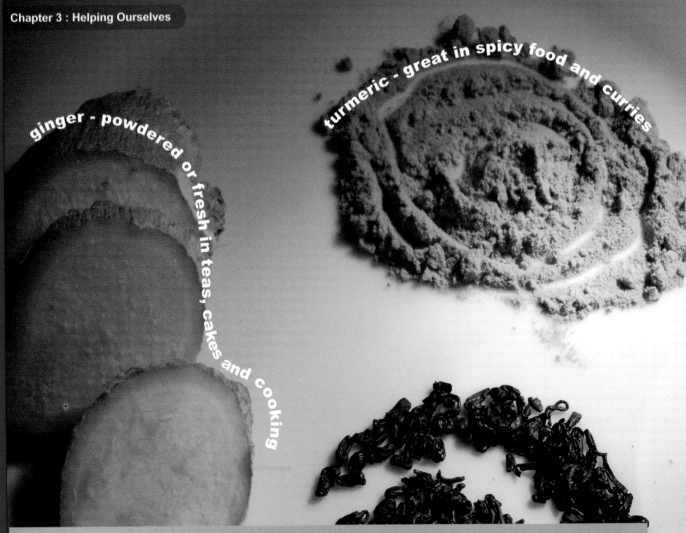

ginger - powdered or fresh in teas, cakes and cooking

turmeric - great in spicy food and curries

green tea is a natural anti-oxidant

DISCUSS ANY SUPPLEMENTS YOU ARE TAKING WITH YOUR DOCTOR

DIET & PARKINSON DISEASE

There are many theories on diet and its impact on PD including low blood sugar, the timing of medicine, the type and amount of food you eat, high fat diets, supplements, antioxidants, fava beans, etc. It is an area within our control, needing no prescriptions, special materials, or licensing. You might consider investigating an approach that appeals to you, but remember experimenting can have consequences. Before making major changes in diet, do your research (public libraries and their interlibrary loan progams are a great resource.) As always, remember to consult with your physician first, because even herbs can conflict with some of your medicines.

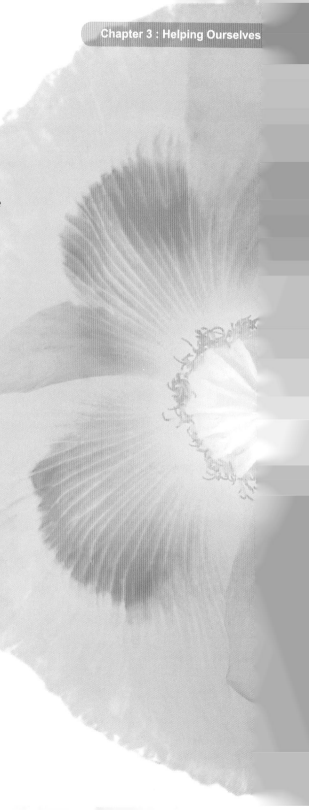

PwP who come to the forums have tried practically everything they can find in the search for things that will help slow the progression of their PD and help them live well with it. While we make no recommendations for any of these do-it-yourself remedies, the following are three ordinary, easy to find, and freely available foods that come up in discussion time and again.

It is interesting to note that scientists are also studying the potential benefits these foods may have for Parkinson disease. If you are interested, please do further research using the research guide at the end of Chapter One of this book.

GINGER

Ginger has been used traditionally in cooking and in medicine for many centuries, both in the East and the West. It is sometimes recommended for the prevention of pregnancy sickness and is useful in PD for its anti-nausea properties and for relieving stiffness. In either fresh and powdered state, it can be added to food or made into a tea.

CURCUMIN

Long used in South East Asia in cooking, the spice turmeric also has a place in traditional medicine, notably in the Ayurvedic tradition of India. Curcumin is an extract of turmeric.

GREEN TEA

Many PwP choose to use green tea as a part of their daily self-help routine, both for its anti-oxidant properties and in the hope that it will provide some form of neuroprotection. Some report that it has helped with ongoing symptoms and that they feel better while using it.

Scientists are interested in the possibility that some of the chemical constituents of green tea in particular catechins and l-theanine, may have beneficial effects on a range of conditions including PD.

CURCUMIN STUDY

Curcumin prevents dopaminergic neuronal death through inhibition of the c-Jun N-terminal kinase pathway.

Yu S, et al., Rejuvenation Res. 2010 Feb;13(1):55-64.

The authors demonstrate that curcumin treatment of mice with PD significantly improved behavioral deficits and enhanced the survival of neurons in the substantia nigra. The mechanism of action of curcumin is via the inhibition of the JNK pathway and is independent of its already established anti-inflammatory and anti-oxidant properties. These studies suggest that curcumin treatment can be neuroprotective.

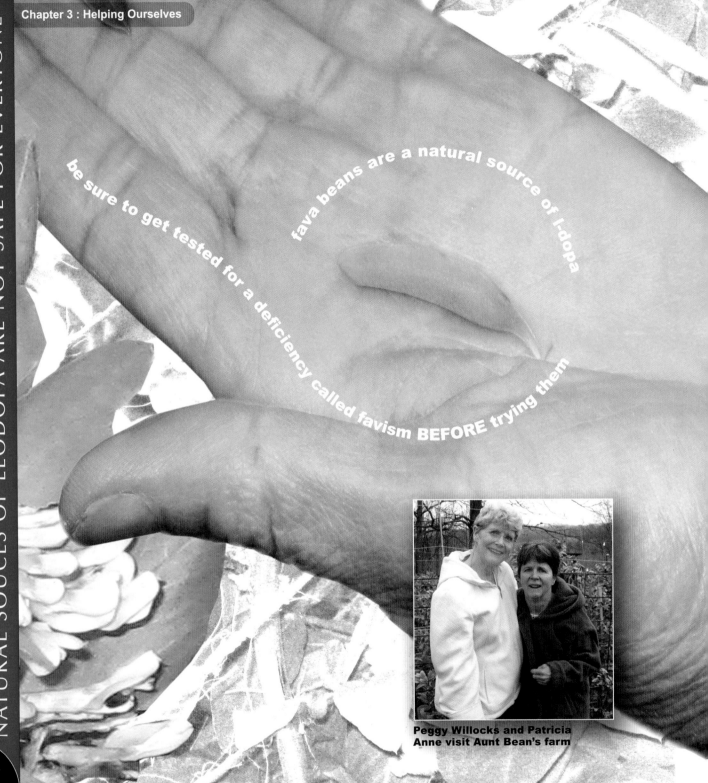

NATURAL SOUCES OF LEODOPA ARE NOT SAFE FOR EVERYONE

fava beans are a natural source of l-dopa

be sure to get tested for a deficiency called favism BEFORE trying them

Peggy Willocks and Patricia Anne visit Aunt Bean's farm

4 ACRES OF FAVAS

In search of natural remedies that could help combat Parkinson disease symptoms, I came across the book, **Green Pharmacy**, by James Duke, PhD, published in 1997. Here are some excerpts:

> "Fava beans are one of nature's best plant sources for L-dopa. The sprouts contain ten times more L-dopa than un-sprouted beans."

> "They are high in fiber, which helps constipation, a common problem in PD."

> "Favas contain choline and lecithin which researchers suggest might have a positive effect in preventing or relieving PD symptoms."

Duke states that although he had discussed the potential of the beans with dozens of people for several years, that he knew of no one with Parkinson disease who had taken the food approach seriously.

He also writes about mucuna (velvet bean/hairy vetch),which I am also attempting to experimentally grow this year.

Via computer, we found Ken Allan's website and began communicating with him. He has PD and has grown favas for many years to help in alleviating his symptoms. We are so grateful that he shared his experiences with us.

Seeds were purchased and planted in March 2009.

My friend and I took the G6pd blood test to make sure we did not have the enzyme deficiency that would make using the favas harmful to us.

Our plants began producing in June and I will always remember what a change they made. I usually had to push my friend in a wheelchair at the Earth Fare Market, but for her birthday she was walking around, visiting and feeding herself and looked 10 years younger than the weeks before. (After just eating favas for a few days, her on times were longer, her posture straighter and out-look brighter). We found, like Ken Allan, that the young pods (about 2 1/2 inches long) should be picked before the bean develops. We steamed them for about 6 minutes and froze them in single layers in ziplock freezer bags so they were easy for my friend to get out as needed. A fall crop was started in August (hoping for our usually moderate TN winter). They grew well despite the summer heat. In September, I began to wonder if we could also use another part of the plant for its L-dopa content. The stem, leaves, flowers, beans, all contain this product that our bodies were a little short of. I had been making echinacea tincture from my homegrown plants for years; why couldn't this be done with the fava plant? Upon going to the garden and carefully studying the plants, I chose a part of the plant top, collected a few and dried them. Then they were placed into brandy and shaken for a month. During this month and into October, I started experiencing a few more PD symptoms. The one that bothered me the most was urination frequency, becoming worse, until it was about every 45 minutes. I was even incontinent twice. I had not been using the beans, but saving them all for my friend, because our crop had been small and she was benefiting so much from them. I wished now that I had managed to plant a lot more.

The tincture was finally finished/strained and ready to test. I was the perfect guinea pig for the experiment. I took about 1/4th teaspoon of the tincture, put it into a glass and poured hot water over it and drank it. Tasted OK. No sudden effects. About an hour later went out to my car for something and upon coming up the front steps noticed that I didn't halt on my right leg . . . like I always did. Strange, try that again . . not my imagination! Tried standing straight up from a chair . . . didn't have to 'propel' myself, like I'd done for years. 'Tapping' was quick and then we had to go somewhere in a car. Now, driving was a REAL TEST; it had always been hard, even scarey, for me to be behind the wheel of a car. My reflex times were very slow and I had never wanted to learn to drive in the first place.

Amazingly enough, driving was easy, I was relaxed and even enjoyed it for the first time in my life! PD seems to run in our family (my grandfather, his brother, my brother all have PD, and many others in the family - along with my father - have Essential Tremor). My first symptoms showed up after a diving accident in 7th grade . . .which I attributed to spinal injury all these years. Interestingly, though, stress makes the symptoms re-appear.

Anyway, I started taking the tincture the end of October 2009 and now in May 2010, it is still keeping my PD symptoms under control. The fall crop of the fava patch came up and was beautiful. We started harvesting a few beans around Thanksgiving, and dried lots of the part I had selected to make tincture. The plants were not frostbitten until the weather reached 26 degrees Fahrenheit. However, they were not dead and started coming back up from the roots after about a week of really warm weather in February. Then 26 degrees came again, this time killing the roots. I think with protection, they might grow all winter in the East Tennessee area.

Now I have moved from the city to an almost 4-acre farm with wonderful soil. I have planted over 7 pounds of fava's along with some mucuna's to experiment with this year. God has been so good and will guide us as to how these beans can benefit many people with Parkinson disease . . . my extended family. God Bless Us Every One.

Aunt Bean posts regular updates on her fava crops on the NeuroTalk Forum.

Ayurveda, Mucuna Pruriens and Parkinson Disease

Ayurveda is the traditional medicine of the Indian subcontinent, developed over many centuries, and practiced in everyday life by millions of people all over the world. It is the "veda" (knowledge) of "ayus" (life & longevity). It is a holistic medical system, aimed at treating mind, body and self and does not focus on treating any specific symptom. In Ayurvedic therapy, each patient's treatment is custom designed. A combination of treatments that include diet, herbal medicines, exercise and various spiritual practices are incorporated into daily living to bring a person back into balance.

Dr. Ram Manohar, Director of Research for the Arya Vaidya Pharmacy (AVP) in Coimbatore, India, describes the differences between Ayurveda and Western Medicines as follows:

"I think Ayurveda and Western medicine originated in entirely different cultural paradigms, which nurtured radically different world views. So, the basic difference lies in the epistemology, the very approach to knowledge building.

I would say the most primary thing is that Ayurveda looks at the human personality as composite of the body, mind and self. This is very central to the approach of Ayurveda.

The human personality is considered as a dynamic manifestation of interactions between the mind, body and the self, whereas Western medicine seems to be more focused on the body. The mind is just an epiphenomenon of reactions that take place in the body, and the self is almost a nonexistent entity. Whereas in Ayurveda, the mind is given much greater importance than the body. The body is the shadow of the mind, as far as an Ayurvedic physician is concerned. So, this makes radical differences in the way an Ayurvedic physician approaches a patient and tries to understand disease and health."

Parkinson disease is known in Ayurveda as "Kampa Vata." Treatment protocols were described centuries ago in ancient Indian literature. At an Ayurvedic center in India or in other countries, the therapies are tailored to the individual person.

Max Lafontaine's Experience

Max, a NeuroTalk forum member, posted a detailed account of the Ayurvedic treatment he tried for PD.

He said: "I would like to share with you my experience of going through a "Pancha Karma". This was a 10 day cleansing to remove toxins out of my body at an Ayurvedic center in California. Pancha Karma is considered the single most powerful healing therapy utilized in Ayurvedic medicine.

While I was there, they explained to me how important it is to remove the accumulated toxins (ama) from my body and to do my best in preventing it from building up again. Ama is toxins caused by what and how we eat, pollutant/toxins in our environment, stress in our life, from how we think, live and act, etc. They believe, for PwP, that ama is really in there deep. It has to be, in order to effect the nervous system that severely.

Marc, my Ayurvedic doctor, believes that if I change my lifestyle, my diet, way of thinking, habits, etc. that my PD will stabilize and could even start reversing itself. So it is really up to me now. It's a lot more than just taking "mucuna".

They talked about how important it is to meditate, do yoga, respect and appreciate the food you eat, proper breathing exercises, how to live in the present with joy, avoid stress, etc.

I'm just about finished with my cleansing diet now, I'm in my fourth week. I lost 15 pounds, never realized how full I was of it. They also gave me my "Vata/Pita" (my constitution) food program. So it's been a couple of weeks now since I finished my Pancha Karma. Has it been worth it? Definitely, I feel a whole less toxic, my skin is healthy, no longer have cravings for McDonald's or Starbucks. I feel GREAT.

My meds are a lot more effective, last longer, my mind is calmer and I'm enjoying life more. I'm even able to do my morning walk unmedicated now, couldn't do that before. Oh one more thing, Marc is having me take two additional herbs, listed below, to help rebuild my nervous system. He wants me to take it with my mucuna.

Ashwaganda: A well-known rejuvenating tonic used in Ayurveda for stress-induced fatigue, nervous exhaustion and general debility. Strengthens and nourishes both mind and body.

Brahmi: Traditionally used in southern India as a rejuvenate for the nerves and brain. Believed to increase mental clarity, promotes memory and intelligence. It's only been a couple of weeks, but I can already notice improvements in my mental capacity and clarity.

Marc gave me lots of info to read. This is my favorite and it may be the most valuable: How you eat your food is even more important than what you eat. In fact, Ayurveda understands that eating is one of the most sacred experiences we have. After all, when we eat our food, we are taking in the atoms and molecules that have been around in different forms since the beginning of time and asking them to become part of us. If we eat our food properly, with awareness and respect, the food joins well with our bodies. If we do not, the food has difficulty joining with our bodies

causes gas and other digestive disturbances. The end result of poor digestion is ama (toxins formed from bad digestion) and this leads to disease. Hence, in Ayurveda, we try our best to make eating a form of meditation (to eat in peacefulness and with awareness).

This Pancha Karma treatment really wasn't that hard on me. I had to rest and take it easy. No TV was allowed during these 10 days. Marc wanted me to keep my mind, spirit & body calm and relaxed. I meditated, did proper breathing exercises, read calming books, Yoga, peaceful walks in the forest, etc. He even had me do "NO TALKING" a day of silence. It was a very pleasant experience. It has helped me turn to a new page in my life."

Girija Muralidhar's Experience

Just as Max did, I too went through Ayurvedic therapy for PD in 2007, five years after my diagnosis. I felt great after the therapy. I tried to incorporate Ayurvedic principles of life in my daily routine. Sadly, I could not continue with it for very long as my day-to-day activities of modern, urban life took most of my time.

Upon recent enquiry, I learned that Max was also unable to continue with his Ayurvedic regiment for personal reasons.

As of 2013, almost 10 years after my diagnosis, many PD symptoms are slowing me down. I think about various alternate therapies.

I wonder, would PD be different for me, if I had continued with Ayurvedic treatment???

MUCUNA PRURIENS

Mucuna pruriens is a tropical legume grown in many countries, and is commonly known as the velvet bean, or cowhage. It gets its botanical name in part from the severe itch produced by contact with its hairy seed pods. It is widely grown for forage and for fallow fields and as a green manure. The seeds contains high concentrations of levodopa, which is a precursor to dopamine in the brain, and in a powdered form mucuna pruriens has been used in the ayurvedic treatment of Parkinson disease for centuries. It also contains traces of seratonin and nicotine.

MEDITATION • RELAXING MIND AND BODY

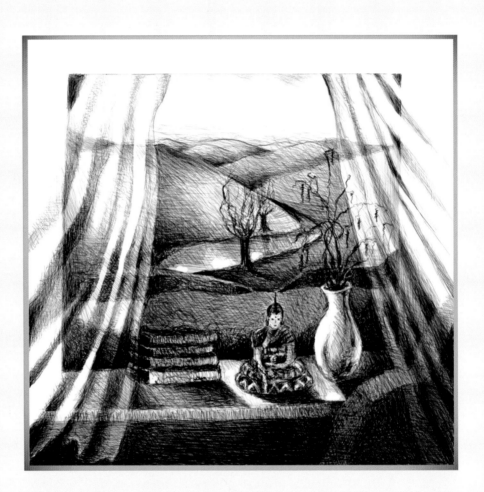

Meditation and Contemplation
Coming to terms with loss of wellness

A diagnosis of long-term illness can create a sense of inner unease that goes beyond the way we feel physically and mentally. It can be a challenge right at the core, where our world view, belief system, trust, hopes and fears lie. With it can come conflicting emotions, thoughts, inner stress. In most faith traditions the supports of the inner self are meditation and contemplation. Increasingly science and medicine are recognizing that these activities can help improve our quality of life. The oldest techniques in the world for finding peace can even be observed on a brain scan!

A simple exercise in contemplation

Make a quiet comfortable space for yourself for a short time. Imagine yourself in a comfy chair by an open window. You can put anything you want into the view you see through the window and anything you wish on the window sill beside you. In your contemplation you can look at the thoughts that rise as you observe your surroundings, the objects beside you, the world beyond the window. You can observe your feelings towards everything in this picture. Your feelings, what things remind you of, why you have chosen the things on the sill, the view, the color of the sky. You can let your thoughts rise, look at them and let them go. Don't engage with them too much, or hold on to them. Just observe the thoughts rising; and let them pass.

You might decide that there is something in this picture that you would like to look at deeper. Do the same with these thoughts. Look at them and observe your reactions to them and let them pass. When you decide to finish your contemplation let everything gently dissolve. Sit for a couple of minutes more before you get back to everyday living.

My picture has a road that leads to a river, just out of sight are friends and family, down by the tree that is somehow related to me. In the vase are willow twigs, which remind me of childhood. The books are my past, I can open them and take a look if I want. There is a tree across the river almost out of sight. A long view of hills. Some of my picture is about difficult things. All of it is about coming to terms with who I am. I can use it to examine difficult thoughts safely in a way that does not cause me stress. It is also about the things that give me strength and the things that bring me joy.

A very simple meditation

Make yourself comfortable, sitting cross legged, or in a chair, or if you are not comfortable sitting, you may lie down. Whichever you choose, ensure that your spine is straight but not tense and that you are relaxed. Let your eyes rest on something a few feet away from you. You can chose something inspiring like a flower, but you do not have to have an object to look at, you can just let your gaze rest in front of you, with your eyes very slightly lowered. Breathe normally, gently and as you do so, focus on your out breath. If a thought arises, don't fight with it, just let it come to the surface and without hanging onto it, let it pass. Observe your thoughts as they come and go, but don't attach to them. A minute or two at first is enough. You will be surprised at how long it will seem! Do this several times a day and gradually extend the time till you are doing about 20 minutes a day. Meditation masters describe the mind as being like a glass of muddy water, if you let it settle the water becomes clear......

Linda Ashford

GETTING MOTIVATED

BE INSPIRED EVERY DAY
The Davis Phinney Foundation

Davis Phinney, an Olympic medal winning cyclist diagnosed with young onset PD, started the **Davis Phinney Foundation for Parkinson's** as a way to promote and fund innovative research and provide programs that improve the quality of day to day living with PD. The Foundation funds research that demonstrates the effect and importance of exercise, speech and other elements that are critical to quality of life. The Foundation states its "mission is to help people living with Parkinson's to live well today."

The Victory Summit® symposia series organized by the Foundation brings together as many as 750 people in local communities for a day of inspiration and learning. In presentations by internationally and nationally recognized researchers, clinicians, and physical therapists, The Victory Summit symposia deliver up-to-date information and practical tools that people with Parkinson can use immediately. The Victory Summit is free to all members of the Parkinson community. Here are some reviews by PwP.

"I was at the DPF Victory Day conference in San Diego in 2011. It was one of the best one-day conferences I attended in a long time. Very informative, excellent speakers, good topics and extremely patient-oriented. I came back feeling good about my ability to do things I can still do, rather than focusing on what I cannot do anymore. I, for sure, need that kind of positive thinking these days!

Davis Phinney was there, among the patients, talking and answering questions about DBS. Check out their website and attend their one-day conference if you can." Girija

"He was the lunchtime speaker at an NPF/APDA YO meeting I went to in Reston a few years ago - 2006, I think. He had us throwing our hands in the air (like a winning cyclist) at every little accomplishment, such as getting out of bed that morning. He told his Tour de France stories, revealing courage and character that were inspiring. To this day, if I successfully navigate steps with no railing, or mail the bills on time, I shout "Another victory!" Davis Phinney believes in celebrating even the little achievements, not necessarily in competition, but sincerely and often." Jaye

BE INTENSE
John Baumann

I am writing a book. The title came from something an elderly neighbor said as I stood by my house, holding a shovel, wearing a new suit and new shoes, trying to decide how to compassionately euthanize a mouse unhappily discovered in our house by my wife. After it occurred to me how ridiculous I looked, I felt the presence of someone staring at me and I locked eyes with an old lady in a rocking chair on her front porch. After a short, understanding exchange, she said something that I will never forget: "If it ain't dead yet, it ain't gonna die."

I often think of this exchange. What it means to me is: whatever happens in your life, you need to realize that "you ain't dead yet."

You are alive. You are a survivor.

A principle I live by is, "Be so intense that you can feel a rush of adrenaline." I have felt the rush of adrenaline more in the last 3 years than ever before in spite of, and maybe because of, my Parkinson. My biggest symptom is fatigue. I have found that while my body is releasing adrenaline, my fatigue is counteracted, or, at least, postponed. I pay for it later, but, for a while, I feel normal again - empowered, strong, full of energy.

Following my first speaking engagement for the Houston Area Parkinson Society, I received a handwritten note saying, "You came, you thrilled, you brought people to tears, you brought people to laughter, but, most of all, you inspired." I was on pure adrenaline during and after this sixty-minute talk before almost 500 attendees. I felt like a faith healer.

I had a hard time, at first, seeing how having Parkinson was for the best. But it is. I am living a much more rewarding and purposeful life now and it all has to do with Parkinson.

Be intense about something, anything. It is what makes life exciting.

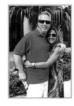

Diagnosed in 2004 at 43, John Baumann left a corporate law department to become a speaker and author.

KEEPING MOTIVATED

Vivian Morgan is an example of how to deal with a Parkinson diagnosis and use it as motivation to improve your health. An active grandmother with 17 grandchildren and 2 great grands, this strong woman, who has survived breast cancer and many other challenges isn't going to let PD get her down.

The early symptoms were non-motor – her mood became uncharacteristically depressed. Then the retired hairdresser noticed her hands cramped, she couldn't do a shampoo massage and there was tremor. When the neurologist told her she had Parkinson, she fell apart briefly. She now thinks it was due to the way the news was delivered. He told her to have her daughter go online to get information, gave Vivian pills but nothing else. That wasn't helpful; so her daughter did find resources online and the local National Parkinson Center for Excellence, where Vivian had a very different experience. Doctors and nurses answered her questions showing her that people can survive with Parkinson. She felt that the staff cared about her. It made all the difference. "The more information I got about PD, the more comfortable I was with it. Getting the information made me feel better."

In addition to medication properly timed for her life, her new doctors suggested exercise. Vivian enrolled in water aerobics and group exercise for PwP – now she's in better shape than ever, works on her balance, is more flexible, has less pain and takes fewer doses of arthritis medicine. Independently, Vivian has chosen to resign from some stressful leadership roles to devote more time to her health.

In all areas of her life, Vivian says she'll do all that she can for as long as she can. She says it happily, after receiving the support and information necessary to live well with the diagnosis.

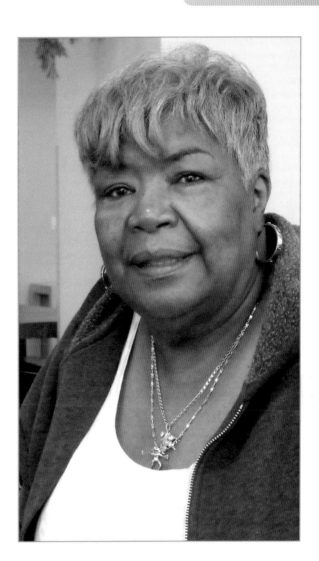

VIVIAN'S ADVICE TO NEW PWP

Vivian's advice to the newly diagnosed:

- Find out everything you can about PD.
- Don't feel that it's a death sentence; it's not.
- Open your mind to different possibilities but don't give up.
- Find a doctor who you can work with.
- Use PD as motivation to do more.
- Exercise - you'll feel better.

POETRY: DISTILLING EMOTION

BLISS

I sit at sea and face the stinging salt.
"Another day in bliss," you'd posted here
When I still saw this illness as my fault.
I shook, and slept, and raged with loss and fear.
I read your words and asked if they were true.
How could they be? I mused in disbelief.
How far I placed myself from your purview.
I never guessed my mind could find relief.
Today I can't recall if you replied
But if I could, I'd thank you even more.
For bit by bit the waves of grief decide
To go their way and leave me to the shore.
I watch my boys who chase white birds around.
In bliss, I note beach roses root, abound.

End Stage
an attempt at haiku

we are long shadows
the mountain will meld into
black at loss of day.

Pam Kell

GDNF
Mind Mist - Cure Kiss -
Dismissed
Misdirection Disinfection
Hope Lost – Great Cost
No Sound – Profound. . . . .

Some mice were
Chewing on an allegory of
The plasticity of time
While playing with elusive
Dream-strands within the mind
About chemicals of passion, sloth,
Curiosity and drive
Mixed, pondered, listed,
Discussed, survived.

And how brains whose complexity -
Patterned from Divine
Conceal strength & purpose,
A true measurement denied
This annoying patients and baffling
Scientists alike
So earnest doctors must tip toe
A labyrinth of land mines

Contemplation waning, was this
Illusion, ruse or muse?
Banquet attendees vanished.
"They'll start to notice, soon"
As the haunting of emptiness
Begins to fill the room.
These words like a ballad waft
In cadence to this tune:

Weevils supped at a table with
Grasshoppers and swine
In chambers owned by flies
Elegantly dressed "to the nines"
A menu of bacon maggots was
Toasted to, with locust wine
And they all said these placebos
Are the best on which to dine.

The following is one person's approach to managing her illness. Remember to always check with your health team before you initiate any new treatment approach.

ONE ALTERNATIVE APPROACH

By Cyndy Gilbertson

I was diagnosed with PD on April 26, 1988, about 24 years ago. At that time, the general consensus in the Parkinson community was that a cure would be discovered within 10 years. But twenty plus years later, we are still waiting for the cure that was supposed to have been found more than ten years ago. Research seems to proceed at a snail's pace as scientists follow stringent methodologies intended to protect us. Their results must insure safety and indicate statistically significant benefits before the FDA will approve a new treatment, which takes time.

As a patient, my perspective is very different from that of the research scientist. I'm looking for something that is going to help now, not in ten years. As a result, I'm willing to take some calculated risks, both financial and physical, in order to try complementary treatments that are outside the standard allopathic framework. My goal is to gain time: an extra hour, day, year or five or 10 until there is a cure.

At the time of my diagnosis, I had an advantage. I was already familiar with alternative medical approaches. I had a working knowledge of basic supplements. I was studying Chinese medicine, Polarity massage and using homeopathic remedies with some success. I sought the most reputable, licensed practitioners in homeopathy, nutrition and acupuncture to complement the services proved by my neurologist.

I surveyed research articles about Parkinson and determined that I would base my approach on the premise that environmental toxins are highly suspect as a causal factor for Parkinson disease.

I concluded that I would:

- avoid further exposure to incriminating toxins
- detoxify the body of accumulated toxins
- rebuild the body with supplements and a healthy diet
- attempt to support and perhaps restore neurons in the substantia nigra

The first thing I did was to make an appointment with a nutritionist.

Based on my knowledge and his recommendations, I began to take an assortment of supplements that included antioxidants and amino acids in the dopaminergic chain.

The second thing I did was to purchase a high quality water filter. I discovered that I had intestinal parasites, so I found a doctor who specialized in that area and followed his recommendations to expel them.

I also located a dentist who specialized in removing mercury amalgams and replaced them with a safer alternative.

I used chelation to help remove heavy metals from my system.

I found an acupuncturist from Beijing who specialized in Parkinson.

There is no way for me to prove what has worked and what hasn't. Perhaps my approach contributed to the fact that I did not require the use of sinemet until 15 years after my diagnosis.

What worked for me may not work for you, but one thing is certain: if you take a chance, you open the possibility for success.

Empower yourself by taking action.

Be responsible for your own health.

And please, without delay, buy yourself a high quality water filter.

PD, Procrastination, & Loss of "Want to......."

There are some inherent symptoms of PD that I don't hear mentioned much, but I believe they are nonetheless real. I have no scientific evidence to back up my theories. I may or may not, get around to investigating resources to substantiate my hypothesis. If, of course, I remember just what it was I wanted to look up.

I also seem to have a "focusing" problem. For example: My eyes may water when watching TV or reading, or they'll be so dry I have to repeatedly use eye drops. I seem to go back & forth, neither condition allowing me proper focus to function well enough to see with clarity much of the time.

Then there's my brain. I can't seem to stay mentally focused either. My mind jumps around like a bee during pollination season, going from topic to topic without purpose.

I cannot seem to complete the simplest of tasks because of interruptions in my mind, or lack of motivation because I can't remember why I started the project anyway. I used to tackle most any task, if I had a manual and/or a schematic. Now I hesitate to tackle anything. I received a "Therapy Controller" from Medtronic for my DBS, and I haven't even put in the battery that came with it.

Desire, motivation, interest, "want to," all add up to the same thing. When the results of an expended effort are worth more than the cost of said effort, one moves into action. However, when the effort required to achieve a goal is greater than the goal once achieved then one starts to think, "what's the point?" The point is that almost everything's more trouble than it's worth, these days.

In conclusion, if I do nothing, I get nothing, but then nothing's expected if I do nothing, so at least I'm not disappointed in the results. However, I strive to push on, by realizing that too long of a hesitation is actually a stop, & too long a stop is actually a regression. It's like paddling a canoe upstream. Your effort, or lack of it, determines your direction.

Just something to ponder that took me two months to complete.
Jimmie "Toad" Cuzler

It's like paddling a canoe upstream: Your effort, or lack of it, determines your direction.

SAILING
Pam Kell

When our sons were three and five and I was pregnant with our daughter, we bought a catamaran. That first summer we sailed every week-end. We packed up kids and food and life jackets and drove three and a half hours every Saturday to the closest lake suitable for sailing. We were on the water from as early as we could manage until the dark drove us out.

As soon as we were free of moorings, both boys would fall asleep and we would sail with only the sound of the wind lufting the sails to disturb the tranquility of the moment. The silence was a welcomed and needed balm for our busy lives. We were in love with sailing.

The next summer our daughter was an infant and fears for her safety kept us from the lake all but a few week-ends when we opted to swallow the prohibitive cost of child care and return to the soothing pleasures of running with the wind.

The following summer we didn't put the boat in the water. It sat, neglected, until it slowly became an eyesore and we junked it, but not the lovely memories.

Several years later we began an annual summer trek to Florida. That first summer, my husband rented a catamaran to try and keep our three teenage and near teenage children occupied. We fell in love again.

Before our next trip south, we bought a catamaran (for approximately the cost of renting one for a week) and towed it down with us. It was our pattern for several years and a wonderful investment.

Of course our children got older and our annual trip ceased and ultimately we gave the boat away.

This summer my husband was taken sailing and was smitten yet again. We began talking about getting another boat. One early October day, we drove to see a boat on a lake some hours from our home. It was larger than we had planned but we were only looking.

The owner took us out and we sailed for three hours in the quiet splendor of a perfect Autumn day on an empty lake. I could feel the stress and worry of my life drain out of me. I was powerless to stop it and all the better for having no power.

When we got back to our car at around 4:00, I realized I had taken no medication since early that morning yet I was moving easily and smoothly. I have been diagnosed for ten years.

I can't guarantee it will work for anyone else, or even if it will continue to work for me, but just for that little while, I felt as if I were cured.

We bought the boat.

GLOBAL HEALING REALLY

After revelations about conflicts of interest in the medical world - it just seemed like the more I became informed, the more grotesque and unbelievable it was.

It was starting to look like everything on which we had based our trust and our feeling of advancement as humanity in the technological age, even the development of civilization through scientific materialism, suddenly seemed horribly undermined by corruption, by bias - cultural, market, and otherwise......

I kind of fled the country feeling overwhelmed with uselessness and a simultaneous serious decline in my own condition - and this was before the economic crisis truly hit. Although I could feel its inevitability in the winds before, because it was starting to look like everything on which we had based our trust and our feeling of advancement as humanity in the technological age, even the development of civilization through scientific materialism, suddenly seemed horribly undermined by corruption, by bias - cultural, market, and otherwise.

Our feeling that we could find wisdom through objective observation, through applied technology, and the sophistication of technique, seemed to add up to nothing when so easily thwarted by dishonesty, clumsy inefficiency and its cover ups.

I looked at my father, who had worked on the world's first computer back in the 50s, and said "What hast thou wrought?"

Just the very revelation that many of the different brand-name products that we buy and are advertised to us are actually all exactly the same thing made by a couple of plants in China, affixed with different labeling and different marketing schemes, was somehow really a disorienting and mind-boggling concept for me.

I feel somewhat different now. Most of that has come from realizing that at my core, I have to determine my own reality. And that thought and intention do determine action and result. And that healing does come from within. I have 'known' that for a long time, but it wasn't until the last few months when, far away from all that I knew and loved, I lay there and thought "Well, who am I really? What would it feel like and who would I be if I was a person who had more than enough serotonin and dopamine in my body? whose sense of life energy was not impeded? After all, energy flows through our universe constantly around us...why shouldn't I have enough to be able to live and walk around and do what I was meant to do?".

I realized that the answers lay nowhere but within myself. Some kind of mysterious process occurred in me after that, where there became some part of my core that could feel and depend on its own strength with a sense of certainty and a determination that I could wield my own strength against whatever it was that was out to vanquish me. It's hard to explain.

A feeling of inner certainty and truth started to become more than an attitude, more of a real experience that I could absolutely rely on.

Some of this I achieved for myself by turning to ancient and traditional wisdom as imparted through my contact with some very special indigenous peoples. This was a very strong experience for me that gave me a sense of continuity beyond the parameters of what we think of as our times. Some was by connecting to the love and good intentions of many people who are still out there, who are sincerely doing their best to do good despite a corrupt system all around them and a world in shambles. That love IS real and there are still good works being done and many people I think have gotten inadvertently caught in a system, that when they stop and deeply examine themselves, they realize has compromised them greatly.

I think this whole process of examination, of profound disillusion, is very necessary for humanity as a whole as part of the process of - at the risk of grandiosity - but global healing really. The transition to a new paradigm that respects our planet and the people on it - all life on it - and realizes that there are more important things we should be cultivating than the ability to consume at a more and more relentless and ultimately heartless pace. I think that's why I have thought of PD as a profound disease and one that is strongly emblematic of our times, because it concerns the very core of life energy in a way. Movement is life.

So what we are confronting physically is the depths of what it means to be alive, to take action, to be real. Our struggles and suffering, I feel, are tremendously important to the world's progress, because our experience can resonate in an exponential way as the rest of the societies around us come to terms with illusion, the limits of how we thought we could define and experience the material world.

I realized that if I was going to live, I needed to change something about myself so that I was not that person who would be sick in that way - I can't find other words for it. But I needed to change, to admit the mistakes of my past, to take responsibility for my actions, to live utterly sincerely and to accept when I feel I have done my best and then trust another power to take care of my destiny.

To discipline myself to think positively, more even-handedly, especially in moments of hysteria and anguish. To humble myself and appreciate everything around me with great intensity and live fully as possible in the present moment. The present moment - that's what we have as our only reality - but paradoxically to balance that with the realization that the seeds of change too are in every present moment and that what we do now will shape and define the reality of the future.

I do feel different than I ever have in my life. My family says I seem totally different than I have ever been in my whole life and I do find that I am more and more easily restructuring my responses to life. I have no doubt that I am in recovery from this disease. On a practical level, it has meant being somewhat protective about my own energy and sharing that - at least for the moment. But also it has meant just accepting that I have to do my own research, trust my own instincts about things and make as informed decisions as I can, based on what I know.

It's quite a journey though and I salute my stalwart and valiant PD knights errant who accompany me, whether I have found you in flesh or spirit. *Fiona*

Who would I be if I was a person who had more than enough serotonin and dopamine in my body? Whose sense of life energy was not impeded? After all, energy flows through our universe constantly around us... Why shouldn't I have enough to be able to live and walk around and do what I was meant to do? And I realized that the answers lay nowhere but within myself.

I think that's why I have thought of PD as a profound disease and one that is strongly emblematic of our times, because it concerns the very core of life energy in a way. Movement is life. So what we are confronting physically is the depths of what it means to be alive, to take action, to be real.

IT CAN GIVE YOU AN OPPORTUNITY FOR PERSONAL GROWTH

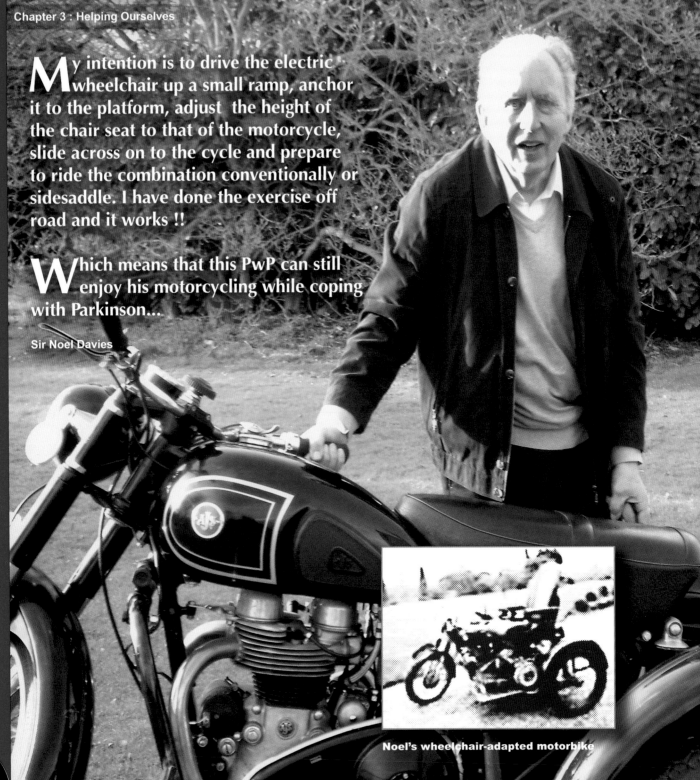

My intention is to drive the electric wheelchair up a small ramp, anchor it to the platform, adjust the height of the chair seat to that of the motorcycle, slide across on to the cycle and prepare to ride the combination conventionally or sidesaddle. I have done the exercise off road and it works !!

Which means that this PwP can still enjoy his motorcycling while coping with Parkinson...

Sir Noel Davies

PD DID NOT MEAN GIVING UP ENJOYMENT

Noel's wheelchair-adapted motorbike

Nan Little, diagnosed with Parkinson disease in 2008, successfully climbed to the summit of Mt. Kilimanjaro in 2011 in a group that included 14 people with either Mulltiple Sclerosis or Parkinson disease. Physically, 11 of the 14 reached the summit.

NAN

Climbing this mountain was the most difficult physical thing I have ever attempted. My husband and I trained for over seven months with packs laden down, climbing thousands of steps and going up and down local mountains, hills in comparison with Kili. Enabling me to even think of making such an effort was the strength I had gained through Pedaling for Parkinson's (an offshoot of Dr. Alberts' research). By biking at high rpms several times each week, I had essentially eliminated my PD symptoms.

Many people have told me that this effort has inspired them to think of themselves differently even though they have PD. I never thought of myself as an athlete, but after being diagnosed with PD, I am stronger than I have ever been. Prior to the climb, my doctor told me I'm probably one of the most physically fit 65 year old women in the United States. It still astonishes me that I'm physically stronger with PD than without it. Cycling changed my life with Parkinson disease.

WENDY S

I did a two day 50 km hike in the mountains awhile back - I was asked to go when I was really going downhill … and had to train like crazy to be able to go - and it let me think of myself as an athlete instead of a patient. I've felt better about everything ever since. I'm very proud that I'm in better shape than a lot of people my age who don't have PD.

NAN

If I, or you, or any of us, can inspire another to take that important step to think of ourselves as more or other than a patient, then our efforts and communications are all worthwhile....

 Already I'm very close to being back to where I was in terms of both health and cognition, only stronger and more determined to share Imad's message that "nothing, not even PD, can rob us of our pride and determination to reach the top."

I hope that you (PwP) realize you climb a mountain higher than Kilimanjaro every day you get up, go to swimming or tai chi or whatever you do to get past your barriers. I trained for months and completed a most challenging task, but the climb, up and down, took one week. You do this every day for your life.

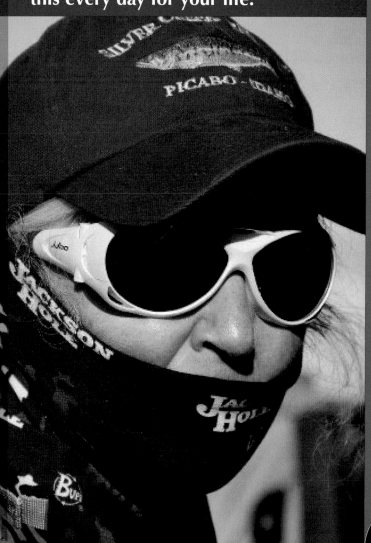

EXPLORE YOUR CREATIVE POTENTIAL

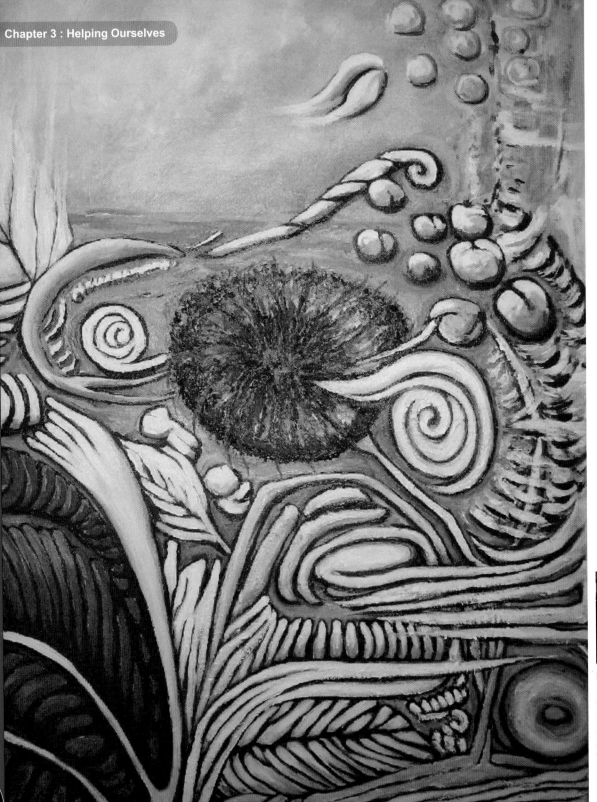

possibilities

Carol McLeod, multimedia artist and co-editor of YOPD e-zine Virtuality.

SING FOR JOY !

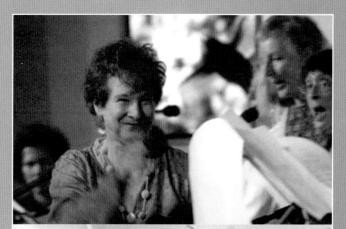

When Nina Temple invited me to work with a group she was setting up for people with Parkinson disease, I was immediately interested. I spent some time at the National Hospital for Neurology, Queen Square with the speech therapist Elina Tripoliti and soon discovered that both the physical and creative aspects of the singer's and vocal facilitator's life, which I knew well, worked wonderfully with some of the symptoms that the group were struggling with.

So, muscle tension and rigidity, shortness of breath, loss of vocal strength and stamina, monotonic speech patterns, imprecise articulation, a closing down of facial expression, low self esteem, tremor in jaw, lips, tongue and body, disturbed swallowing patterns, fatigue; all these symptoms and more seem to be helped considerably by the singing and breath work.

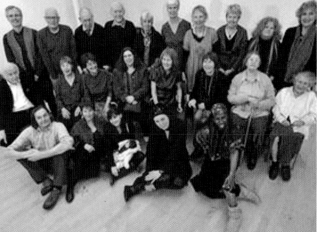

There are no musical criteria for joining the choir. Most of the Sing for Joy members had never before performed in public or even sung in a choir or group. A few people had sung with amateur choirs, but most had not sung since school days.

At the beginning of each weekly session, whether rehearsing or not, we work with a warm-up using breath for respiratory support, resonance, vocal pitch practice, harmony and rhythm, singing loud and soft and in between, muscle exercises for the mouth and the face, all put together with a gentle physical movement. These skills have clearly helped in soothing some symptoms and building vocal strength and breath control.

We have found that you can live a fuller and more valued and pleasurable life as a disabled person if you have friends, community, music and a purpose, than if you are able-bodied but living a lonely, driven and essentially meaningless life.

We can name four essential qualities which people gain from the choir and its practices:

1) relaxation, or release of a variety of stresses and tensions.
2) gain in vitality, including feeling a wider range of emotions.
3) companionship – freedom from the paralysing and silencing isolation of illness, an experience of having things in common, of other people looking out for you, of not being judged but just accepted.
4) a sense of purpose, structure and routine.

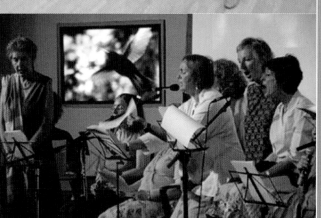

Sing for Joy as a structure and a group of people has its own problems; it is a work in progress. But a common work in progress is, I think, the best that humans can aspire to. Carol Grimes

WHAT'S SO FUNNY ABOUT PD? I'LL TELL YOU!

I'm Mark Solomon. I've been a TV Writer/Producer for over 25 years, which means I'm pushing 30!

I've written and/or produced scripts for such hit shows as "ALICE," "GRACE UNDER FIRE," "DIAGNOSIS: MURDER," and "NEWHART." I was nominated for an EMMY Award for writing the now famous Last Episode of "NEWHART." I lost out to an episode of 'THE WONDER YEARS" about the death of a teacher. The category was "Outstanding COMEDY writing!" Go figure.

I live in Ojai, CA with my wife, Cary, three birds and a smelly (but affectionate) dog.

About 4 years ago, I found out I had Parkinson disease. I'm still at a very early stage, though I do have tremors in my right arm and leg. Like Michael J. Fox, I tried to hide it. I sucked at it! People could tell something was wrong with me.

I'm also a singer/songwriter. I noticed that my vocal chords felt tighter and I couldn't hit those falsetto notes. So much for singing along to the Bee Gees! I was also having difficulty playing the piano and guitar. Especially the guitar. I'd be playing along at a nice clip, the song would be over and my right hand would still be strumming! ARRGGGHHH!!! Frustrating to say the least. Cary told me not to get discouraged. Keep practicing! Easy for her to say. She then suggested that maybe I should write a new song!

About what!?

She said "How about Parkinson's".

WHAT!? I'm a comedy writer and that's way too depressing! She said it didn't have to be a sad song. Make it funny! I was ready to have her fitted for a straightjacket, then I thought "Hmmm… she might be on to something!"

I picked up my guitar and started playing a few chords… poorly.

I pushed onward. After a few minutes I came up with a cute hook for the chorus. Suddenly, the words and the melody started to fall into place! VOILA! Within a half hour I had the song!

Then I started to worry. I just wrote a jaunty little number about a DISEASE! What was I thinking!? So I played it for Cary. She said it worked! WHEW! I then played it for a musician friend of mine, Sean Fullerton, over the phone. He said he loved it, but the guitar playing stunk! Sean can be brutally honest, damn him! He said he would record a new guitar track and send it to me over the internet and I could record the vocal track to it on my Mac computer. I said, "Wow, thanks! And while you're at it, could you also add piano, drums, bass and organ tracks to it as well?" I tend to push the limits of my friendships! Sean, however, being the pussycat that he is, agreed! Three months later, after recording about 500 versions of the song, we finally did one version we were both happy with!

The reaction to the song has been amazing! Recently, I have been performing the song at various PD symposiums here in California. Some people laugh, some cry, some tap their feet (That could be a side effect from the Mirapex!) At a recent event, I decided to auction off a CD of the song for charity. I started the bidding at $36,000! Okay, I admit that might've been a teensy bit high! I had no takers, so I lowered it to $10. About twenty hands went up! $15! More hands went up! $20! Even more hands! Yikes!

Suddenly a woman in the back of the room yelled out "$500!" Heads turned to see who this crazy lady was!

"SOLD!" I quickly screamed! I ran over to her and asked her "why?" She could've downloaded it on Amazon for 99 cents! She smiled at me and said the song was so uplifting, she wanted to give it to her brother who happens to have PD. She wanted to see him smile again. I started to get choked up… in a good way! I kissed her and quickly grabbed the check before she changed her mind!

Anyone who has PD or knows someone who has it or can spell "PD" will identify with the song. Thanks to his daughter May May, Muhammad Ali heard the song one Thanksgiving and his response was "Nice!" That was one of the highlights of my life!

It's a very uplifting song about a terrible condition. Very few diseases have their own theme song! I think I've cornered the market!

"THE PD SONG" is now available for download on Amazon mp3, iTunes, CDBaby, and Rhapsody. It can also be downloaded from my web page www.markssolomon.com.

All proceeds from each download will be donated to the Michael J. Fox Foundation

Photo: Cary and Mark

AND A WAY OF RAISING FUNDS FOR PD RESEARCH......

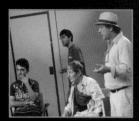

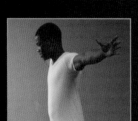

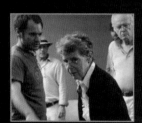

Filmmaker Faizan Uzma inspires others through his film and PD testimonial project, both named "My Angel My Hero".

Paula Wittekind, PwP with advanced PD, was the focus of his "Pool Party with Parkinson's" (water exercise helps, see https://www.youtube.com/watch?v=lXIBRzlh6Uw).

See more at his website, www.myangelmyhero.com

My Angel My Hero

Faizan works more than 12 hours a day at Wall Street but today, it is only mid-morning on Tuesday, as he unlocks the door to his apartment. He enters quietly and sits on a sofa. He is in deep thought about how to unlock his own future having just been laid off from job. However, he is not as distressed as one might expect, as he feels God has a greater work for him to do.

After lengthy contemplation and much later that evening, he nervously asks his parents about beginning work on his passion; something he truly loves – making films. His parents may call him an entertainer, a story teller, a dancer, an actor or even a film maker but they truly know him as a dreamer; a man who believes dream is the foundation of everything. He reminds them that his dream was to begin by making his first film.

Now, two and one half years later, he has done just that! He has fulfilled his dream with the completion of his 'ambitious' first project; a project about hope, love and how to prosper even in hard times.

His film "**My Angel My Hero**", entertains through its dance sequences while conveying a strong message; How dance helps people with Parkinson. This disease is such a dire one that a patient struggles each and every day with even the simplest of tasks. And Faizan recalls how he struggled each day of these past two and a half years; a struggle to change the thinking of the world. It was a struggle to tell the world what art and love can bring forth. A struggle to convince everyone around him, that this project is not only important to him, but to millions of those who suffer, everyday, with this disease.

CHECK OUT FAIZANS PD PROJECT....

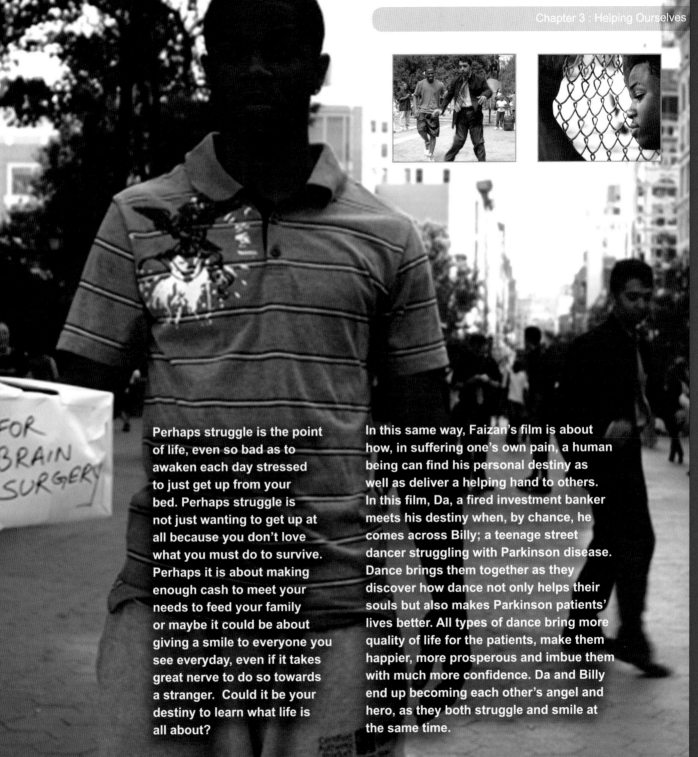

.....AND LOOK OUT FOR HIS FILM.

FOR BRAIN SURGERY

Perhaps struggle is the point of life, even so bad as to awaken each day stressed to just get up from your bed. Perhaps struggle is not just wanting to get up at all because you don't love what you must do to survive. Perhaps it is about making enough cash to meet your needs to feed your family or maybe it could be about giving a smile to everyone you see everyday, even if it takes great nerve to do so towards a stranger. Could it be your destiny to learn what life is all about?

In this same way, Faizan's film is about how, in suffering one's own pain, a human being can find his personal destiny as well as deliver a helping hand to others. In this film, Da, a fired investment banker meets his destiny when, by chance, he comes across Billy; a teenage street dancer struggling with Parkinson disease. Dance brings them together as they discover how dance not only helps their souls but also makes Parkinson patients' lives better. All types of dance bring more quality of life for the patients, make them happier, more prosperous and imbue them with much more confidence. Da and Billy end up becoming each other's angel and hero, as they both struggle and smile at the same time.

SERVICE DOGS & PD
A Decade Of Tilting At Windmills

Over ten years ago I embarked upon a most enlightening voyage. My omnipresent companion Parkinson disease had settled quite nicely into my life. It was enjoying the shakiness, off balance and general upheaval it could create.

I had seen and read about 'service' or 'assistance' dogs and the positive impact they bestow. My neurologist had reservations; he thought a dog would interfere with my gait and cause more problems than benefits with my walking. He did, however, consent to my getting one and in October 1999 the call came, and I went to train with MY dog.

There were five of us in the training group. MY dog burst out of the door like a bronco in the rodeo! Leaping, airborne, twisting, bounding, alive and wild in this freedom! Over the next two weeks, with many mishaps/mishandlings and laughs, Squire and I became a cohesive unit.

Some of the dogs were 'puppy raised', others pound rescues. In our group, Squire and Lucky were the pound rescues. Riding in the van to go to the mall, the three 'puppy raised' dogs looked around casually and gawked out the windows. The two reformed felon's with ears, lifted and heads swivelling, checked the parking lot and entries for cigarette butts with a few puffs left on them to save for later. While hanging out by the dumpster they could smoke, and tell the goody four paws about life in the joint.

On Graduation Day we received the certificate proclaiming Squire and me a certifie Team. During the ride home I took the ribbon off and unrolled Our certificate.....?!?!?.....it was a blank piece of paper! I called the training center the next day and I was told it would be mailed, as some dogs in the past were over-zealous and had eaten the diplomas.

This dog continues to amaze me. When we got home He wasn't trained to break freezes. How was I to train Him for that? No need. When we stopped to talk to a curious passersby, after a couple of minutes, He would begin to paw my leg. I soon realized that by pawing my leg when I stopped He was breaking any forming freeze. Then He began to teach me! Much to my distress while driving He would at times reach between the seats from the back and paw my shoulder. I'd tell Him to quit but He wouldn't listen. He kept pawing until finally I began to pay attention. Shortly before I could tell my meds were waning, Squire would start the pawing, like a seizure dog who can sense changes in the brain and alert his owner of the on-coming

seizure. Did Squire sense the chemical changes in my brain and alert me to stop driving? I don't know for certain; I'm not a scientist or professional trainer, but experiencing this 'cause and effect' is good enough for me.

Along with the 'pluses' of Squire picking up dropped objects, 'fetching' items for me, having Him also has kept my voice going. Living alone you don't have much conversation, Squire has seen to that. It is hard to be a couch potato when the dog HAS to go out. More importantly, He has taught me about unconditional love and devotion, that life has many twists and turns and if given a chance, people and dogs can change.

He has also taught me that if I don't let go of the retractable leash, a 75 pound dog can generate enough speed and force to pull a 225 pound man off his feet and if I do fall, I'll have a furry face peering down at me, head tilted, with a "why'd you do that" look on it. I also swear He's developed the ability to snicker on these occasions.

Over time my gait has gotten worse, Squire has adapted to that too. One winter day I fell in the road on the ice and snow. When I landed I heard a whoosh beside me. There, tucked under my armpit, Squire lay giving me a dirty, surprised look. Fortunately we were both ok. It was shortly after that He began to step from my side to in front of me at the most inopportune times. I grumbled for Him to stop and heel. I was having trouble walking and I thought He was going to cause me to fall but, in fact, He was preventing my gait becoming a head long dash into trouble.

It hasn't all been serious though. Soon after I got Squire, I was in a super market when a friend I graduated high school with saw us and came over to say, 'Hi'. He was behind me and said, "Hi Al, it's me, Rick." I said, "Hi" and added, "I know who you are". He said, "I saw the dog, and thought you might have trouble with your eyes." I said, "Oh, the dog - I'm not blind, I'm deaf!" His voice from behind me said, "I'm sorry I didn't know." After a chuckle I explained about Parkinson and how the dog helped my balance.

Another time, in the drug store, a young lad asked quietly, "Gramma, why does that man have a dog in the store?" Not bothering to lower her voice, she told him and the whole store, "That man is blind, the dog helps him to walk around, and not bump into things". At the checkout they were in line behind me. They were just leaving the

If you happen upon a service dog team, please ask the person if it is OK to pet the dog. 99% of the time it will be fine. We're glad to talk (brag) about our dogs. By asking, you can be sure you're not interfering with any work the dog may be doing at that time. Plus, it makes us pretty proud: you're respecting our dog and the jobs they do so well.

store as I drove by them - through the car window I heard, "Gramma, how does that blind man drive the car? Does the dog help with that too?". I looked at Squire and said, "let her explain THAT one!".

Windmills were used in lowlands as a source of power to turn the wheels to grind the grains. As a cure for Parkinson disease still hasn't been found, as our brain cells still die off, the Parkinson windmill still grinds on.

In Massachusetts, Seeing Eye Dogs and Dogs for the Deaf were exempt from the licence fees. We were told the town or city clerk could waive the fee for our Service Dogs. My town clerk of course wouldn't. That would be against the law he told me - so after a trip to my State Senator's office, and a call to my State Representative, we submitted a bill to amend the law to include any dog trained to assist a handicapped person. Four and a half years later the Governor signed it into law.

Parkinson disease softens and steals our voices, trying to rob us of the ability to speak for ourselves. This is why we must speak up now and advocate for research, for funding, for a cure, for ourselves and those who follow, else we are left to the whims and fancies of others. Change comes, it might take time but it does come. It just needs someone to step up and start it in motion. Everyone reading this can do that.
Alan Labendz

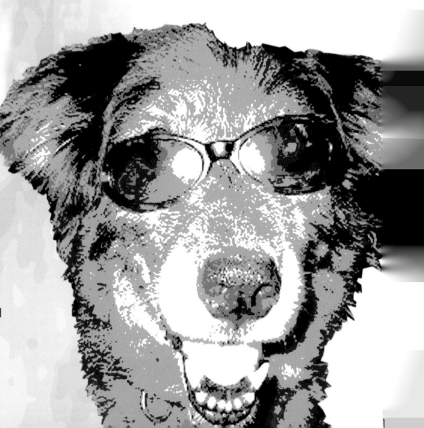

TOP TEN NUTRITION TIPS FOR PEOPLE WITH PARKINSON DISEASE

FISH - Did you know that 20% of the gray matter of the brain is composed of DHA, found in fatty fish? Especially fatty fish, like salmon, sardines, herring, anchovies, and halibut. They contain the omega-3 fatty acids EPA & DHA, which protect against dementia and depression. Some evidence suggests a high intake of fish (and omega-3 fatty acid) is associated with a lower risk of developing PD, and may even be neuroprotective.

TEA - Black, green, white, and oolong teas contain substances called "polyphenols" which appear to protect against Parkinson and Alzheimer disease, and may also help reduce or prevent PD symptoms.

NUTS - Rich in all the forms of vitamin E, as well as fiber - good enough reasons by themselves to eat nuts. One study indicated that foods high in vitamin E (but not supplements) seem to protect against PD. But there's more - nuts are a storehouse of hard-to-find trace minerals like selenium, which works together with vitamin E as an antioxidant.

BEANS - Dried beans of all kinds are not only rich in protein, they are among the foods with the very highest sources of fiber, helping to prevent constipation, which frequently occurs in folks with PD. Besides this, they contain B vitamins and magnesium, important to the nervous system.

HONEY - Folks with PD often develop a 'sweet tooth.' If so, choose honey over sugar every day. Sugar has no nutritional value, whereas honey contains as much antioxidants as some fruits, along with trace minerals. It's even used in wound healing.

BERRIES, CHERRIES - PD is a stressful disease, and stress produces free radicals; antioxidants destroy free radicals. Cherries may be better free-radical scavengers than vitamin E. Blueberries may protect against dementia; cranberries are remarkably high in antioxidants and help protect against urinary tract infections; blackberries, raspberries, strawberries, all are rich sources of powerful and protective phytonutrients.

TURMERIC - Contains a substance, curcumin, that is used medicinally to prevent and/or treat diabetes, heart disease, cancer and liver damage; it is currently being investigated as a possible treatment for PD.

GINGER - Helps with the nausea that often occurs when starting PD medications; also helps speed stomach emptying, for those with gastroparesis.

FLAX SEED, GROUND - Very high in two kinds of fiber. One helps control blood sugar, the other keeps the stool soft and bulky, which relieves constipation.

VITAMIN D - Studies have shown widespread deficiency of vitamin D among folks with PD; whether it contributes to the development of PD is not yet known. But deficiency is associated with falls and fractures, diabetes, cancers and autoimmune diseases. It is strongly recommended that people with PD have vitamin D levels checked and take supplements if needed. Foods rich in vitamin D include fatty fish such as salmon, mackerel and tuna; egg yolks; beef liver; and sardines.

 Kathrynne Holden is a nutritionist who specializes in the science of nutrition for PD. She moderates the email forum "Ask about Nutrition" at www.parkinson.org. Her books, **Eat Well, Stay Well with Parkinson's Disease**, **Cook Well, Stay Well with Parkinson's Disease**, and CD **Parkinson's Disease and Constipation**, are the first to provide practical answers to PD-related concerns such as levodopa and protein, constipation, swallowing difficulty, and unplanned weight loss.

EATING WELL IS VITAL FOR PWP

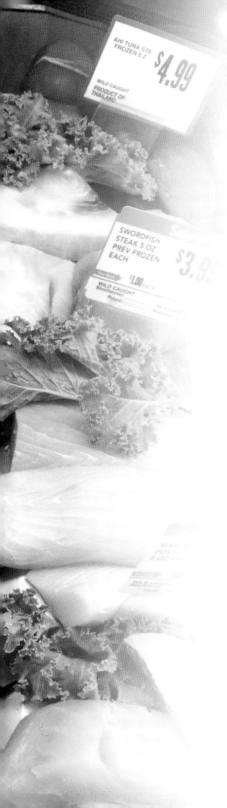

DIET, NUTRITION AND FOOD

Does what, how and when you eat affect your Parkinson symptoms? Most doctors and researchers would say "yes" on the issue of protein interfering with l-dopa absorption.

There are theories on how food and nutrition may interact with PD including low blood sugar, the timing of taking medicine balanced with the type and amount of food you eat. Some suggest: high fat diets, fasting, brain healthy food, supplements and antioxidants, while others say nothing you eat will cross the blood brain barrier. Current research in neurological conditions seems to promote healthy eating to enhance brain health.

So how to begin? You might consider investigating an approach that appeals to you. That doesn't mean that you can experiment blindly without consequences. Before beginning any change in your diet, do your research. PubMED online or your local public library or an interlibrary loan program are good places to start. And again, please consult with your physician.

You can find resources and information to evaluate on NeuroTalk and other reputable web sources. In a 2009 thread titled 'Parkinson's disease - the importance of nutritional management' - people described books by Lucille Leader and her anesthesiologist husband who run a PD clinic in London.

Rick Everett, one of the most thorough citizen scientists on NeuroTalk, said the Leaders, "have written some of the best books on PD that I have found".

Look for **Parkinson's Disease: Reducing Symptoms with Nutrition and Drugs,** Denor Press; 2nd Revised edition (January 1, 2009) by Geoff Leader, Lucille Leader and Leslie Findley. This book presents much science and nutrition information and detailed ways to test your body's reaction to your PD medications so that you can fine-tune your timing of drugs and food for optimal results.

If your approach to nutrition and PD takes the direct route to your stomach, look for **Take Charge of Parkinson's Disease: Dynamic Lifestyle Changes to Put You in the Driver's Seat** by professional chef, Anne Cutter Mikkelsen, written with Carolyn Stinson. It contains brain healthy recipes rich in nutrients and antioxidants and low in inflammatories that also appeal to PwP who may be losing the ability to taste food. The book also provides positive encouragement for carers and PwP by telling the personal stories of the family's life (Anne's husband Mike has PD).

Visit the **Parkinson Disease Foundation's Resource Section http://www.pdf. org/en/resourcelink/category/Nutrition** where you'll find thirteen listings under "Nutrition." It includes free pamphlets, programs and information about finding a consulting dietitian, or use National Parkinson's Foundation, **"Ask the Dietitian"** forum where questions asked anonymously are answered by Kathrynne Holden, a registered dietitian.

Personally, I've found my most interesting, useful diet, supplement and nutrition information on NeuroTalk posts. Being an empowered patient means taking the time and effort to read the supporting journal articles. Thank you to all the citizen scientists who have helped me on this journey called PD.
Katherine Huseman

MAINTAINING GOOD GENERAL HEALTH IS ESSENTIAL

CREATIVE SOLUTIONS

Few products for people with medical conditions are inspiring or even interesting, even when they are helpful or useful. Good design, plenty of imagination, and a vision for a great product, can make a big difference to the life of someone who would rather not be limited by PD. Here are a few of the better ideas we have seen:

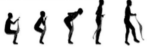

FLO
Fed up of getting stuck.....

Being unable to get up from an armchair easily is something that can be embarassing and stressful on our bodies too.

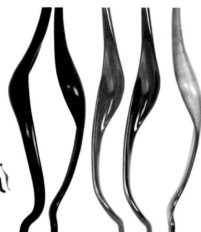

Flo is an ergonomic standing and walking aid that addresses this problem with its curvy lines that support you as you rise from your chair. While is is quite pricey its sculptural lines are functional and it is made of carbon fibre giving it extra strength.

MAKING LIFE EASIER

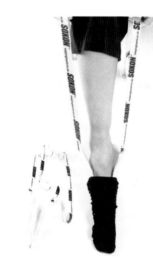

SOXON
Even small tasks can feel huge

Soxon is simply the best and kindest of the gadgets to help people with the task of getting their socks on. Many of us have this difficulty and it can be the first difficulty for which we ask for help.

Soxon will put this off for a while and help us maintain independence. Unlike similar devices which are usually made of plastic, it is made of soft washable fabric on a flexible frame with two sturdy long tape handles, and will not scrape your legs or damage socks or tights.

Check the internet to find more details about these aids.

THE COUNTRY FLYER
Could it keep you moving?

NeuroTalk's Max19BC, a Canadian with Parkinson disease, surprised fellow forum members with The Country Flyer recently.

This amazing machine, designed by Max Lafontaine, has gone through several revisions as he brings it to mobility perfection, in the quest for a truly patient designed mobility device that will improve mobility and help those with walking difficulties enjoy the freedom to get out and about. The Country Flyer can be used as a traditional walker offering a high level of support, but also provides an adjustable seat that allows the user a more proactive means to exercise. In addition the seat can also be used as a body support to walk, helping those with weak legs or impaired walking ability, giving the user a flexible 3-way aid to better mobility indoors and out, on a variety of surfaces.

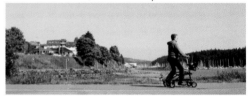

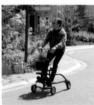

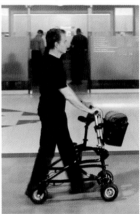

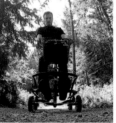

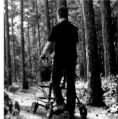

HOW TO BE A PARTICIPATORY PATIENT

The author is a Canadian health educator and reformer. She developed these guidelines for herself after a doctor speaking in medical terminology gave her a diagnosis that she interpreted as terminal cancer when in fact she had the "best" type.

MY 8 POINTS OF PARTICIPATORY MEDICINE

1. I want to learn about my health issue(s).

I feel I have sufficient skills and capabilities to be participatory. I understand that, along with the learning and empowerment process, come stresses, disappointments, irritation, frustration, and exhaustion.

2. When I don't understand something, I ask for an explanation.

In the doctor's office, I seek strategies to improve meaningful communication, and ask that jargon be written down so I can do my own research. Before a doctor's appointment, if I'm fearful, I research my symptoms and conditions to the best of my abilities, and bring my questions with me.

3. I've learned to do my own research.
Using a combination of keyword searches, seeking out communities of interest online, talking things through within my communities, real and virtual, and, when the appointment comes, consultation with my primary care physician and/or another appropriate healthcare professional (eg, chiropractor, pharmacist, or occupational therapist). If I'm referred to a specialist, I repeat the above process.

4. I get copies of any and all laboratory reports.

I likely will not understand much of what is in the report, so when reading something that worries me, I try to keep the anxiety at bay until I go over the results with my primary care physician. Waiting until the doctor's appointment can be stressful, but I consider it an opportunity to learn something about my body, and to learn what to watch for in the next report. Where electronic health records (EHRs) allow, I ask that my comments be noted in my health records.

5. I do my part.

I maintain a healthy lifestyle, and try to do all the "right things." If I have issues (eg, with various meds or side effects) I move quickly to try to get them sorted out and to resolve them. I'm willing to accept help. I make sure to keep my primary care physician in the loop, and ensure that my comments are incorporated into the EHR.

6. Sometimes I don't do, sometimes I can't do.

I make choices that aren't/may not be in the best interests of my overall health. I accept responsibility for these choices and expect them to be respected. I accept that when I'm not feeling well enough, I can't be as actively participatory.

7. My health care team.

I try to establish rapport with my team of health care professionals, establishing a relationship that is mutually respectful and provides me with the best possible care, as well as caring. I recognize that trust is gained over time. I rely upon my health care professionals because of their training, knowledge, and perspective. My communities, real-life and virtual, are also part of my health care team.

8. I trust in myself, and to the extent possible, in my ability to make good decisions about my health care.

©2011 Kathy Kastner

BEING PROACTIVE IN YOUR HEALTH CHOICES

TOP TIPS FOR SURVIVAL

TOM ISAACS
Co-founder and President
The Cure Parkinson's Trust

1) **ENGAGE WITH YOUR PARKINSON**
Understand it, study it. There has been research which shows those people who get involved and who face up proactively to their condition have a far better quality of life than those who don't.

2) **BE SELF-AWARE**
Monitor your own physical symptoms as much as you can.

3) **LISTEN TO YOUR BODY**
When it tells you to rest - rest, when it tells you to go home - go home. I do not practice what I preach.

4) **NEVER...**
sit on the left hand side of someone with a broken left arm on a train when you have bad dyskinesia in your right arm.
They don't like it!!

5) **TRY TO SEE THE SAME PERSON...**
each time you visit your doctor, neurologist or geriatrician. Strike up a rapport with them. Some of them are quite nice.

6) **SLEEP...**
is fundamentally important to overall quality of life. For some people it is impossible to sleep without medication but for me I have found that sleep without the use of medication seems to give the brain a break and makes me better in the mornings.

7) **BE OPTIMISTIC**
We are cracking this thing. Massive progress is being made. We need to hang in there and soon our hope of new therapies will convert to belief.

8) **IN THE BAD MOMENTS**
Always remember that tomorrow will be better.

9) **EXERCISE, EXERCISE, EXERCISE.**

10) **HAVING SAID EXERCISE, THERE ARE EXCEPTIONS TO THIS RULE...**
for instance, if you do not want to be the subject of ridicule, don't, under any circumstances, enter an egg and spoon race - you will lose.

11) **TAKE YOUR PILLS ON TIME...**
or when you need them and always take them with plenty of water; otherwise they don't work.

12) **KEEP MENTALLY ACTIVE**

13) **COMMUNICATE...**
tell people how you feel and don't keep things bottled up. People with Parkinson are like fizzy drinks, they are best when they're opened up quickly but leave them too long to fester and they are likely to lose their sparkle.

14) **TRY TO LOOK AT THINGS FROM THE POINT OF VIEW OF THOSE AROUND YOU**
You are not the only one who is affected by Parkinson - in fact others around you may be affected by your Parkinson even more than you are.

15) **BE UP-FRONT ABOUT YOUR PARKINSON**
Spread awareness. I have become so upfront about having Parkinson that I have been known to tell people when I am first introduced to them and then those same people tend to call me Parkinson for the rest of the evening because they think it's my name. So on second thought, don't be that up-front about Parkinson.

16) **KEEP PROPERLY HYDRATED...**
and do not drink much alcohol.

MANAGING YOUR PD

17) AVOID EATING LATE...
and try to eat easily digestible foods.
Also avoid too much protein during the day
if you are taking l-dopa - have your main
protein meal at night.

18) PAY GREAT ATTENTION TO YOUR DIET
You are what you eat. Diet is more
important than our medication.

**19) KEEP YOUR GUT IN GOOD
WORKING ORDER**
Keeping regular is crucial.

**20) AH YES, AN IMPORTANT ONE THIS.
DON'T GO TO A FINE ART AUCTION.**
There is no more dangerous place for PwP.

21) TAKE REGULAR MASSAGE
It does wonders for releasing all that
tension and stress.

22) NEVER ACT WEIRDLY AS A JOKE
People will think you are genuinely
weird. There is no benefit of the doubt in
Parkinson. I am all too often a victim of
this particular mistake.

23) IF FINANCIAL HARDSHIP STRIKES YOU
Burglary is not the answer. To be a
successful burglar, you need to have stealth
and with Parkinson it is nigh on impossible.

**24) IF YOU ARE EXPERIENCING SEVERE
'ON' 'OFF' FLUCTUATIONS....**
as I do, it is a good idea to try to
"compart-mentalise" your life.

Almost make yourself into two people so
that one's misery does not impact on the
other's joy of living.

25) FINALLY, TEAMWORK
Don't be afraid to use all the services
out there that are available.

PWP LIVING WITH PD

When you speak to others about what it's like to live with Parkinson, you may need examples beyond your own experience.

Here are some that Peggy Willocks received from PwP on NeuroTalk.

It's like drowning. You sink beneath the dark water with fear and despair. You bob up into the sunshine with exhilaration and hope. Over and over every day.
Rick Everett

It's like being on vacation without an itinerary. Never knowing what the next day [or hour] will bring.

Dyskinesia is like being a clown in a side show. One provides entertainment of everyone around. .. It can eliminate the need for a diet.because we lose weight without one.

PD allows me to test my ability to pick things up off the floor, since I spend so much time putting things there...aka dropping things due to clumsiness.
Carolyn Stephenson

PD is like old age. You no more say "Get well" to people with PD than you say "Get Young" to old people.
BEMM

PD is a fresh challenge every day. You have to win every time by telling yourself you are improving. Where else can you have such an exciting daily challenge!!
Ron Hutton

I try to see the "blessings" behind having PD. It truly does help me keep my priorities in order.

I have tremendous faith that I was given this disease for a reason ... look at how many people's lives I'll be able to impact between now and then.
Proudest Mama

What I find is the most difficult aspect of PD... struggling to live in the moment and not to project.

I work hard to enjoy and celebrate everything I can do today, and to avoid thinking about the things that may become impossible down the road.

PD is a road you want to cruise not race down.
Sheryl Jedlinski

Taking family, work and the rest of your life into account

In spite of all her research, she was continually surprised that PD affected so many different parts of life. After a few years, she could no longer work at her job and had to apply for disability. Leaving work felt like losing a part of her identity.

Family and friends tried to understand, but she worried about them and they did the same. The question was: how could she live as well as she could, with the reality of PD, 24/7?

She read, talked to others and created a new life. She discovered you could choose your reactions to PD, even if you couldn't choose the outcome.

In this chapter you will find how we have learned to live differently with PD and improve our quality of life.

If you're as strong as those living with PD, read on.

CHAPTER FOUR

Quality of life

Pretend you are the doc. The PwP are your patients. They take the drugs, they follow the science. But also they make use of art and exercise, in this case dance and music....

And it all becomes more liveable; and the condition their condition is in will be visibly improved.

Science and art/spirit/hope/beauty are all needed.

Bob Dawson

CHAPTER FOUR

Quality of Life is all of those things that make getting up in the morning preferable to staying in bed. It is the result we hope for when we take hands full of medication several times a day. It is the essential ingredient in our appreciation of family, friends, nature, beauty and faith.

Quality of Life is different for each of us and is made up of what is to us, individually, most important. While we cannot define it for one another, there are some factors that most of us agree diminish our Quality of Life.

"**Quality of life is the degree to which a person enjoys the important possibilities of his or her life.**"

QUALITY OF LIFE

Tom Isaacs

Parkinson disease is a journey and like all journeys it is not about the destination, but about how you get there. Quality of life (QoL) with Parkinson disease varies depending on where you live and who you are. It is all very well to say, as I will later, that attitude is everything, but if you are stuck in a fine art auction room with uncontrollable tremor, a good attitude will not help you. Although stated lightly here, this point is a serious one; QoL varies from country to country and from situation to situation to an alarming degree. Quality of life varies depending on where you live and who you are.

Symptoms and QoL

I was diagnosed at 27 years of age.
• I have been frozen-rigid to the spot in the middle of a busy street.
• I have had flamboyant dyskinesias that have led to taxi-drivers thinking I am either drunk or deranged and refusing to pick me up.
• I can have long, hot and sweaty sessions of bat-wing tremor while the pills kick-in or wear off, and when the muscle spasms are so painful, all anyone can do is scream for help.

The psychological effect that the diagnosis of Parkinson disease has in the early years, the more recent lack of sleep, the inability to organise oneself, and periods of obsessive behaviour, are all real problems that many people with Parkinson disease encounter.

The combination of these problems would, one may expect, have a profound and negative effect on my QoL during the last 15 years since my diagnosis. And yet, it may surprise the reader to learn that my perception is that my QoL is currently better than it was 15 years ago – indeed it is probably better than it has ever been.

Perceptions of QoL

So how could 15 years of Parkinson disease have improved somebody's QoL? One person's perception of QoL is likely to be entirely different to another person's. When I think of QoL, I think of traveling, enjoying my work, playing golf, seeing friends and sharing good-times with my wife. In general, I measure my own QoL in terms of a sense of fulfilment or a sense of worth in what I am doing.

Undoubtedly the best definition I have found is by researchers at the University of Toronto's Quality of Life Research Unit, who say, "Quality of life is the degree to which a person enjoys the important possibilities of his or her life". Their Quality of Life Model is based around the categories '**being**', '**belonging**', and '**becoming**' – in other words, who one is, how one is connected to one's environment, and whether one achieves one's personal goals, hopes, and as-pirations, respectively. The three different values of who I am, how I interact with the world and my sense of what the future holds define my attitude to living.

There is a lovely saying, "The greater part of our happiness or misery depends on our dispositions, and not our circumstances" (Martha Washington, 1731-1802). The severity of my Parkinson disease symptoms can be shocking to those not used to them, and yet my perception of my life and QoL is probably as positive as anybody reading this article.

My positive perception can be explained if we return to the concept of '**being**', '**belonging**', and '**becoming**'. After 15 years of living with Parkinson disease, I have got used to the idea and have become accustomed to the symptoms. The negative effects of these symptoms have been offset by immersing myself in the business of Parkinson disease. Before I had the condition, the only purpose of my day-to-day work was to make money for already wealthy people - now I have a far greater sense of fulfilment in my working life, which in turn gives me a greater sense of identity and greater belief and commitment in everything I do. Therefore, despite living with an incurable degenerative and highly disabling movement disorder for 15 years, I feel good about who I am (about '**being**').

Parkinson disease is an isolating disease with an associated stigma. People with Parkinson disease get stared at and are treated differently as a result of this pronounced movement disorder. This is not an enjoyable experience, but I have overcome the feelings of isolation by engaging myself in all things related to Parkinson disease. By working in the world of Parkinson disease I am not ostracised. More than this, the Parkinson disease community embraces me as one of its own and it is a place in which I can thrive – perhaps even flourish. Through this, I am connected to my environment and my sense of '**belonging**' is satisfied.

With the diagnosis of Parkinson disease, there comes uncertainty in one's future and a sense of having no control. By co-founding an organisation which seeks to cure Parkinson's disease, I know that there is science out there that will soon bring improved treatments. Armed with this information, I can drive on with optimism, belief and a sense of purpose, because The Cure Parkinson's Trust has a role in accelerating a brighter future, not just for me, but for everyone with Parkinson disease. This optimism satisfies the '**becoming**' aspect of my QoL concept.

These three aspects of life, along with other more personal influences, result in a good QoL.

Leaving work does not necessarily equal bad QoL

For many of us leaving a career is more than quitting a job. Because of the culture in which we live, we may define ourselves by what we do. Giving up what we do can be tantamount to losing our identity. The process of redefining ourselves, our worth, our goals, can be difficult. The common thread is that we all make sacrifices and adjustments because no matter what our financial position, our lives change. Parkinson disease does not respect money or status, education or breeding, race or religion. It is an equal opportunity thief. Financial considerations are almost universally a major concern. Loss of income, along with the expense of regular medical care, huge pharmacy bills, medical equipment, home modifications and later possibly residential nursing care can leave a person financially depleted.

Sometimes it's surprising where the best things come from. Leaving ourselves open to possibilities and remaining willing to risk failure for a chance of success may once have been daunting. Given a PD diagnosis, we may not define failure the same the way as before. "Taking a shot" is no longer out of the question for those of us who may never have committed an impetuous act. We now have so much less to lose by venturing out, that we may feel a sense of freedom we didn't feel before.

COPING IN THE WORKPLACE

Do you tell your employer or not? There are advantages to the open approach. Employers may make accommodations that improve our working conditions, and even extend the length of time we are able to continue working. Some are willing to reduce hours, or alter responsibilities to better fit the skills we have lost and the ones that remain. But one disadvantage that may occur is being passed over for advancement. Keeping our situation secret has advantages as well. We continue to be judged by the work we do, unaffected by pity or expectations of failure. However, keeping such a secret is exhausting.

DISABILITY & WORK

Many countries have legislation that protects the rights of workers with disabling conditions which contain suggested accomodations that employers can make to ensure people can continue to work. Such laws are subject to ability to carry out work effectively. Check out the legislation that applies to your country if you have concerns about your employment. Maybe you could join a campaign for disabled workers' rights and help improve conditions.

FINANCIAL PLANNING FOR A NEW REALITY

When you were first offered disability insurance you probably said no. Hardly anyone at forty-two,or even fifty-two does. The best advice is to take the insurance. By the time you realize you are disabled, it is usually too late. When you are not longer able to work, in the US, you can apply for Social Security Disability and, after a waiting period, healthcare benefits.

ASKING FOR HELP

There are professionals who can help for a substantial fee, but you can apply for disability on your own. Social Security personnel can often be very helpful in expediting the process. Help may also be available from experienced people on forums, PD organisations and support groups and especially your local Congressman's office.

Nothing is written in stone; changes that come as a result of our PD may bring opportunities for living well that we never expected. **NEUROWRITERS**

TIPS FROM A NEUROLOGIST WITH PARKINSON

May Griebel, MD

As a neurologist, the only way I have been able to make sense of this disorder is to use my background and training as much as I can to assist fellow patients.

It is now thirteen years since I was first diagnosed. I thought I was handling things well until recently when I had to quit giving lectures in front of large groups, something which I had always enjoyed, because my dykinesias increase with stress, and I have to wiggle my way through a presentation. My vanity raised its ugly head; I don't like looking out of control. I don't want someone to "feel sorry" for me. Yet as I have been asked more frequently to become involved again, I have realized that I can address this issue up front: "Before I start, I have an apology. I have Parkinson disease and the medication side effects make me wiggle. It's always worse in front of people, so I may dance my way through this talk. But hey - it burns calories." People laugh, the air is cleared and then I begin, with far fewer problems than I might have had, had I attempted to suppress everything.

I handle clinic visits with new patients the same way, up front. That is, after I found a patient staring at me, toward the end of a visit I told her what was happening and she signed in relief, "Thank God. I thought you were on some type of drug." Well, I am, but not what she was imagining. Now I address the issue immediately, and again, the problem becomes no problem at all. Also, I pull out my pill trays when I am trying to stress the importance of a regular way to take medication or when patients complain about the quantity of pills they have to take. I acknowledge that I dislike that too, but that they are better off than I. The complaints shrink away when I pull out my pills.

Some ideas:

• Use a weekly pill tray from the start, so that you can be absolutely sure that you are being precise with your medications.

• Keep a list of your medications, including vitamins, over-the-counter and herbal medications too, with you on your person or in your purse. That way, if you are involved in any sort of accident, health care workers will know your needs.

• Read about the medications and their potential side effects. For example, it can be dangerous to stop Sinemet abruptly.

• Be careful with supplements. Many are potent and may interfere with your ongoing prescriptions.

• Be sure your physician is completely on top of things. A truly skilled movement disorders specialist knows how to use older medications in different ways and combinations.

• One of the best signs I know that you need to consider seeking a second opinion is if a physician tells you that you don't need to see a specialist.

• Don't be ashamed of being depressed or scared. Get help - fast.

• Do something to make you feel empowered, to be doing as much as you can to be helping yourself.

• For your body, become involved in a regular exercise program; get a bowel program for the constipation; give yourself breaks when you are tired.

• For your soul and brain, take up piano lessons or painting, Sudoku or crossword puzzles. Be of service to your community, learn about the non-motor aspects of Parkinson disease and face them head-on.

• For your peace of mind, schedule important meetings/activities at times when you will be at your best if possible.

• Just for fun, do the things you have always wanted to do. When the diagnosis of Parkinson disease was stamped onto my forehead formally 12 years ago, I knew I was going to die. I became maudlin. I even pulled out my short-list bucket list: I wanted to sky dive, para-sail, go up in a hot air balloon, and get a tattoo. People want the weirdest things. Why a tattoo? Is it the 60s rebel that never got expressed? I made the mistake of asking my husband about the skydiving. I got in return a resolute and frankly loud, "NO, no, no. Not only no, but h*** no." I gathered that he was against that plan. We agreed on the parasailing and the hot air balloon and did each over the next couple of years. I didn't ask about the tattoo. I figured if he didn't know, he couldn't say a thing. And yes, I have a lovely butterfly tattoo. Just don't ask where!

• Finally, make a plan for leaving work. I fought it tooth and nail for a few years, but then had to cut back to half time and a less demanding practice. Turning over the care of my patients to another neurologist felt like ripping a hole in my heart. I grieved deeply. Ultimately, it was almost like a death. However, there is a flip side to many life decisions. I am surprisingly content. The decreased stress and increased time have been extremely valuable, allowing me time to deepen family relationships and become more involved in my community. I appreciate that I am also extremely blessed to be working in a nurturing system, which values me and has allowed these changes.

GRACE

Grace has several definitions: **(1) seemingly effortless beauty or charm of movement, form or proportion (2) a pleasing characteristic or quality (3) skill at avoiding the inept or clumsy course (4) good will, mercy, clemency (5) Divine love bestowed freely upon mankind.**

I generally use a cane if I am going to walk any sizable distance and so I run into all those situations in which people try to make life a little easier - they make way; they offer to reach something; they try to make sure you have what you want so you don't have to get up; if you are having trouble cutting your food, from tremor or weakness, they may offer to cut your food for you.

Some of these acts or offers of generosity are gratefully accepted; others are unneeded and some can be embarrassing or even humiliating. Assuming they are sincere attempts (as most are) to help for the sake of helping another in need, then it seems to me that they all involve the question of "grace," in its several senses. I am beginning to think that grace is a word that holds a key to dealing successfully with Parkinson.

Parkinson disease, in its outward manifestations, has everything to do with the loss of grace. As our disease progresses, seemingly effortless physical beauty or charm of movement, form, or proportion, as well as many of our most pleasing physical characteristics and qualities, are lost. Skill at avoiding the inept or clumsy course becomes dulled and ultimately is almost completely lost. In this sense, Parkinson in its most reductive form is all about the loss of grace in the world. To lose this grace, smooth and accurate movement in relation to the world around us, is a devastating loss. The ability to walk smoothly, to swim or run, to use utensils effectively, to speak easily, are all measures that so many of us use to place ourselves, to define ourselves, in the world. What teenager has not spent countless hours wishing to look different, be better at a sport, have the charm and ease that contribute to a sense of being part of the larger normal world and all its rhythms and swirling currents, and of bending every effort to avoid being an outsider. What man or woman has not carried in some form these same measures of who we are, along with us into adulthood and even old age?

To slowly lose this physical grace, the ability to move smoothly and accurately, is a catastrophic disability for most persons. Everything you learned to do accurately and smoothly as a child may be lost and cannot be relearned.

Grace also means good will, mercy, clemency and divine love bestowed freely. Here is where people with Parkinson cannot only find a key that unlocks their cages and helps set them free in the world, but also gives them a special opportunity to bestow that grace upon others, by way of example. In the course of a life lived 'normally' these are often not high priorities. We are too busy getting to the next goal or obligation or pleasure.

But I think the loss of physical grace gives us an opportunity to more completely acquire this second, and to my mind more important, spiritual grace. With it, we can accept the loss of physical grace, making our own adaptation to our disease easier to bear. We can also impart to others, through our own acts and attitude toward our loss, a sense of who we now are in the world and a different sense of the world itself and what is important to know and what is not important.

The struggle to find this kind of grace is not easy, I know. But if we can achieve this ability to live our lives in the light that shines from within, then merely by being in the world we demonstrate to others that the most important attainments in life are concerned with the "spiritual" (however each of us defines that word) aspects of grace. By struggling successfully to learn the difference and the profound importance of the difference between the grace that comes from without and that which comes from within, we can embody the concept of good will, the meaning of mercy and even grant a kind of clemency to others, because we can then give to others the example of how life can be lived fully under even the most difficult of circumstances.

When we have unlearned the lessons that the world tries so hard to teach us, that to live fully and in harmony with ourselves and others we must be attractive, move with charm, be financially well-off, in other words to be good consumers of modern culture with all its meretricious charm and instead look within ourselves, without reference to those outer and misleading forces, to our hearts to find the definition of who we are, then our very existence becomes an example of true grace.

When we have found that inner grace of being in the world, we can also accept the assistance of others with both humility and dignity. We shouldn't bristle that 'we can do it ourselves', thereby embarrassing a well-meaning person who we could not reasonably expect to intuit our real needs.

We will not be as likely to act with embarrassment or humiliation when we can't do certain things for ourselves, because we will know that not being physically able doesn't reduce or even substantially affect our sense of who we are. We also, I think, will diminish that terrible sense of otherness and being 'out of step' in the world. The sense of ourselves as being "normal" no longer depends on a definition of ourselves with reference to the outside world of physical grace.

I think if we can come to a real understanding that grace and our humanity abides not on the surface, not in the ability to put a spoon in one's mouth or swing a bat or walk unassisted, but rather in making our souls the touchstone of our experience of ourselves and others, then we will be able to live with our Parkinson with some sense of inner peace and calm. We will also be able to feel true goodwill to those around us, to have mercy and act with tenderness towards others and to forgive the failures of others and of ourselves to sometimes deal easily with what it is to have become people with Parkinson.

See you at the dance,

Greg Wasson

Parkinson disease, in its outward manifestations, has everything to do with the loss of grace... not being physically able does not have to reduce our sense of who we are.

A Poem For Chloe

Come here my little one.
Sit upon my lap and wipe away my clouds
so I can absorb the warmth of your sunshine.
Wrap your arms around my rigid frame
and show me your wonderful smile.
Today I will feel the joy of being your Grandma.

I long to watch you romp through my garden,
then join you to pick flowers when your legs tire.
There will be some to fill the vase
that is waiting for your magic touch on my table,
and a bouquet of your favorites
to bring home to share with Mommy.

When my body aches we will go in the house.
I have your blanket ready on the bed,
so we can lie comfortable as you tell me of your day.
If the pain closes my eyes,
I know you will not be afraid.
You will sing a beautiful solo to soothe me to sleep
and then join me with your head on my shoulder.

I will dream of being the Grandma I long to be.
My shuffled gait would not hinder us at all
as we run along the ocean beach
flying a colorful kite high in the sky.
The sandcastles we build will be magnificently huge,
full of seashells for doors and pebbles for windows.
When I awaken you still are dozing with contentment.

I look to you and whisper a thank you in your ear.
The love that is shown in your innocent gestures
keeps everything fresh and in perspective.
You show me how blessed my life really is
each time you spend a day with me
and say to me, "I love you Grandma."

Laura Jeanne Dean
© January 2002

BECOMING BARBARA

I was diagnosed with Parkinson disease in December 1995, at the age of 45. I was a wife, mother of 2 teenagers and an academic librarian. After working part time jobs for many years, so that I could be home with our children part of the time, I finally landed a full time, tenured position at a local college. I thought I was going to have a smooth ride from there on. As I learned, life has a way of littering smooth roads with unexpected potholes, such as Young Onset Parkinson Disease (YOPD).

I needed to know more about my new, uninvited life companion, but found little patient-friendly information available, especially about YOPD. While surfing the web, quite by accident I came across the Parkinson's Information Exchange Network (PIEN), an online, international discussion group, based at the University of Toronto. Through PIEN, I met Barbara Blake-Krebs, who was working to get her two Kansas Senators to co-sponsor the Udall Bill, as I was doing in New York State. Getting actively involved politically was therapeutic. I couldn't change the fact that I had PD, but I felt that doing something to help fund the research would give me greater strength to fight the disease and maybe I'd find some positive meaning to my fate. As a newbie, it felt safer to communicate with other PwP (often more advanced than I) through my computer, rather than meeting them in person. I was not yet ready to meet my future.

Barbara Blake-Krebs was fifty-five when we met on PIEN, ten years older than me and eleven years into her disease. She was the founder, administrator and producer of a Kansas City community radio station. During the early 1990s, her symptoms worsened and she was forced to reduce her workload at the station, as well as other activities. Barb said she, "grappled with a growing state of dependency and isolation . . . and became increasingly housebound." Her husband Fred Krebs brought home a Mac computer for her and encouraged her to learn simple applications. Barb said she was, "soon happily able to expand her horizons online" - the day in April 1996 when she joined PIEN was one of "pure joy!"

Through online discussions with another PIEN friend, Jeanette Fuhr of Missouri, we realized that PwP were often isolated from the world. The public knew and cared little about the people hidden **Behind the Masks of Parkinson's** (the original title of our book), especially those diagnosed in their 30s, 40s or even 20s. Most of us with early onset PD in those days had heard similar pronouncements from our doctors . . . "You have all the symptoms of Parkinson, but you're too young!" This lack of awareness about PD and its medical, social and economic impact on individuals,

families and communities, was one of the causes of inadequate research funding.

In 1998, Michael J Fox came out as a PwP and suddenly the world became aware that this cruel disease could strike at any age. His announcement became a catalyst for us. From our interactions on PIEN, we knew many list members had compelling stories about living with PD and it became our mission to get them heard. As we added the voices of other PIEN members to our own we concluded, "Why not a book?"

Barb and I, with Jeanette's help and encouragement, worked for two years on the book that eventually was published as **When Parkinson's Strikes Early** by Hunter House. It included a compilation of e-mails, poetry, letters, PIEN postings, etc. from contributors around the world, woven into a global conversation on living with young onset PD. Facts about the disease and its treatment were interspersed between the first-hand accounts.

I called the two-year process a "labor of love." Barb wrote "The last two years of compiling the stories of our fellow PwP and documenting the rise of patient advocates - nobodies - has been one of the richest times of my life." Yet there were numerous difficulties between us. Although I respected and cared about Barb, it became increasingly difficult and frustrating to work with her. More than once, our disagreements threatened the completion of the book. If I knew then what I now know about advanced PD I would have better understood what she was going through; how difficult the writing and editing process had become for her; how important it was to her that her voice be heard. If I had listened better we might have found better ways to work together.

I understand her behavior now, because you see - in my 15th year with Parkinson - I am becoming Barbara.

In November 1999, Jeanette and I traveled to Barb's house, outside of Kansas City, to meet in person for the first time and work out some details for the book. By then, Barb was in a wheelchair most of the time. She was having problems caring for herself. Her husband Fred had pieced together a patchwork quilt of caregivers for Barb while he was at work – friends, neighbors and paid home health aides, but they did not always have the needed coverage, and costs were mounting ...

Despite her progressing physical challenges, Barb wanted to remain an equal partner in completing our book. She was especially adamant that we include the stories of advanced PD patients. While I worried about scaring newly diagnosed readers with too many depressing details, Barb's mantra was ... "No sugar-coating ... tell it like is ...", so we did.

In July 2000, the book was accepted by Hunter House, a small publisher focused on health and self-help books. The book would go through two major edits, and they wanted us to include more factual information about PD. We were now on our publisher's time line with pending deadlines.

Barb didn't seem too concerned with meeting the deadlines and though she said she wanted to assume half of the workload, she was often late or unable to complete what she had promised. Keyboarding became more difficult and her speech was difficult to hear and understand.

I understand now the cognitive challenges of PD because I experience them first-hand: problems with organization, time management, how the act of writing itself becomes slow and laborious. I know now what it means to be "off" - when I can do little except wait until my meds kick in. I know how badly we want to make a difference; we often promise more than we can physically deliver. I'm learning to say, "No" to people, but I'd still rather say, "Yes."

I should have been more patient with Barb, but at the time the most important thing to me was finishing the book and helping to educate the world about PD. It had become a mission for both of us.

When Parkinson's Strikes Early was finally published in September 2001. Holding the book in my hands felt as if I had given birth again - after 2 years in labor. Barb was equally thrilled and looking forward to working on publicity - one of her strengths. However, a few months later she was hospitalized with blood clots in her lungs and respiratory infections. She was placed in a nursing home when she left the hospital; she stayed there for most of her remaining years. She no longer had the use of her beloved Mac and it was nearly impossible to understand her on the phone, so our infrequent communication was through her husband. Her physical condition continued to deteriorate.

In September 2005 (nearly 4 years to the day **When Parkinson's Strikes Early** was published) Fred Krebs called to tell me that Barbara had died of pneumonia. She was 65 years old and had battled PD for over 21 years. Her husband told us she had always wanted to write the "next chapter" about life with advanced PD, documenting her physical decline, the difficulty finding good home-based care, the financial burdens and her life in the nursing home. I can relate some of Barb's story, but it is not adequate.

It's now been 15 years since I was diagnosed and I often think of Barb these days. Everything is becoming more difficult and takes too much time. Now it's me who cannot keep up with the work I've promised to do. I have to ask others for the patience I often lacked myself. I wonder how many more years of independence I can hope for.

The cure did not come in 5 years as promised when I was first diagnosed - nor in 10 or 15 years. Today, in 2010, scientists are just beginning to realize how much more they need to understand about PD before they can cure it. I may be too far gone to benefit from today's most promising experimental treatments such as stem cells or gene therapies.

In spite of all the setbacks and roadblocks, the disappointing failed clinical trials, the political battles for funding stem cell research, Amgen's halt of the phase II Glial Derived Neurotrophic Factor trial and their shelving the molecule for

some 4 years, I am trying to remain hopeful. Any day a new discovery could significantly move the science forward. PwP are now a recognized force in Washington, thanks to the Parkinson's Action Network and its grass roots national network of advocates.

We insisted that **When Parkinson's Strikes Early** end with a chapter about hope and I will end similarly.

I have learned so much about PD and about myself in the last 15 years - most importantly, I learned that we must live with hope, because we cannot live without it. Linda Herman

COPING ALONE
by Patricia Davies

After the initial shock from my diagnosis, I bought all the books on Parkinson disease I could find, and started reading and Googling. I began to notice a word that was always mentioned alongside "Parkinson Patient" … "Caregiver". Everywhere I looked there seemed to be the assumption that all PwP had caregivers, and I could find very little written for people like me who live alone, have no family, and hate asking for help.

I am fortunate that I have good resources, and live where excellent specialized medical care and information is available. I am also fortunate that my disease is progressing slowly and, so far, I can live a normal life. Even so, as a PwP, my future is uncertain and unpredictable. Things can change quickly, and my condition could deteriorate at any time, so I have put in place some safety nets to enable me to try and retain my independence for as long as possible.

MY SURROUNDINGS: I have moved to a house with a bathroom and a small bedroom on the ground floor, and space for a live-in caregiver. I have to decide where that caregiver will come from, but I know that there are reputable providers in my area, and I hope that my long term care insurance will help cover the costs.

I have visited retirement communities and selected one I might consider moving to in due course. In the meantime I have joined my local neighborhood "Village" which provides volunteer assistance to members to enable them to stay in their own homes and "age in place".

MEDICAL AND ALTERNATIVE TREATMENTS: For a long time I resisted taking medication. I dread getting dyskinesia and I heard that this could be caused by prolonged use of some of the Parkinson medications. Eventually I decided that my quality of life was more important, and I began taking PD medications. My handwriting is back to normal and I feel pretty good most of the time. I transferred from a regular neurologist to a movement disorder specialist. I know that in some areas it's difficult to see a neurologist, let alone a movement disorder specialist, but I recently heard a presentation about telemedicine which, if developed, may enable PwP in even the most remote locations to consult with specialists.

Exercise is essential. I adopted a dog to get me out walking several times a day (and provide companionship). I practice yoga twice weekly, which is invaluable for easing joint stiffness and helping maintain good balance.

I am a huge advocate of physical therapy, especially the BIG and LOUD programs. I have done both of them and cannot speak highly enough about their benefits. Now if only I had the self-motivation to keep doing the exercises at home!

I find acupuncture and massage beneficial, as well as occasional visits to a psychotherapist who specializes in patients with chronic illnesses.

THE PARKINSON COMMUNITY: I have become active in the Parkinson community and have met some wonderful and inspiring people. I attend a monthly support group, and as many conferences and other events as I can.

Above all, I try to maintain a positive outward focus and keep busy. PD is an isolating illness and I get concerned about what the future might hold, but I know that I am doing my best to plan for it, and I hope that I will recognize when I can no longer cope alone.

To: Paula and Peg
From: April.

I have walked those roads with you. I have seen your courage, your instincts - as you put it, your patience, your anger, your highs and your lows. But always, I have seen you give of yourselves for the good of others. Granted, there is the hope of the cure dangling out there for all of us and the recognition that comes from those who see our lives as a cause. But mostly - you gave your time, your heart and you still do today so many years later.

I wrote this poem for Paula, after first experiencing seeing her go through dystonia. It was frightening and inspiring. This poem could be said to a lot of people here on this site that fight day by day, hour by hour the unseen enemy - Parkinson. Here's to you!

You are the heart inside the candle
Passionate
Jumpy with giggles and laughter
Smoldering after spending
Yourself – selflessly
Bright burning – darkness-defying

You are a flame
Refusing to be doused
Stubborn
In silence loud
You re-iterate
Your refusal to become cold
And though you may seem alone
You entice others
To hold their candles high
And twinkle boldly
Sharing, sizzling
Chipping away – purging the dross
To reveal the pure beauty
of your soul – my friend
In my eyes
You are a hero
Paula

SHARING THE BURDEN

Recently, I received a call from the rehab facility where our Parkinson support group meets. The lady gave me the name of a person who "needed to be contacted" and showed an interest in joining our group. I took the number and forgot about it until I started making plans for our annual picnic. I saw the sticky note on my roster of members and decided to give "Bobby" a call. I am so glad I didn't pass up this opportunity.

A child answered with a lengthy pause before speaking to my intended party. Bobby's voice sounded weak and nervous. After a few of the "formalities" of informing him when the group met, membership, and programs; we got to the meat of the conversation. I shared first, "I'm 49 - honestly- and have been diagnosed since 1994,". But it was Bobby's response that left my mouth gaping.

At 27, Bobby was diagnosed, and he was now only 38. He had been through DBS (deep brain stimulation) and was still having difficulty with tremors and dyskinesias. He was also in the midst of a divorce and custody battles.

"Bobby!" I lamented, "You've been enduring this battle all alone?" He shared how he had become somewhat of a "recluse" for the past 11 years. For 11 years Bobby had been trying to fight the war of severe tremors plus all the other PD symptoms, was disabled and having financial difficulties and was now fighting the losing battle of divorce . . . all of this alone! What's so sad is that Bobby lived within 10 miles of my home.

After swallowing the lump in my throat, I shared some online sites with him for information and support. Then I invited him to our upcoming picnic and we exchanged e-mails. My heart melted as he told his story - one that needed to be shared immediately after his diagnosis was given . . . not 11 years later.

In our story comparison, I was an elementary principal - in the limelight of the community's eyes. My symptoms, diagnosis, and battle with Parkinson had been followed by many from the onset until my disability retirement. Even then, my network of support was insufficient to prevent the depression that followed. It has only been the past year that I felt that I had control of the inevitable monster.

As I hung up the phone and immediately sent a follow-up e-mail, I wondered how many other young onset victims were out there. How many were becoming a "recluse" as Bobby had described himself? How many could or would have benefitted emotionally from being able to share their battles of job security, raising children, weathering relationship changes or treatment options? I shuddered to think. Although I was thankful that I had opened this door of opportunity, I still shed a tear of remorse for not finding it sooner.

Peggy Willocks

PD Blues

I don't want to be a negative person
I want to DO things
Solve problems
Work with inspiring things and inspiring people
Make a difference
But sometimes the walls in my way are too hard
The bruises and bumps hurt too much
And I feel alone, afraid

Afraid of what? Loneliness?
Not being alone but fighting alone
Afraid of being wrong
Afraid of making mistakes. But mainly
Afraid of PD

Afraid of losing my independence, my strength, my intellect

Above all my intellect

I don't think like this every day
Not even once a week
Not even once a month
Most days
I'm just happy
That my body works reasonably well
And my brain

That I'm still way smarter than my daughter
And just a little bit smarter than my husband

As far as my daughter Frida is concerned, I have always had Parkinson disease.

I was diagnosed with PD in October 2003, when I was 32 years old and she was 9 months old and she was just starting to learn how to walk. Prior to my PD diagnosis, I had another diagnosis which turned out to be wrong, but luckily it was also treated with l-dopa, so I have been taking l-dopa since April of 2000.

Starting l-dopa really gave me a new life. I felt strong and in control of my body, I could walk long distances, something I had been unable to do for a long time. I started to hear my 'biological clock' ticking and I can honestly say without l-dopa I would not have felt strong enough to have a baby.

Frida is now 7 years old and a very active, quick (both in body and mind) and loving girl and of course the pride and joy of her mother and father. She has always been early doing things for herself, like dressing herself and eating by herself, perhaps because she was also aware of my PD.

Having PD and raising a child poses a lot of challenges. There have been times when I have had to tell Frida that at that moment I just didn't have the energy to carry her home or help her learn how to ride her bike. That makes me value the times when I do have the energy all the more.

The hardest part about PD is the unpredictability. One day I can run around all day doing what I like and being very active and the next day I can be a very different person, with the strength and energy of a 90 year old.

I have a lot to gain from planning ahead and I try to make sure my 'good times' occur when they're really needed, like when I'm picking Frida up from school. or taking her to track and field practice.

Although strict plans don't mix very well with the spontaneity of a 7-year old, improvisation and plenty of good humour are good skills to have.

Sara Riggare

No one in her right mind would wish for her family to be struck by Parkinson but, hey, these things happen... and I'm absolutely sure that my husband and daughter, as well as myself, have been made stronger by it.

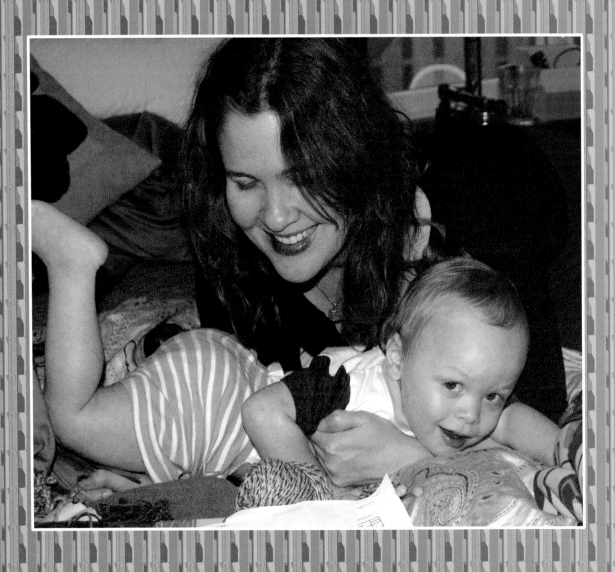

ACCEPTANCE

Acceptance for me means that, paradoxically, as the illness slows me down, I must work faster than ever before to complete knitting and sewing projects while Sinemet and my body still have a solid working relationship. PD has given me a time line; I either accept and adapt now to savor doing what I still can, or I end up losing even more in the long run, given an uncertain future. Beyond this rather pragmatic observation, I realize that acceptance means different things to each of us reflective of our cultural or fundamental beliefs; it's an essential part of how we experience life. Do people, as young adults, really put pen to paper and develop a guiding philosophy of life? I never did, but no time like the present to mull it over and loop together some ideas while I knit.

I've always been drawn to Eastern philosophies and wondered how acceptance of my PD might look through the lens of the I Ching. In this sense, one might view it as a balance between dualities; wellness/illness as two sides of the same coin; a yin and yang, so to speak. Acceptance is like breathing. Without the sun, the moon has no light. Without disease, we cannot truly know wellness; without grief, we cannot have joy. Lau Tzu said, "Foregoing... separation, one enters into the harmonious oneness of all things." I understand this duality intellectually but have not been able to grasp it on a spiritual level which is where it counts most.

I see PD from an existential viewpoint; we have no explanation why; for me it is simply like being, accept it as such. The Gallic in me expresses it with a cosmic shrug of the shoulders. The French have a singular talent for this expression. I've observed, in Paris, things that really tend to work us into a frenzy, like rush hour traffic woes; there they seem to elicit a calm reaction of acceptance. This was epitomized by a taxi driver who, when confronted with impenetrable traffic on a cobbled medieval relic of a street, abruptly shifted the van into park, hopped out, and lit a Gauloises. Taking a deep drag, he shrugged and calmly said "Ç'est comme ça"- it's like that. Accept it; why not make the best of it? While a traffic jam is a far cry from struggling with PD, in reflecting back, this expression of acceptance suits me. I can't change it, so why not seize the moment, enjoy what I still can? One thing that has been hard to accept is the loss of control I once felt I had over my body; by figuratively shrugging my shoulders, I am gaining control in a sense because I am now more consciously defining my self, my life, in the moment.

Please note, a cosmic shoulder shrug does not in the least mean that I am resigned or apathetic. Quite the contrary, I'm here on this forum and have jumped in with both feet to volunteer and make a difference. I'm on another forum educating other new PwP about the need for research participants. I can and will write to all web sites that continue to archaically describe PD as "the shaking palsy". I will write to pharmaceutical companies asking them to redefine how they depict PwP in their advertising; we're not all yet in our golden years. I will educate the ignorant acquaintance, who after seeing a film that stereotypically depicted PD (shuffling older man with dementia), exclaimed that he would kill himself if diagnosed.

I can't single-handedly change research models or convince the world of neurology that we need a new scientific research model that goes beyond using placebos, but I can try to affect change by continuing to probe and ask for change, to help fellow patients achieve a respected, prominent role in the search for a cure. Please, I know many of us are more comfortable with quietly sitting behind the scenes and reading, hoping, immersing ourselves in faith, looking for acceptance and seeking answers that don't exist. As much as we'd like to believe it, hope is not going to bring about change.

Please consider that without more of us becoming a louder, squeakier collective wheel, we're resigning ourselves to not only accept, but to "be okay with" having PD, to be okay with having no real drug improvements in over forty years, let alone a cure. In our inaction, we are nonetheless making a choice to passively sit on the sidelines letting those with fully cooperative neurotransmitters, in the absence of anything else to go on, define what PD is for all of us, how it looks and how it is treated.

Laura Brooks

KIDS, PARENTS & PD:
Some thoughts

Girija:
I was diagnosed with PD when my daughter was five years old. I had symptoms prior to that. She is eleven now and has a fair idea of what PD is (thanks to internet) in biological terms. Last year we both participated in a Parkinson Walk. It was her first exposure to the world of PD and PwP at different stages. She talked with several PwP and was comfortable among them. Did I do the right thing by accepting my PD and making it part of her life? It seems so . . . and she still sees her mom and not a PwP when I say 'Hi' to her. That's what matters to me, assures me and motives me to go on fighting PD with all my might.

Soania:
I was first diagnosed when I was pregnant with my first child at the age of 27. For my children 'Mama's shaky hands' and 'Mama's medicine' are part of life and the norm. This condition has not defined me thus far.

My primary concern as a parent was not to place any stress on them. We've raised them to be sensitive to the situation and needs of others but I didn't want them to worry about my health and future. Thankfully they do not. The evening that we put a label on my symptoms, my very perceptive 8 year old essentially finished the sentence for us and my 10 year old was completely surprised. My sweet 4 year old just went on playing with her toys and obviously didn't understand a thing, which is exactly the way it should be.

Both older girls announced that the money they give from their allowances to charity would from now on go to Michael J Fox Foundation to 'find a cure for Mama' and after hugs and kisses we went on with our bedtime routine.

Laura:
I've been diagnosed for a year and I have a little one who is only 4 months old. I fear not so much telling him or being symptomatic around him, but I do fear seeming 'weak' around him. I really fear having my meds wear off, not kick in or worse - not work well when I have to do things like register him at school or pick him up after soccer practice. Seriously, I go to bed at night worrying about this stuff though it's a ways down the road. I fear that he will not feel safe or that I can't care for him. I know that children are incredibly resilient and compassionate, but it's for him, that he'll even have to deal with this stuff, that I feel most angry at PD.

Soania:
Those of us with Young Onset Parkinson Disease have gone through the same feelings that you are expressing, I know I can completely relate!.

Cherish every moment you have with your newborn son. Through your strength, your son will learn perseverance. Through your challenge, he will learn empathy...concentrate on that!.

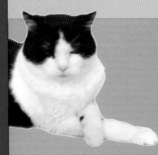

We often worry about our children's reaction
One thing I learned from my own children, now 20 and 24, is that they're far more resilient than our fears. They will adjust, although perhaps not happily, to the new norm. If we're lucky they will be there for us, and if not, our PD alone probably won't change the two-way street of love between parent and child. **Katherine**

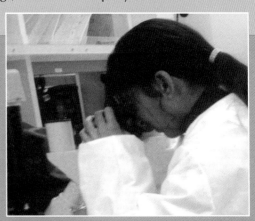

Your daughter sounds like a sweet girl - a researcher in the making! Soania

A TWO WAY STREET OF LOVE BETWEEN PARENT AND CHILD

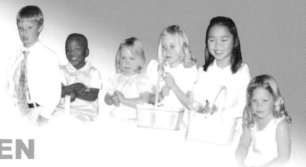

CHILDREN

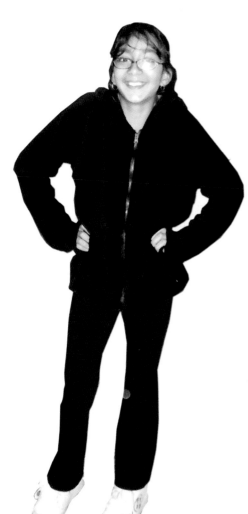

Children, while the main focus of our lives, can be a very difficult issue to deal with when we have a serious disease. Children, if we are completely honest, represent both the most joyous and the most demanding aspect of our daily lives. Small children require energy, compassion and unwavering attention, not to mention feeding, clothing, cleaning and a myriad of other tasks, on a daily if not hourly basis. For someone whose energy level has been severely diminished by illness, pain and adverse drug reactions, the demands can be overwhelming.

Children are our reason for living, for struggling against the draining forces of Parkinson disease and our reason for not surrendering to all the ill effects of our condition.

In dealing specifically with children, there are a unique set of issues that must be addressed, probably more than once, as they grow and mature. They must be told, which may be easy or difficult depending on their age, level of anxiety and understanding. As time passes, they will require additional information. Some children will simply ask, others will require observing to discern when the information is appropriate.

Children, regardless of their ages, often understand far more than we realize. Sparing them the difficult details may not be a kindness, it may leave them unprepared for what they must, themselves, deal with. Even for children, knowledge is power. They will be stronger for knowing in advance what to expect. The conversation may be a difficult one for us to initiate but the faith it demonstrates in the capacity of each child to cope will benefit the entire family. **Pam Kell**

It's like living in a glass house and watching the world live its life.

It's like the Tin Man in the Wizard of Oz. Squeak, squeak, FREEZE.

Just a little dose of drugs and lubrication is in gear...until squeak, squeak, FREEZE.

Even down to the frozen lips of the poor Tin Man who can barely say "o..i..l".

TxLady

161

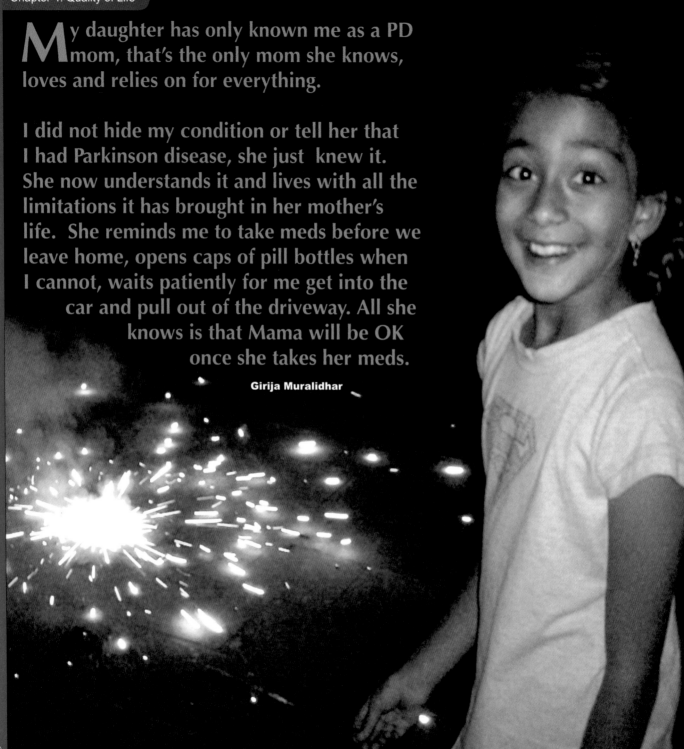

My daughter has only known me as a PD mom, that's the only mom she knows, loves and relies on for everything.

I did not hide my condition or tell her that I had Parkinson disease, she just knew it. She now understands it and lives with all the limitations it has brought in her mother's life. She reminds me to take meds before we leave home, opens caps of pill bottles when I cannot, waits patiently for me get into the car and pull out of the driveway. All she knows is that Mama will be OK once she takes her meds.

Girija Muralidhar

CHILDREN

GENERATIONS

I became a grandmother at 51 and I became a PwP at 53; becoming a grandmother was more fun. In the early days I didn't worry about genetics. No one in my family had ever had Parkinson.

I was sure my children and grandchildren were safe. As I read the new research some of the certainty has faded. Fear is a great motivator and there is no fear that compares to that of your children or grandchildren being put in danger. My only weapon is advocacy, so beware anyone standing in the way of discovering a cure for Parkinson disease. THERE IS A GRANDMOTHER ON THE WARPATH. **Pam Kell**

My mum has Parkinson disease

This is our house and I like living here. I live with my mum and my dad. In my family I don't have any sisters or brothers and my mum has Parkinson disease. Parkinson is a disease that you can get if you're young or old. My mum is pretty much like other mums even though she has Parkinson. She takes medication sometimes and sometimes she gets really tired. You can get sick in other ways too, even if you have Parkinson, like get a cold or stomach flu. But the other ones go away.

My dad is very good at taking photos and my mum makes the world's best pancakes. I drew the whole family as dogs because I am better at drawing dogs than people. I also drew the kinds of dogs that we are most like. Dad is a bulldog because he is strong and has a large face. I am a cocker spaniel because I have long curly hair, brown eyes and do a lot of mischief. Mum is like a Yorkshire terrier because they have straight hair, are curious and stubborn, kind and quite obedient and they like sleeping.

Frida

LIFE IN THE SLOW LANE

Once upon a time, I would have been at the head of the queue

When I took early retirement from teaching on the grounds of ill-health, I was very apprehensive about what lay ahead. I was full of resentment because Parkinson had stifled and killed my career prospects. Making the best of a bad job was the most I could hope for. I spent the first few weeks sulking in some kind of convalescent state of self-pity. I did not know how to start retirement, I had not received training for that and it took weeks to get out of the routine of waking up at 6 am and worrying. Gradually as I started to make up for a huge sleep deficit I began to see things more positively. In fact, I began to see things from an entirely new perspective.

It was June when I retired and the garden was looking its best. Until now I had never explored its beauty close-up. I had never appreciated the subtle shades between the petals of a rose nor the dedication of the bee as it moved from one flower to the next. I could develop photography as a hobby and start to observe things close-up and over a period of time such as a flower opening at the start of the day.

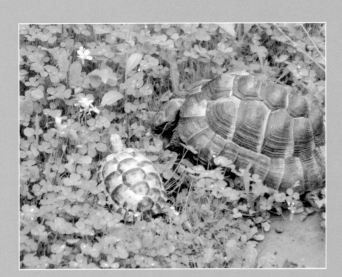

One mellow September afternoon, I decided to behave badly and sat in the sunshine overlooking the garden from the rockery, eating the most extravagant ice cream the local service station could provide. I looked ahead and watched my tortoises plod slowly across the grass and I thought about the other world; the one I had left. September would be stressed by the scrutiny of exam results and the enrolment of students. Would we fill the classes? Would we keep our jobs? How glad I was to be out of the rat race and to be plodding along in the slow lane like my tortoises.

Now I was at the back and it didn't matter one bit

To have time to think, explore and express how I felt was a privilege.

This change in attitude did not come overnight and I still thought every day about life in college and how I missed the students, but gradually as winter replaced summer these thoughts receded. One day in December I went to London to meet up with my daughter. The train arrived around 10 o'clock but was still packed with commuters. As we drew into Paddington, instead of queuing anxiously by the door to get out first, I stayed in my seat and slowly gathered my possessions and waited. When I eventually did get off the train, I looked down the platform ahead of me and watched the sea of commuters filter slowly through the barriers. Once upon a time, I would have been at the head of the queue, but now I was at the back and it didn't matter one bit. I had left the working world.
Briony Cooke

165

FROM A HUSBAND'S POINT OF VIEW

When my wife was first diagnosed with Parkinson, over ten years, ago my first reaction was that of concern but also fear. The fear was because my mother died from the disease at age 65. As it turned out, my mother probably had a host of other problems that contributed to her death. Nevertheless, the very real concern was, and is still, there.

It took several different doctors to come up with a Parkinson diagnosis. At the time I don't think we really discussed it very much; we just accepted it and decided we would deal with problems as they arose, a pattern of many years.

The first major decision resulting from PD was when to retire from practice as a CPA. She had spent a considerable amount of time and effort getting to the level, in her professional career, that she was when she was diagnosed. She had obtained several advanced designations and developed a respected practice and partnership. Her practice entailed a lot of work in the field of litigation that was very stressful.

As her PD progressed, she got to the point she did not feel she could perform at the level she felt necessary to give her clients her very best and we made the decision it would be best for her to retire. As it turned out, the timing worked out great for us. Her parents had moved in a couple of years before. Her retirement allowed her to spend some quality time with her father before he died, which she would not otherwise have had.

From my stand point, my life has not changed much. That is entirely, and I mean entirely, due to my wife's insistence that she is doing everything within her power NOT to let the disease affect her daily life and especially the lives of those around her. I must say she has done an absolutely outstanding job. I still work every day, go hunting and fishing and enjoy most of the same things I have always done. I did quit smoking and more recently lost about twenty five pounds. Watching her confront her problems inspired me to try to get a little healthier and take a little better care of myself.

We recently purchased a sailboat that we have enjoyed immensely. I truly believe the boat, along with working on this book, (certainly not in that order) have given her a new purpose in life. The boat has been something we can do together and really, really enjoy. It has become an ongoing

weekend project we look forward to all week. Some weekends are work weekends, but now more and more of them are just fun sailing weekends. We have not had a lot of similar shared interests throughout our marriage. She doesn't like to duck hunt or fish and I don't care much for theater or the symphony; so the boat has been a true blessing. I like to tinker with things. There is always something to tinker with on a boat and the relaxing effect it has on her has been almost miraculous.

I would encourage each of you, if you do not already have a common interest/hobby/activity which you do together, to find one as soon as possible. Not only will it benefit your relationship, it may well help slow down or at least make the effects of PD on you partner disappear for a while. (A word of caution, set your timer so you can remind your partner to take her medicine, she is likely to forget when she gets relaxed.)

I just want those in my position who may be coming to grips with the reality of living with someone who has this disease to know that life will go on. You can go for several years with only minor changes to your life. My wife doesn't get around as well or fast as she once did, but much of that may be attributable to having both knees replaced and then having one knee replaced again. I do find myself doing things for her that I know are difficult but that's not a big deal. It use to bug her because she is so independent, but she has come around a little and has decided that sometimes it's just easier to let me have my way.

I don't mean this to sound like our lives have not changed as a result of her having PD. Hers certainly has - but she plays the cards as they have been dealt to her and we are coping with it. We are more fortunate than many of the people afflicted with Parkinson as my wife is what she calls a 'slow leaker'. She claims it is a real term, at least among those who have the disease.

Because of this, her symptoms have developed slowly allowing her far more freedom than those with the more severe symptoms. For this we are very grateful and hope her 'slow leaker' status continues until a cure is found. Until then, we will continue to follow her lead; living and going about our daily live as normally as we can and believing tomorrow will be the best day we will ever have.
Dan Kell

A HUSBAND SPEAKS

NOT LIFE THREATENING
JUST LIFE ALTERING

You still remember that moment. Your mom and dad sat you all down and had some news. Somewhere in between "you're getting a new sibling" and "someone died" kind of news. I had never heard of the disease before, only knew it in the vague spaces in the same sentence where it lived between Cancer and Alzheimer. So I learned. I did the research; "degenerative" it says, not "life threatening". Just life altering.

There was a moment in a parking lot once, listening to the sound of a President on the radio as he simply denied funding for stem cell research. That sinking feeling, thinking that the hope for an answer to this question was slipping away as I heard the words of his disembodied voice.

You tell your friends eventually, given time and they understand even less. They don't see what is different and there are some times you don't either. There are times you forget, until a drag of a foot or the need for medication rears its head. You sometimes feel that things haven't changed at all and then you feel guilty it hasn't affected you more. You feel that you should have that expected anguish when in reality things are really pretty reasonable. Manageable symptoms. Not great, but things could be worse.

There are times when you think about the future. When things will be worse. Whispered conversations with a sibling about the times to come, the care that might be needed, the plans to be made. Where some children wonder about what life will look like at a certain age, you are at least given some assurance, some warning of the times to come.

So you relish this calm before the storm. These times when it really doesn't matter. When it is still that vague word floating around these precious moments. When they are more than their disease. When they are just your parents and you love them. **Meredith Rich**

So you relish this calm before the storm. These times when it really doesn't matter. When it is still that vague word floating around these precious moments.

When they are more than their disease. When they are just your parents and you love them.

Dealing with tough issues

When she first became a PwP, she was scared.
Eventually, she realized that progression was gradual.

She had imagined a person drooling, demented, sitting in a
wheelchair needing full-time care - all within a short period of time.

What if she had to go to the hospital? Were there things to be aware
of or do if one were hospitalized? Yes, there were. She watched PwP
friends age and deal with issues she could only imagine.

What about home care versus nursing homes, caregiver burnout,
writing a living will and hospice - what does it mean?

She wanted to prepare for an uncertain future.

**In this chapter you will find issues that PwP and their carers often
face late in the disease. You may wish to defer reading this chapter
until you feel you need the information.**

If you're as strong as those living with PD, read on.

CHAPTER FIVE
The difficult bits

Time is not neutral for us

CHAPTER FIVE

The title of this chapter is a warning: an admonition not to go forward if you are not ready to confront some of the hard parts.

The Difficult Bits

COMMON LOSSES

When you have a serious illness, invariably there are losses. Big losses that are obvious to any observer and smaller losses that may not be apparent to anyone but ourselves. It is possible for the diagnosis of Parkinson disease to be an opportunity for personal growth, but that doesn't prevent the losses.

I'm finding lately that I am losing things more often: coordination, confidence, poise, faith and friends. Sometimes it matters to me, sometimes it doesn't. The culprit is the disease, or perhaps the medication, or perhaps it's only me - my lack of attention and discipline. I used to be quite vain (not that I necessarily hold that to be a desirable characteristic) but lately I find it almost impossible to care enough to even attempt to fix up or dress up. The reason could be that there is no place I am really interested in going.

I don't know when the fading of my zest began, I don't know if it is permanent or temporary. I don't care. Maybe it is all symptomatic of a chronic, incurable, debilitating neurological disease, or perhaps it is just my reaction to having Parkinson, or maybe there is no difference in the two.

Sometimes in the dark, late at night when sleep eludes, thoughts turn to those small losses and how they steal bits of me when they go. Their names don't all come to mind at once. Some happen trying to button little dresses, or comb hair into tidy pony-tails. Some emerge in social situations when I want to dance and have Frankenstein feet, or I am trying to prepare dinner for friends and cannot manage the knife, or when I need to type something and it's stroke, stroke, back space, back space. Sometimes, often the worst times, I am alone and wondering if I can make it back to where I started, or if I will ever again be able to put mascara on just my eyelashes, or do my hair without lumps that will not be combed out.

There are things I know intellectually: I have physical limitations that don't interfere with my mental acuity, I have good friends and steadfast family who are not burdened by my illness, and until it's over, hope remains. On an emotional level the entirety of the previous statement is complete and utter drivel. Emotionally, I feel as if all those people in the "normal" world can see is my dragging foot. My lack of dexterity and stumbling gait are evidence of total decline and undesirability for filling any critical position - or even being useful as a friend.

The losses, taken one at a time, are insignificant mostly, even trivial, but in the aggregate they are the difference between being normal and not. Then I remember, today is probably as good a day as I will ever have again and I had better get up and enjoy it because who knows what tomorrow will be like. Losses are losses, we all have them. Bad - but not as bad as those of others. We can muddle through or surrender, or we can attack. Either way we survive, we go on growing, contributing, taking, learning, loving, hating and accepting the losses, because there is no other choice. **Pamela Kell**

I've found that the great majority of my old friends are now avoiding me, whether they understand anything about PD or not, whether I can remember their names or not.

When I look up across a large room and see someone that looks familiar, I have to stare at them for several minutes while my eyes slowly focus for that distance and I can recognize them and wave. If you stare steadily without blinking or smiling it will make most people nervous, especially if your face was scary even before PD gave it an evil expression as if made up for Halloween.

Some of my family and my very close friends do understand my situation and still dodge when they see me coming. I think they want to remember me as I was 15 years ago, or maybe I remind them of their own mortality. Whatever the reason, it really hurts to see them scatter as if I were contagious. I can't catch up and I can't yell "Hey, wait up!" as I once did. My voice is so soft and weak that I can't even be sure of calling the dog for dinner.
SLOWBOB

The Patient with PD Collides with Hospitalization

Many PwP report receiving poor treatment in hospitals, nursing homes and rehab centers. We think this is because staff, at all levels, do not understand the special needs of PwP. Our medication and timing of dosage is similar to that of a diabetic. It's important to advocate for ourselves, but when you're sick or in pain, your ability to do so is often compromised. Following are two accounts in different cities plus some advice from an MD with PD.

TWO TALES FROM THE HOSPITAL
A Fractured Leg Nightmare

In October 2011, I fell playing Pickle ball and fractured my leg. That fall took months from my life, and I remained in pain with more healing needed. It took an MRI to find the fracture, and I was in such excruciating pain that I had to be anesthetized for the MRI, and again the following night for the surgery. Was this too much anesthesia for me?

Within the week, I had my first psychotic episode with memory loss plus 3 days of post-op delirium, probably due to the anesthesia plus heavy duty pain killers.

When I finally started thinking like a PwP, I realized I was full of drugs, but not my PD drugs, which they had cut way back. The doctors thought that Sinemet made me have hip and leg movements. But that's not the way it works for me. I have off dykinesia. It was turning into a real mess. I don't remember getting any of my normal drugs in the hospital - drugs that shouldn't be dropped cold turkey. I was given sedatives, which I don't take, to keep my leg still.

I was transferred to rehab where I stayed for a few months and had a similar series of problems. Now, looking back, after I learned how many drugs I had been given and not given - I wondered, how did I come back?.

Paula Wittekind

NPF Hospital Toolkit

In response to many complaints about hospital care, the National Parkinson Foundation created a new program in 2012. It aims to help people with Parkinson disease get the best care possible during a hospital stay, including receiving their medications on time. (Order a tool kit from NPF on their web site or by calling : 1-800-4PD-INFO (473-4636)) http://www.awareincare.org

PWP in Hospitals : BYOD (bring your own drugs)

Thank you NPF for creating the Aware in Care program. In August 2012, I was in a local hospital undergoing surgery. I had my "Aware kit" by my side the entire time. I thought I was prepared.

I tried to talk to the nurses about the fact sheets, although few of the nurses had enough time. They seemed to know very little about PD - its symptoms (one thought it just caused shaking), drugs (most only knew about Sinemet), special hospital needs (getting meds on our schedules, needing to move after surgery). They said they dispensed meds every four hours and they couldn't accommodate individual schedules, like mine.

The official hospital policy is that no meds can be brought from home, but I was very glad I brought some anyway (with their original bottles, as advised). I had checked in at 6:30 AM, filled out yet another medication form. Still, the hospital's meds did not get to my floor until 9:30 PM. When I asked if I could take my own meds, the first response was "Absolutely not!" But they didn't take my meds away and I quietly used them. Later, I complained to another nurse and she finally agreed that since the pharmacy's supply had not arrived, I could take my own meds, under her supervision. I had my full day's supply arranged in a pill container, which I gave her.

After dispensing one Sinemet pill she gave the pill holder back. I told her i needed all my other meds too. She then emptied the section containing my Sinemet for the ENTIRE DAY into a pill cup and gave it to me. Did she think I was to take all at once? It was lucky I was still alert.

The kit points out how important it is for PWP to get up and move as soon after the surgery as possible. It wasn't until the following late morning that someone helped me to get out of bed and sit in a chair. By then I was stif, immobile and in pain. I hadn't slept all night. The doc came later and said I could go home that day - - one day post-op. It was music to my ears - i did not want to stay there one more night.

The NPF kit can be very helpful in advising you what to expect, and how to protect yourself, but it's going to take a lot more than that to change the system. Hospital staff need pro-PD policies, education and training to provide better care for PwP. Until then, If at all possible, - stay out of hospitals.

Linda Herman

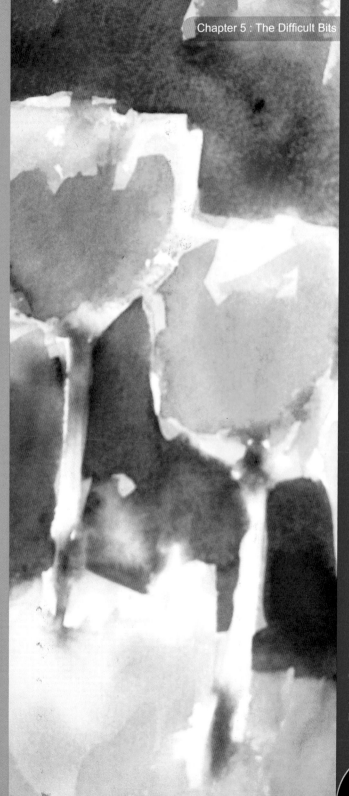

HOSPITALIZATION :

1. Take two medication lists with you: one which lists each medication by name with its dose and the time you take it, e.g. Requip-XR 6 mg at 8:00 am and 2 mg at 8 pm, Amantadine 100 mg at 8 am). On the second list, start with time and drug name for each hour of the day the meds you take and their doses, e.g., 8am: Requip-XR 6 mg and Amantadine 100 mg. Give exact times, and don't just say "twice a day." In hospital lingo, twice a day does not equal every 12 hours.

Be sure that the admitting MD writes the exact times you need dosages in the admission orders.

2. Take all of your medication in their original, pharmacy-labeled bottles.

3. If at all possible, be sure that you have an educated advocate with you at all critical times. The person needs to know you, your medical history, your level of functioning, and your medications. Then, if you have someone willing to go tell others your needs and urge action, you might have an easier time than Paula did (see Nightmare story). Check each pill every time you are given meds; ask why? if you are given a new med.

4. Some medications are clearly contraindicated and dangerous combined with meds for PD, for example, Demerol. Other medications block dopamine and can cause problems, e.g., haloperidol (Haldol), metoclopromide (Reglan) and promethazine (Phenergan). I have them listed as "allergies" in my medical records. When asked what kind of reaction I have had, I state simply "that they mess up my PD meds."

The entire experience can be better or worse, depending mainly on the people who really matter for your care: the nurses.

May Griebel, MD

PLANNING AHEAD FOR HOSPITAL • HAVING AN ADVOCATE

PROCESSING OUR EMOTIONS

NAVIGATING THE EMOTIONAL PASSAGE

In 1969 Dr. Elisabeth Kübler-Ross wrote a book called **On Death and Dying** in which she outlined the five stages of grief one goes through after being diagnosed with a terminal disease, or suffering a catastrophic loss such as the death of a loved one.

While Parkinson disease is not terminal, as such, it is a catastrophic loss and the stages provided by Dr. Kübler-Ross make a good framework for understanding the transitions we go through beginning with diagnosis.

These five stages have not been scientifically verified by double blind studies but they, nevertheless, represent the procession of emotions that most of us experience. We have adapted Dr. Kübler-Ross' broad categories but not necessarily her reasoning. Everyone does not go through every emotion nor does everyone spend the same amount of time in each place or go through the emotions in the same order. But for most everyone there is a process that parallels Dr. Kübler-Ross' five stages and makes them relevant to our journey.

DENIAL
Ah denial, the favorite condition of Parkies. Some of us begin denial at or even before diagnosis and simply stay there, forever looking for some excuse to continue to believe that an awful mistake has been made and will be discovered in time. In time, however, the evidence becomes yet more convincing and sooner or later we are forced to relinquish denial and move on.

ANGER
Nothing collectively pisses PwP off like being forced to give up our denial. In the darkness, late at night, sentiments rarely spoken in the light or in company, sneak into our reverie: Why me? What did I do to deserve this? Why isn't anyone working on a cure? What will happen to me? Anger is a dangerous stage because of the damaging effects it can have on relationships. Spouses can be the innocent recipient of our misdirected anger, as can children and friends. Some will manage to overlook and forgive the undeserved ire, others will not.

The anger can also be difficult for us to cope with because we are so often told, "we're lucky to have PD". While it's rare that we feel lucky the statement itself implies a level of ingratitude on our part and that may make us feel the need to hide it, consequently exacerbating the feelings of anger. Well-meaning family and friends may try to lighten our spirits by telling us to, "buck up, things could be worse", thereby invalidating the anger that is not only appropriate but necessary for us to improve.

BARGAINING
If we are religious we bargain with God, "I will never lose my temper again", "I will live a life of service to others", "I will be in church every Sunday, if only you will let my diagnosis be a mistake." If you are not religious, you may still bargain with God or perhaps just the cosmos. The bargains remain pretty much the same; an effort to trade future benevolence for present health. There is a certain desperation in the bargaining. Denial and Anger are both within our own control; bargaining calls upon an outside force and places us at the mercy of something (someone) else.

DEPRESSION
Whether situational or clinical, depression is a condition that few of us manage to avoid entirely. As a rite of passage, depression can be mild and temporary. As a brain chemistry malfunction, it can be long, serious and severe and it may require medication to resolve it.

Recognition of clinical depression will most likely come from outside ourselves, either by family or friends or physicians. Many of us are reluctant to admit to the feelings inherent in depression. From childhood we are taught to "walk it off", "get hold of ourselves", "keep a stiff upper lip", "quit whining" and "go do something for someone else, it will take your mind off of it." Men probably have a harder time owning up to feelings of worthlessness and hopelessness, not because they are less likely to have them, but because traditional male upbringing tends to denigrate feelings, resulting in their ability and desire to conceal them.

Depression often goes hand in hand with the sense of having lost ourselves, of no longer knowing who we are. The loss of career, the loss of family or spouses, the loss of agility, all these things can lead us to believe something fundamental has changed within us. There is no doubt, once we become a PwP, we feel different in many ways, but we are still who we are. At our core we don't change. We may adapt, we may look different, we may even feel different but we remain ourselves. We may require help to find that self again, but we are still there, and are wiser and more compassionate than before.

Ultimately, when depression resolves, whether on its own or with treatment, we arrive at the final stop.

ACCEPTANCE
The duration of each of these phases is entirely dependent on the facts and circumstances of our individual lives. Some of us remain for years in denial, some can be stuck endlessly in depression, due to lack of treatment or resistance to it. For many, our time of acceptance is the shortest of all, arriving at it only on our deathbeds. Prior to that, acceptance can represent, in our minds, capitulation to illness or surrender to invalidism, when actually, it is only the realization that the rest of our lives will be lived on a different plane. Priorities will likely change, not necessarily for the worse. Choices may be colored by the tint of chronic illness and the future will probably be filled with less adventure and more contemplation.

Loss is not unique to the chronically ill, but among the chronically ill it is universal. Recognition of loss and the ability to cope with it, is not information you will get in your doctor's office. The community of PwP is wide and varied and dedicated to helping show others, coping with this affliction, that it does not have to be the single determining factor in our lives. We may not be able to overcome Parkinson disease, but we can with help, outwit it, at least for a while, and what we can accomplish in a while can be astounding.
Pam Kell

For me PD is the uninvited guest, the unwanted visitor that has very much overstayed its welcome...one which I never offered in the first place! Its funny (or not) how you can feel like a prisoner in your own body as PD relentlessly does its thing. Hour to hour, you never know how you're going to feel or be able to function.

And yet, it has given me a new purpose. I am dedicated to speaking out about this dreaded and devastating disease wherever and whenever I can. Educate, advocate and make people aware. We can't sit back and just assume people will understand or relate to what we deal with every minute of our lives. So I plan to talk (and then talk some more) to attempt to create that understanding as best as I can.

What's it like living with PD? For me, it's the same as you and yet so different. It sucks, I hate it, it makes me angry and sad. Yet it also reminds me of how precious and fragile life is and that we should do everything we can to not only improve our own quality of life, but that of others.

The bottom line for me is, I've decided that if PD wants a fight, then I'm going to give it one. I hope it's ready for me...
Todd
PDTalks.com

There is no doubt that once we become a PwP, we feel different in many ways, but we are still who we are. At our core we don't change. We may adapt, we may look different, we may even feel different but we remain ourselves.

We may require help to find that self again, but we are still there and are wiser and more compassionate than before . . .

175

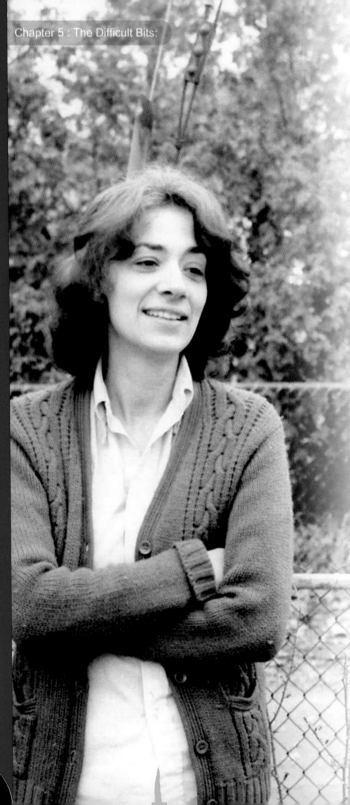

ADVANCED PD • MILLY'S STORY

THE REALITY OF ADVANCING PD

My late wife, Milly, did not have classic Parkinson disease, so readers who do (and their families) should not be overly alarmed by what I am writing about - planning for the worst kind of decisions a family can make.

Milly had one of the various Parkinson-plus syndromes that her doctors finally just labeled "multi-system atrophy." It did what the name describes: attack all her "systems," including mobility, balance, swallowing and cognition. She fought it for 17 years until her death in 2004.

People with classic Parkinson may suffer from one or more of these and, in later stages, may face the kind of issues we did - but not as rapidly.

The first was whether to move from the beloved three-story home where we raised our children to a one-level apartment. This was a simple decision after Milly's balance problems caused her to fall backward downstairs - miraculously not injuring herself. We moved within weeks.

Next was the decision whether she needed to stop trying to walk, or use a walker and settle for life in a wheelchair. That came harder, and often she'd try to dispense with the chair. We spent enough time in hospital emergency rooms for treatment of cuts, bruises - ultimately, a broken nose - that she submitted to the inevitable.

Then there was the decision whether to install a feeding tube when she could no longer swallow. She'd often said that she wanted to die rather than live with Parkinson. It was the most painful part of my life as a caregiver - trying to determine whether she really meant this or whether it was a product of depression.

I finally decided that the moment of truth would come at the point when she needed a feeding tube. I consulted Hospice of Washington and was told that, if she refused the tube, she would die peacefully and without pain. The absence of nutrition and liquid results in a chemical process, ketosis, that actually produces a low level of euphoria and suppresses discomfort.

I did not want her to refuse the tube and, thankfully, she did not. It involved a relatively simple surgical procedure to install it and for four years she got liquid nutrition and water through the tube.

I cannot stress enough the importance of doing three things. One is talking about life and death to determine what your loved one wants - how much "heroic" hospital care he or she wants to be performed (or inflicted) to keep life going.

The second is, consult hospice and do so as early as possible so that you understand what services this God-sent institution can provide for you both. It's a matter of individual choice, of course, but - having seen both "bad deaths" (where needles, surgery and tracheotomies are employed to keep a patient alive) and "good deaths" (where the death comes peacefully, at home, with the patient surrounded by family), there's no question which I favor.

And Milly favored it, too. So the third important decision is to have a "living will" or "advance directive" instructing medical professionals what your wishes are - basically, whether you want to have "heroic" measures taken when death is inevitable, or not. At the end of her life, Milly was bed-ridden and had lost the ability to recognize others. She spent about six months in home hospice care, with nurses coming once a week to check on her and see if she needed doses of morphine to ward off discomfort, which she rarely did.

Probably later than I should have, I decided that in August, 2004, I would accede to her wishes - have our children come home to be with her and me, stop her feeding tube and "let her go." Even though she could not communicate any longer, I am convinced that she sensed that I was ready to "let go." She died peacefully in her sleep on July 20.

Morton Kondracke, Executive Editor of Roll Call, Washington DC and former Fox News contributor. Morton is also author of best-seller: **Saving Milly: Love, Politics, and Parkinson's**, which was also made into a television movie.

Milly and Morton Kondracke testifying before Congress.

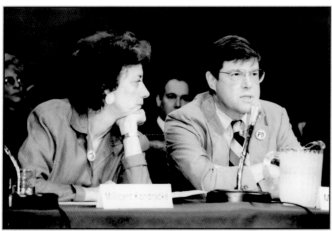

HOSPICE

When there's nothing more that medically can be done to improve your condition and your mind is ready to say enough, it's probably time to call hospice.

Hospice is about comfort oriented care. Its intention is to assist in providing care for people who are at the end of their lives - to bring them physical comfort through managing pain aggressively and to assist them and their families in this transition.

Too often, people enroll in hospice much later than their situation warrants.

Besides nurses visiting and doctors available for consults, most hospices also provide social workers to help with the emotional aspects and other details to aid the family.

In most cases hospice's role is mainly as a consultant and educator. It provides support to the family members and friends who do the direct care.

As in any relationship, some hospice providers are better than others.

If one of the professionals involved does not work well with your family, consider requesting to be reassigned to another person.

In some locations, residential hospice is available on either an indefinite or short-term respite basis.

To enroll in hospice ask your doctor or your local hospital for a referral. In the US, hospice services will be paid for by Medicare and most insurers.

If your health improves you can leave hospice and resume it, if necessary, later.

IT IS NEVER TOO LATE TO BE AN ADVOCATE FOR PD

TEMPUS FUGIT

I was recently asked why, at age 78, I wanted to volunteer as a collaborator in writing this book. My still long term memory immediately thought of my high school days recalling a Latin phrase still seen in literary works today. The English translation "time flies" is probably overused these days but I'm going to use the Latin version because it's an attention getter!

Tempus does indeed Fugit. I can't remember most of my life as an infant. I do however, remember getting my bottom spanked from time to time. To the best of my recollection, the word "NO" was prominent in my vocabulary and produced the expected response. I suspect these incidents triggered my first real advocacy. To this date, I'm an advocate of no spank.

The remainder of my youthful years passed quickly also. As quickly as I can say my favorite baseball player's name - Jackie Robinson - I was 17, in the Navy and an antiwar advocate. When discharged from the service I vowed that I would serve mankind instead of annihilating it.

Thanks to the GI bill, a university education helped redirect my advocacy to reformation of the political process. I was, I believed, well prepared to take the world's problems on my shoulders. I did not realize there were people like Joe McCarthy in the business of character assassination. I scrapped my application for foreign service duty, was retrained as a trust administration officer and devoted the next 50 years to protecting the rights and property of fellow human beings.

I recall being identified as a character in Ayn Rand's bestseller **Atlas Shrugged**. The book's title refers to the mythical Atlas, said to have held the weight of the world on his shoulders. A trust colleague once presented me with a paperweight image of Sisyphus, another mythological character, said to be continually rolling a stone up a steep mountain, only to have it roll back down as it reached the top. My Karma?

In December 2006, I was diagnosed as a "late onset" Parkinson disease patient. The stone was back at the bottom of the mountain and I started pushing again. I became an advocate and champion trying to establishing a patient voice that would be heard by those involved in searching for treatments and a cure for this deadly disease. At first I merely posted to several forums for patients. I discovered a caregivers forum that cried out for patient input. As a commentator and contributor to this forum, I hoped to make another unique approach to advocacy.

In 2008, an inspired group of NeuroTalk posters began to discuss creation of this book. While in my twilight years, and despite time continuing to fly by, I firmly believe I will be allowed to complete this cycle of my karma.

BOB CUMMINGS

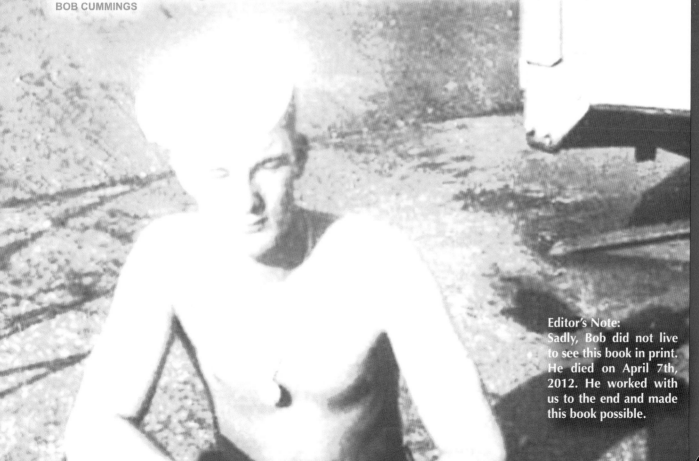

Editor's Note:
Sadly, Bob did not live to see this book in print. He died on April 7th, 2012. He worked with us to the end and made this book possible.

TIME IS RUNNING OUT FOR MANY HOPING FOR A CURE

179

THOUGHTS ON MY FATHER'S BATTLE WITH PARKINSON DISEASE

My father has always been a sensible man.
An intelligent man.
A funny man.
I am lucky to have such a father.

Born in 1931 during the Great Depression, he learned at a young age about harsh realities and realistic expectations.

He turned out to be a success story, pulling himself up from modest roots into the shine of accomplishment using his wits and a strong work ethic.

He likes to dance. His wife Jeanne likes to dance. He made sure that after a long career there were plans for a retirement filled with traveling and dancing.

Parkinson had other plans for his well-earned golden years. Endless medications. Daily humiliations. Looking into the mirror and wondering who that is staring back. An inability to even lace on the dancing shoes, much less tripping any light fantastics.

I can only say that for me, my father's situation would put reality itself into question.

A Vice President in a large banking concern, he had an unpredictability in sharp contrast to his conservative vocation.

I remember him teaching me a series of dirty limericks when I was ten - on the promise that I wouldn't repeat them to any of my friends. Predictably, I repeated them to every kid in my Cub Scout pack. After a series of angry parental phone calls, uh… let's just say that among other punishments, he awarded me a merit badge for Scout With The Biggest Mouth.

On a visit a few years ago, he looked at me across the table and asked me if I'd drive him to the VA Hospital for a routine check-up. PD was still in its early stages. As is his way, my Dad had researched the disease completely. He knew what to expect, when to expect it and didn't anticipate miracle cures. He could get around the house alright, but could only walk very short distances. Jeanne, his warm gracious wife, was having health issues as well.

On the drive out we talked about his days in the Navy. As a kid, I don't remember him telling Navy stories often, but later in life he brought those years up. It was clear to me that his four years traveling the world aboard ship was a happy memory.

At the VA we sat in a lounge, waiting for his name to be called.

"Look. This is how it's gonna be. If I get to the point where I can't lift myself out of bed or if my brain goes sideways and I start getting mean with Jeanne- I'm coming here. I want to stay home as long as I can, but all of that is on the way and I'm not gonna put you or Jeanne or your brother through it. The arrangements are already made." But I don't want any of you to have to make any guilty decisions about me. It's done."

I didn't know how to respond to this.

"Okay." is all is could say.

"If it gets to that point, I want to be here with the boys and we'll sit and talk about Navy days or if we're too far gone we'll stare at the walls."

Three years later his body finally failed him and that's how it went.

This lovely man, who likes a good laugh and wants to dance, has been forced into making a strange journey toward an unknown destination.

My father's mind has always been his strongest asset and I'm thankful that so far it has remained largely unaffected by the betrayal of his body. Everyone who cares about him is thankful that he took a difficult and emotional decision out of our hands and asserted his control over his own life.

Dad taught me other things besides unprintable jokes and rhymes. I picked up life lessons that have served me well over the years. Now he is showing me how to face an awful disease with humor and poise. Yes, someone who can no longer stand up straight is showing me poise.

The disease is relentless. But still the guilt creeps in.

He is only a few years into this journey. None of us know how far it will take him. If the disease progresses and affects his mind, all bets are off. This is a man who has cross-dressed for a laugh, at least twice that I know of. I can't think about what he'd come up with operating with a few less marbles.

If the worst happens, he can rest knowing that he made a bad reality a bit easier for his wife and two sons who love him.

Curtis Cummings

TOP TEN CAREGIVER NEEDS

After many months of participation in an outstanding caregiver forum, I believe I have (from a patient's point of view), determined at least nine major caregiver needs as they have consistently appeared in various threads.

While not necessarily in order, all seem to be on caregivers' lists of questions or comments and perhaps this list will be an aid to the newly diagnosed as well as a reminder to those who have been around for many years.

• A Third Shoulder
A third shoulder you say? Don't you have times when you feel the caregiver burden requires more than just two shoulders? The children will not listen to you, other members of the family are quiet and your patient simply doesn't get it!

So, you turn to the forum. That is why the site was established. Remember, you are the third shoulder of someone else and they are depending on you for good advice.

• Patience
They say patience is a virtue, but if you're a caregiver it is an absolute necessity. Dealing with the PD patient may be the most taxing job you will ever undertake.

• Tough Love
Learning how to dole out tough love is not an easy task. First, you must distinguish between its traditional definitions and the kind of love required of a Parkinson caregiver. Your patient may not always want to hear your reasoning or explanations, especially when you need to take time out for your own needs.

• A long leash
Even after utilization of tough love it may still be necessary to figuratively tie a long leash to a patient. Keeping in mind that PD patients often exhibit compulsive behavior, the leash becomes an important tool for the caregiver.

• Dealing with compulsive or erratic behaviors
Become well prepared for the "worst case" scenarios by scanning the forum posts. Other caregivers have had plenty of experience and can be of great help when you are at your wits end.

• Family related Issues
Distance, denial, disinterest, distrust and disengagement are just a few alliterative examples of what caregivers can expect from other family members.

• Understanding the Symptoms and Stages of PD
There are numerous sources of information on how Parkinson presents and progresses that are available to caregivers. Use your computer's search engine to review sites containing this information

• Caregiver vs. Home Health Care vs. Nursing Home vs. Hospice
Explore all the alternatives taking into account your own needs as well as those of your family member.

• Access to Psychological Counseling when needed
Parkinson disease care giving is both mentally and physically debilitating. Sharing with a good counselor can help sort out the true priorities of care-giving.

• Post mortem support
Many caregivers have remained with the forum to offer advice to those in need. They can help.

Robert Cummings

US VETERANS & PARKINSON DISEASE

If you are a US veteran & have PD you may be eligible for VA benefits. Veterans who develop Parkinson disease and were exposed to Agent Orange or other herbicides during military service do not have to prove a connection between their disease and military service to be eligible to receive VA disability compensation and health care.

Surviving spouses, dependent children and dependent parents of Veterans who were exposed to herbicides during military service and died as the result of Parkinson disease may be eligible for survivors' benefits.

For more information see:
http://www.publichealth.va.gov/exposures/agentorange/conditions/parkinsonsdisease.asp or call your local VA Hospital.

HUMPTY DUMPTY FELL OFF THE WALL

Approximately one year after my diagnosis, a swan dive in our hallway sent me to the emergency room with two black eyes, multiple bruises and a bloody nose. Then, in December 2009, I repeated my swan dive onto our kitchen floor. This time I needed to call paramedics via the cell phone I kept around my neck as a safety precaution. I had two more black eyes, a bloody nose, multiple bruises and a shattered left elbow. Unable to walk following surgery, I spent 2 ½ months in two hospitals and attempted rehabilitation therapy. Still unable to walk, I was discharged and sent home. Unable to secure round-the-clock home health care, I was faced with the prospect of a nursing home and I decided to document my journey through the first months of a monumental change in my quality of life.

EMERGENCY ROOM QOL

Most readers have probably had some exposure to emergency room services. Crowded waiting rooms, excessive paperwork and endless waiting periods are commonplace. The quickest way into an emergency room is by ambulance, as was the case with my Humpty Dumpty fall. Once inside, I was transferred from the ambulance to a rock hard examination table to await the appearance of one of the 'on-call' staff doctors. Meanwhile, my degenerative-disk-diseased back began to notify me it was not happy!

The staff doctor conducted the usual routine visual examination and the inevitable noting of my general health condition, allergies, pain level, insurance coverage, and so on. He ordered x-rays and suggested an orthopedic surgeon who would be able to interpret the x-rays. Approximately one hour later the surgeon appeared, x-ray in hand, and announced that extensive surgery would be required to repair my shattered elbow.

Another hour passed before I was lifted from the examination table to a gurney for transport to a hospital room. I could have sworn my back said "Thank you". I thought the worst was behind me. I was wrong. The six foot long bed would not accommodate my six foot one frame. An extension piece was ordered. An hour later it arrived.

Meanwhile, Mother Nature advised me she was on schedule and it was that time regardless of my condition. So I hit the call button and waited another half-hour for someone to appear. Unfortunately, Mother Nature waits for no one!

Surgery went well, the elbow was put in a cast, but the black-eyed fox-like look remained for several weeks. Unfortunately my Humpty Dumpty fall caused a spinal trauma that left me unable to walk and I spent the next two and a half weeks lying in a hospital bed. They were not my idea of the quality of life I expected to live following my Parkinson diagnosis.

SKILLED NURSING HOSPITAL QOL

My surgeon advised the rehabilitation process would be a lengthy one. Consequently, I was transferred to a skilled nursing hospital. This transfer marked the beginning of a new quality of life experience.

The hospital included a rehabilitation unit as well as routine hospital care. The rehabilitation unit proved to be more than adequate and the skilled nursing staff was competent, responsive, and patient oriented. Hospitals have never enjoyed a reputation as gourmet eating establishments, nor have they been compared to even two star hotels. Mattresses are usually as comfortable as a slab of concrete, rooms are smaller than oversized closets, and you can expect very little solitude.

To offset changes in quality of my life, I developed a tolerance to things that were not familiar. I resorted to humor to counter much of the dark aspects of being hospitalized. For example, I began to assign nicknames to various staff members. Miss America, Miss Sunshine, Macho Libre, Nurse Rachett, Doctor Death, Nurse Lump Lump, Nurse Goodbody, etc. I renamed a section of rehab 'Guantanamo Bay North' and labeled the group known as certified nurse's aides as "underpaid, underappreciated, and understaffed".

Following a two and one half month rehabilitation stay in the skilled nursing hospital I was discharged for reasons which were not clear to me or my family. It was obvious the staff had little knowledge of PD as we were told my elbow surgery had been satisfactory but that nothing more could be expected because of the complications caused by muscle deterioration. Needless to say, we found the nearest exit and returned to home health care.

Unfortunately, there is an important distinction between typical home health care services and that offered by hospice care providers. The former do not provide services on a 24/7 basis. Parkinson patients must be identified as having end of life difficulties before being eligible for hospice around-the-clock care.

In my case, my caregiver was unable to provide for my physical needs, so we turned to nursing home facilities in the area. Several were identified as accommodating Parkinson patients, but in-depth analysis did not support their claims. However, we discovered that the state of Texas supported a retirement home for veterans that currently included several Parkinson patients. After about three weeks on the waiting list I was fortunate enough to obtain a room at this facility. Once again we contemplated the quality of life changes that we may encounter in this new environment.

This veterans' home does provide a semblance of normal life. It includes a barber shop, a beauty shop, dental facilities, two in-house doctors, links to a nearby Veterans Administration-run laboratory, and prescription filling services. Not surprisingly, the staff and administration seem to be dedicated to the responsibilities associated with caring for veterans. While there is truly no place like home, some "no-places" are better than others.

Robert Cummings

CHANGING NEEDS

SLIP SLIDING AWAY........

I was born in Scranton, Pennsylvania, a coal mining region in the north-east corner of the state. I probably had my first exposure to the toxic world when I stood on a bridge overlooking railroad tracks and inhaled coal dust blowing from the steam engine's bowels.

United States Navy X rays indicated I had a black spot on my lung. While in the navy I served aboard the battleship **Wisconsin** and was exposed to asbestos contamination. Firing our 16 inch guns frequently loosened huge chunks of asbestos including dust now identified as a possible source of toxic contamination. Further possible toxic contamination traced to my duties as a radar operator.

In the 1980's I was first advised of what turned out to be a classic Parkinson disease symptom. One morning, walking to work in downtown Los Angeles, I heard a voice calling my name from behind me. When my colleague caught up with me I asked how he knew it was me. His response was "because you always walk like that" He told me my left arm never moved from inside and I always looked like I was about to turn the corner to my right.

In 2006 a dozen other symptoms appeared. Textbooks defined these symptoms as late onset Parkinson disease. After reading up on it, I was shocked. Not long afterward, I began to face reality. My boyhood dream of "living fast, dying young and having a good looking corpse" was not going to happen. Instead, I would have to prepare myself to endure an ugly ending to an otherwise successful lifetime.

To counterpunch this devastating blow, I decided to accept it, fight it as best I could, and devote the rest of my life to helping others while seeking better treatment and a possible cure for this deadly disease.

So here I am,
78 years young,
slip sliding away as a
collaborator for a book
focused on the patient...

Robert Cummings

183

HELPFUL HINTS FOR PARKINSON CARERS

Here are a few hints that will be useful in caring for your person with Parkinson if mobility is a growing problem........

- Avoid buying clothes with either buttons or zippers.

- Use Velcro fasteners whenever available.

- Check soles of shoes and slippers for non-slip treads.

- Install safety equipment (nonslip strips and grab bars) in the bath tub or shower.

- Discourage use of a cane (walking stick), walker, wheelchair or power chair until absolutely necessary.

- If eating meals becomes a problem consider purchasing special eating utensils and non-spill dishes.

- Subscribe to an emergency alert system or hang a cell phone around the PwP's neck with emergency programming for the 911 operator and/or family members.

- Twist off tops, pop-top cans, candy wrappers, and other packaging can be troublesome for a PwP. Be certain whatever is presented to them can be easily opened.

- If your PwP's speech becomes difficult, try to avoid interrupting. Remember that Parkinson disease is a movement disorder. Everything including speech is in slow motion!

- If your PwP's swallowing becomes difficult, keep the doctor informed. There are techniques and medications available to assist.

- When and if cognition problems are present, deal gently with your PwP.

- Stress is particularly damaging to a PwP. Avoid situations that are stress-related wherever possible.

- Encourage daily exercise. It keeps the mind active and the muscles taut. It is possible to exercise gently even if chair bound.

- Read about the side effects of all drugs being prescribed, remembering to include over-the-counter remedies.

THE LEASH

As my PD symptoms escalate, I have begun wondering about when my caregiver will have to put on "the leash". With my typical male ego, I have steadfastly refused to accept help in managing several PD symptoms. Among the earliest was my inability to deal with the collar buttons on my shirt. Shortly after I found I was unable to zipper my jacket. It took me several weeks and a lot of frustration before I realized I needed assistance.

Not many weeks passed before I realized I could not cut my steak. Fortunately, it was at home and I was at ease with my spouse's help. When the waiter brought me a T-bone at my son's wedding, I was mentally prepared to accept help without feeling embarrassed.

Though I am still somewhat stubborn, I am beginning to realize it will be just a matter of time before my caregiver will be more involved with my personal care. I'm not sure how they know, but our dogs take turns watching me enter and exit from the shower. No doubt they are prepared to signal my spouse when they witness a spill.

Other responsibilities my caregiver has taken over include check writing, tax return preparation and the customary personal notes added to greeting cards. What used to be legible handwriting now appears to be 'Da Vinci code' characters. Imagine how difficult it would be to get into our safe deposit box?

At this moment I am at my stubborn best resisting any talk of taking away the car keys. For me it involves independent contact with an "outside world" still available to me; getting a haircut, doctor's appointments, or possibly even stopping for a donut or hamburger. When I am no longer able to drive I will feel just like one of those dogs when they are put on a leash!

Stubborn? YES! Realistic? YES! I have instructed my caretaker to put on the leash when she feels I am endangering myself or others.

If you have not yet dealt with this important decision - think about the consequences of indecision!

"AIN'T NO MOUNTAIN HIGHER"

With an unknown mountaintop facing both me and my caregiver I feel we must learn to accept the unpredictable progression of this disease and accept the notion that there may not be a higher mountain than this one.

Reflecting on my initial reaction when my neurologist confirmed a Parkinson disease diagnosis, I must admit I had no clue as to what to expect. Much of my early research involved references to the time lines involved in various stages of the disease. It was not until I discovered the Parkinson's Disease Caregiver Information Forum that I began to wonder about how long the journey would be. As I began to reviewed posts on the forum it was apparent many of the caretakers had been providing care and comfort to their patients for years. One post suggested an average of 15 years while others spoke of 25 and 28 years! So naturally, I began to speculate on my own time line. I decided to treat my PD "journey" metaphorically. Each PD stage would be a plateau. As with mountain climbing, the task becomes more difficult as one nears the journey's end. Many never make it to the end.

Given my age, the "good news" is that it is unlikely to be 20 more years of caregiving in my case.

The "not so good news" is that I will not be able to provide my spouse/caretaker with even a guess as to how long she must climb the mountain with me. It appears there is no way to measure the patient's stage and then make a judgment as to remaining time.

What is very clear is that mountain is a heck of a lot higher than I originally thought it to be. The Hoehn and Yahr PD staging lists five stages but does not refer to any time frames. I think I am in either stage 2 or 3 after about 2 years following my own estimate of onset PD. Because I am doing as much as I can to offset the effects of the disease I suspect I could have been classified as a stage 3 by now.

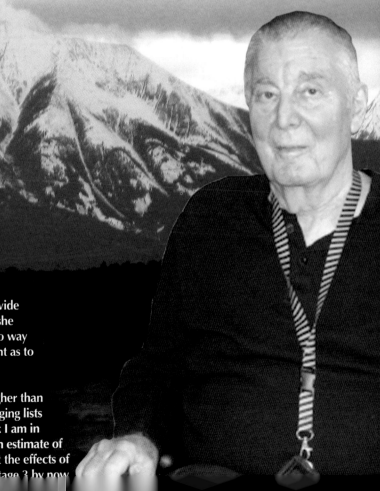

IT IS IMPOSSIBLE TO GIVE OR GUESS AT A TIMELINE FOR PD

OUR JOURNEY WITH PARKINSON DISEASE

Our journey with Parkinson started in August 2001 when Prem was 56. One evening I noticed a tremor in his left hand. My first thought was 'Parkinson!' On checking the Internet I found that he had all the symptoms mentioned, including an early diminishing of the sense of smell. Several doctors we consulted confirmed the diagnosis. He did not realise the gravity of the diagnosis, but I felt as though I'd been hit in the solar plexus.

We chose a neurophysician with a pleasant manner and reputation of being among the best in Calcutta. He prescribed what I now know is quite a heavy initial dosage of Syndopa (local name for levodopa + carbidopa). No alarm bells rang when I mentioned the results of my search saying that Prem had mostly lost his sense of smell and the doctor replied that he knew of no such symptom. We just felt thankful that we had a good doctor. Almost immediately Prem began feeling extremely sleepy, having vivid dreams and hitting out at night. His tremor, however, disappeared and he went into denial. He continued to work at the company where he held a senior managerial position. In India there's often a stigma attached to nervous illnesses, so we kept the diagnosis secret since he did not want any repercussions at work. We decided to travel as much as possible to places we had long wanted to see. We are glad that we did so, as it has now become difficult and we have so many happy memories. In 2006 Prem quit working - he could not cope any more.

I now realise that Prem had some symptoms long before the diagnosis. Constipation started many years earlier. The disappearing sense of smell happened in the early 90s and was soon followed by stiffness in the joints. There were probably some cognitive symptoms too, but it is hard to say with certainty.

Each time we saw the doctor - about three times a year - he tinkered with the medication. He did not like me sharing what I had gleaned from my reading. Prem was soon on rather heavy dosages of Syndopa and in late 2006, he was prescribed an antagonist without the mention of any side effects. In mid-2007 Prem began to have visual hallucinations. They started with cats and dogs, but moved to people sitting about the house, which he found alarming. He found it difficult to manage his own medication. He had two or three episodes of complete disorientation when he was confused about whether he was in our home or elsewhere I was worried, but continued to trust the doctor who now added more medicines. Prem had difficulty sleeping at night so he was on medication for that. He had difficulty in staying awake during the day, so he had medication for that. Late that year our only son returned from studying in the US. I now had someone to share my worries with.

From January 2008, there was a rapid deterioration in Prem's condition. He did not recognise me on some occasions, his hallucinations were constant and vivid and he was paranoid about what he thought was our son's antagonistic attitude to him. We were really alarmed. The doctor sent us to a psychiatrist who upped the dosage of anti-psychotic medication. It was clear that the neuro-physician was floundering. For all his vaunted reputation, he did not seem to have sufficient knowledge about the complexities and ramifications of PD. He advised DBS for Prem, when there is no such option available in Calcutta and when it is not advised for people who are having psychotic problems!

We needed help but Calcutta has no support groups. I sought information and help online. I discovered Parkinson's Information Exchange Network (PIEN) and its sister group for caregivers, CARE. They were of enormous help and urged me to get a second opinion immediately. It was not easy, but we eventually found a young geriatrician recently returned from the UK where he'd been working with PD patients in south Wales. He had a lot of experience with the illness and has proved to be a blessing. He is a doctor who listens and also discusses treatments. He cut back Prem's medication gradually. Slowly the man I had married began to reappear.

Prem has been with Dr. P since 2008. In addition, with his approval, Prem is seeing an excellent Ayurvedic doctor who also has a lot of experience with PD. Ayurveda is the ancient Indian science of medicine with centuries of experience in most illnesses. Its approach to some problems, e.g., constipation, is quite different from conventional medicine. The care of these two experts has helped Prem enormously. He has been relatively stable with hardly any change in medication. He also does yoga three times a week with a personal trainer and tries to walk most evenings. Dr. P has told me that his PD is advanced.

CARE has given emotional support, information and a lot of good advice, which has helped in the management of Prem's illness. Dr. P is supportive of my hopes to start a PD support group in Calcutta but for various reasons, it has not got off the ground. I hope it will in the not too distant future. There is an

CAREGIVERS LIVE WITH THE DILEMMAS OF PD TOO .....

active support organisation in Bombay that has offered help if we can get one going here.

Prem continues to have challenges in his everyday life and my lifestyle has inevitably undergone many changes. I have also learned to have far more patience than I was born with. A cure is not going to happen in our lifetimes, but my hope is that we can continue to ensure for Prem optimal quality of life as the illness progresses. There is a team of us working on this – the doctors, the yoga trainer, the domestic and other help I am fortunate to have, and myself - so perhaps we will manage it.
Moneesha Sharma,
wife of and caregiver to Prem.
Calcutta, India.

Editor's note: Moneesha wrote this in May 2011. Prem passed away suddenly on December 21st 2012

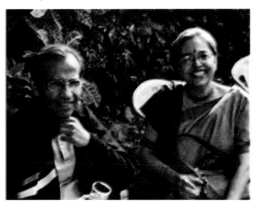

**Prem &
Moneesha**

We needed help but Calcutta has no support groups.

I sought information and help online. They were of enormous help and urged me to get a second opinion immediately.

LIVING WILLS:
WHO WILL SPEAK FOR YOU?

You never thought it would happen: ending up in the hospital with with tubes coming out of every hole in in your body - you can't even talk because there is something filling your throat. Your brain isn't working right and is fuzzy from all of the pain medicine they have been giving you. Where are your PD meds? You are totally off and can't tell anyone! How will you ever convince them how you want to be treated? The door opens and in walks the person you chose to make medical decisions for you if you couldn't. You try to smile, then close your eyes and relax into the bed, knowing your advocate will communicate your needs.

That fictional scenario had a happy ending but many times, without advance directives (which consist of a living will containing your preferences for medical care in certain situations plus a medical power of attorney which authorizes your selected person to act for you) no one speaks for the patient. Without a legally authorized person to make medical decisions for you, the doctors may substitute their own judgment, pursuing treatment beyond your desires. In extreme cases, the hospital might seek a court order authorizing a judge or a court appointee to make your health care decisions.

If you want to decide who speaks for you when you can't, you must follow the local rules and laws to authorize your advocate properly. It is especially important to have these documents in order if you are a single person. Usually any hospital or large medical center will have free copies of the locally approved documents available in their admissions office. You should choose someone who will respect your wishes, voice them strongly and be available to be your advocate when you are unable to speak for yourself. When you've identified the right person, take the time to discuss your wishes fully. Also, make sure your chosen person is comfortable with any end-of-life medical decisions you make.

In addition to these documents, if you are ill at home and want a Do Not Resuscitate Order (DNR), aka Out-of-hospital DNR or Comfort Care Only Order, make sure you ask your doctor for information about the process of obtaining one at home. Usually DNR orders last only until you leave the hospital unless you rescind them sooner. If you want emergency medical technicians who might respond to a call to your house to respect your wishes, you must obtain an Out-of-hospital DNR and have it placed in a very visible position in your home. **Katherine Huseman**

CALVIN'S STORY

In Sickness.............
Peggy Willocks

I tried to help Calvin and his wife several times, but neither of them "got it." They just thought he could take a pill and everything would be better. Calvin has had all sorts of complications from the meds (severe dyskinesia from L-dopa, hallucinations from agonists, etc.). Because of his age, his symptoms had been exacerbated to the point that he needed full-time nursing care. His second wife (his first died of cancer) Sally was the great hostess. She could put out a gourmet meal in a matter of minutes. When Sally was no longer needed to entertain, due to Calvin's deteriorating condition, she went downhill rapidly, losing over 50 pounds which she didn't really have to lose.

I recall Calvin telling me, "Sally is depressed." He and I both knew the main reason. About 2-3 months ago, Calvin, Sally and their families decided it would be in Sally's best interest for her to go back to Ohio to live with her daughter. Calvin, of course, is here in the local nursing home. I haven't seen him in a while, but when I do he is usually covered with food stains, drools, sits humped over with a blank stare. A brilliant man. He has authored several books, and has been published in about every theology periodical known to mankind. He should be writing right now; instead he has Parkinson.

Preparing for brain surgery, I made all of my funeral arrangements; I knew the risk that I was taking. Calvin wasn't just an accomplished author, but an eloquent orator. I wanted him to speak at my funeral. It is highly doubtful that Calvin could still deliver that service for me. His situation causes me to focus on what the future holds for me and my family. After 16 years of living with this debilitating illness, I am certain that my future cannot be counted in decades - maybe not even in months. One bad fall, or choking on food, can bring it all to an end.

I really need to visit Calvin today, on his birthday. If I can give him one ray of hope, or empathize with him, maybe it would help to soften the harsh reality of his life. Calvin was a creative thinker, as was Ralph Waldo Emerson. "Happy Birthday" isn't appropriate; but maybe this quote is:

"The glory of friendship is not the outstretched hand, not the kindly smile, not the joy of companionship; it is the spiritual inspiration that comes to one when he discovers that someone believes in him and is willing to trust him with his friendship."

--Ralph Waldo Emerson

His situation causes me to focus on what the future holds for me and my family.

After 16 years of living with this debilitating illness, I am certain that my future cannot be counted in decades - maybe not even in months. One bad fall, or choking on food, can bring it all to an end.

THE STRANGER I'VE BECOME

Since we are just mortals, sooner or later we come to terms with the fact that we are going to age and die. Accepting that reality is definitely a challenge and sometimes when my peers and I chat, we commiserate on how the unthinkable has happened. We're certifiably old compared to a majority of fellow human beings and we can't believe it!

Do I mind getting older? Of course I do, but what really gets me is Parkinson has greased the slide. Today I was at physical therapy for a bad back and as the therapist worked on me, I remarked how I was not the person I was twelve years ago. He didn't answer and I guess he was thinking to himself, "No duh! Who is?" I realized the futility of telling a temporarily healthy therapist what I really meant. I was not just losing my youth; I had become an entirely different person. This wasn't just an older me. This was an older other . . .

We all have to deal with aging, but sometimes I don't recognize the being I live within. My face still looks like me, but I stand crooked. My shoulders do not line up. Where once I had exercised daily, I can now barely move when I am trying to, and can't stop moving when I least want it. I had been a top student as a young person. Now I panic about my ability to think, taking IQ tests off the Internet to reassure myself. I once had a great interest in my family, but now I am often inattentive to their conversations. Job or task completion once drove me to accomplish more. Now I feel as if I am drifting through life without a sail, or rudder, or navigation tool. I didn't worry about the future back then, but now I try not to even think of it. Although I have a patient and helpful husband, I know that only I get to live every moment of the rest of my life with this stranger I have become.

How am I coping? Well, somewhere I read that Ritalin could wake us out of the apathy that is part and parcel of our disease - but I rely on sheer determination to stay focused on tasks, talking to myself sternly as I do housework, or school work, or bills, or projects, all of which seem to never get completed to the satisfaction of the former me. I try to lighten up when I am with others, because I don't want to become the dullard I fear I might become. I work hard at it, trying to keep not only my body intact, but my personality as well. I am trying to find the person I once was. I am really trying.

To paraphrase Emily Dickinson; uninvited, Parkinson stopped for me even though I never considered such a circumstances as even a remote possibility. Time for the uninvited guest to leave. Time for a cure. **Ann T**

INVITED OUT? NO THANKS - I AM A "PARKIE"

Thanks for the invitation. Frankly I would like to get out each and every day but this disease presents certain obstacles preventing me from doing so.

X **I walk funny. I am bent over like a pretzel. I sometimes fall down and cannot get up without help.**

X **Like a sinking ship, I cannot stand straight and lean mostly to my right.**

X **I drool a lot. Sometimes into my meal. Sometimes on someone else's furniture.**

X **I cannot eat with ordinary utensils. I use a custom designed tablespoon.**

X **I cannot fasten my passenger side seat belt.**

X **Restaurant seating can be a nightmare.**

X **Public rest rooms are equally problematic.**

X **I don't smile much anymore. My poker face prevails most of the time.**

X **I am perpetually in slow motion. "Hurry up" is not in my vocabulary.**

X **I cannot dress or undress myself.**

X **I cannot bathe myself.**

X **I require assistance in getting in or out of beds.**

X **I can neither print nor handwrite except in very large block letters.**

X **I experience extreme fatigue whenever I travel anywhere.**

Bob Cummings

CARING....AND CAREFUL

Nighttime is the worst. My husband lost the ability to sleep soundly or well long ago, and the lack of sleep has taken a toll on both of us. For over 30 years the late hours were for loving, snuggling, listening to the rain, having endless conversations, making plans, and laughing at the antics of, first, our children, and then, our beloved grandchildren. But most of all, Tom was a great sleeper and the night was peaceful and restful.

Like a thief in the night, Parkinson's has had its way with him, though he continues to resist with every ounce of strength he has.

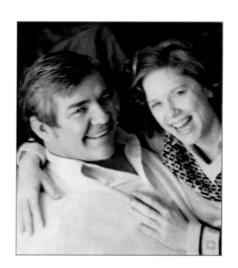

Nighttime now is full of countless trips to the bathroom, restlessness, yelling in his sleep, asking for a drink or snack, and taking medicine. Every move he makes sets off jarring alarm bells throughout my body, and I rise quickly to make certain he doesn't fall, or forget where he is and attempt to wander. Despite my being only inches from him, he falls often anyway. I try to hold back my tears as I get him up, bandage his wounds and help him back to bed. I am not a large person, but I can almost always pick him up by myself! On occasion, I have to call the fire department for help, but they never seem to mind. They are grand people and a great blessing to us.

It's hard to describe how it feels to watch the person you have shared your life with suffer through a debilitating illness. At various times I feel guilty that it is happening to him and not to me, and sad that the marvelous adventure we shared is over, and has been replaced with something else entirely. I am often depressed, lonely, and fearful.

My biggest fear is that it will end badly, instead of peacefully. I simply can't bear watching him suffer.

My second fear is that there was something medically that could have helped him but I wasn't smart enough to figure it out. But this is what I fear the most when I am awake at night – that our children might think I didn't give enough, do enough, love enough, or that I failed him in some way. Daytime is the greatest! A new day brings the possibility of happiness and comfort for my precious husband.

Our children have circled their wagons of love tightly around us, and instead of worrying that I have failed, they worry about me. I do not deserve this grace, but cheerfully accept!

Our children have circled their wagons of love tightly around us and instead of worrying that I have failed, they worry about me. I do not deserve this grace, but cheerfully accept! Friends and family members come over almost daily to check on him and make him smile. For this, I am eternally in their debt.

So many wonderful people make it a point to tell me that they admire my care and concern for him, but that is not the truth.

The truth is that we don't get to choose the role we are cast in, and I am simply doing my best and hoping it is enough. Sure, I'm a little tired and a little cranky at times! But what does that matter compared to the daily struggle my husband endures? He has the disease, I don't. Please just keep loving him and that will be all that we need!

Phyllis Glaze

TELL THEM TO CARE
TELL THEM WE ARE THEM...

Tell them it's like having a tiny bit of the oil that makes it possible for you to move, or not move, or think, or care, or understand, or remember; it's like having a tiny bit of that oil leak out of you each and every day. In the beginning, you don't notice it because you have plenty of oil and even the first symptoms that begin to appear when the oil gets too low go unrecognized, because they are no different from the odd little misfires and clumsiness that we all experience now and again, all the time.

One or more symptoms appear that cannot be ignored and you realize that something is wrong. You don't think it's anything serious, but it is odd, and you go to the doctor or mention it the next time you see him.

A doctor will tell you, or refer you to someone who will tell you, that you have a disease - Parkinson disease - and tell you that there are medications that will control your disease and allow you to live a normal life.

For a while, he or she is almost right. The medications do help you and perhaps for a while you don't even notice those symptoms that took you to the doctor. But the doctor may not tell you that your medications have side effects, sometimes nasty ones, and that eventually your medications will slowly start to lose the war against your disease. Your medications are not intended to cure you, or even to help you slow the progress of your disease, because they can't. They can only hide your symptoms from you and from those around you. They can only do that for a while. You have an incurable, progressive, degenerative brain disease, and that is that.

Gradually your symptoms begin to pop-up again like mushrooms after the rain. You take more medications or different medications and it helps, for a while. Then, after a few years, or many years, or several years, the help they give diminishes and the symptoms that you have become more apparent and continue to grow. The oil is still leaking out at the same rate and the medications simply fool you into the feeling that you are a more or less healthy human being.

Gradually, like a poorly running motor, you have days or hours when your medications don't work at all and you can't move, or you can't stop moving, or you can't think clearly, or speak well enough to be understood, or standup, or walk. Then things get better for a few hours, or a few days, or a few minutes because your medications

are working again. Then they stop.

You learn to accept misery as a periodic companion. A periodic companion who becomes a more frequent visitor with each passing day. Soon it is no longer a visitor but your closest companion, a shadow that inhabits you once or twice or five times a day and doesn't tell you when it's going to leave.

Eventually there's so little oil that the medications cannot keep the motor running very well at all. You cannot walk right, or speak well, or remember things, or stop moving, or start moving, or turnover in bed, or get out of a chair, or feed yourself, or swallow without choking, or overcome your depression or your apathy, or hold your wife's hand, or touch her as a partner needs and wants to be touched, or smile.

Sometimes you decide you have had enough and you kill yourself. Most of the time you simply survive. You hang on, because you never realized how much suffering you were capable of living with. You wait in hope that somebody will find a cure for your disease, but they haven't yet.

After a few more years, or many more years, or next year, you swallow a bit of meat that you can't get out of your throat in time, or you fall and break a bone that does not heal, or you get pneumonia, or you hit your head in a fall and go into a coma and never come out of it. Or you slowly, slowly, slowly lose the ability to do anything and you simply cease to be.

Tell them (the drug company reps) that this is Parkinson. Tell them they are not selling candy or furniture or cars. Tell them they have a special responsibility to understand the world that the people they sell their medications to inhabit. Tell them that they have a special responsibility to understand the courage that the people they sell their drugs to show year after year after year as they get worse and worse and worse. Tell them we are not little profit centers. Tell them we are their brothers and sons and mothers and friends and uncles and aunts and fathers. Tell them to do their jobs in a way that allows them to sleep well at night.

Tell them that we need their help as we fight to save ourselves. Tell them to care. Tell them we are them.
Greg Wasson

CHALLENGES 8 YEARS
AFTER DIAGNOSIS . . . AND A TRIP TO THE PAN FORUM

Dear Family,

Thanks for your good Valentine wishes and the pretty and enjoyable package in which they arrived. Sorry I couldn't get myself together to choose and do the same. After going to the Parkinson's Action Network 13th Annual Forum at a Capitol Hill hotel on Saturday and staying until Monday night, I'm still feeling pretty beat-up, mostly due to the still-recovering hip (replaced in 2006 due to osteoarthritis). I knew I wouldn't hold up for the actual visits the next day to Congress to lobby my Representative and Senators - the Hill is NOT friendly to the mobility-challenged - so in light of the weather forecast, asked hubby to come and get me after his Monday evening class in Baltimore. I might have shared my girl friend's scholarship-funded room for another day, but I'm awfully glad he made the sacrifice of driving so late on a work night. Huge rooms full of loudly chattering people, never much fun for any but the natural-born politician, are getting harder and harder to tolerate and keeping focused on the speakers had about run its course, too. My girl friend is often quite impaired now, but we did enjoy each other's company tremendously. We also spent some nice, relaxed time with other old and new friends, avoiding the bigger parties that the young, even with PD, seem to need.

The highlight of the Forum, for me and I think for almost everyone, was a talk by Dr. J. William Langston of the Parkinson's Institute. You know him, don't you? He spoke on "Parkinsons Complex: the Tip of the Iceberg." He said that by the time the disease reaches the substantia nigra, the brain layer that controls movement, it has already run half its course, and then after 80% of that layer is destroyed, enough symptoms appear that diagnosis is possible. The look of "aha!" on faces all over the room was almost overwhelming to see. Many must have been thinking, "I told you I was sick!", or "So that's what was wrong with me!" I knew bits and pieces of this before, but his thesis was so clear; my whole life flashed in front of me, from being a pokey, inattentive child, to my first husband's frustration that I moved so slowly (some people are just slow-paced, I tried to believe), to not getting a job I wanted because I sat so still they didn't believe I was putting out enough effort, to sitting and sitting while my toddler played at my feet, knowing I should MOVE. I think of the self-help books I bought to figure out what was wrong with me, even though I knew I was saner than most. Doctor after doctor couldn't see the whole picture - seven of them on three continents for my foot problems alone - Who knew to send me to a neurologist? The thyroid tests I asked for all came up normal (and still do). I felt wrong, off, a misfit, even though I was perfectly healthy in any way that can be measured. I feel very sad right now for all the lost relationships and the unclimbed mountains, both literal and figurative. I have always felt like I wasted so much, but now I can proceed with forgiving myself, not that I can blame all my faults and shortcomings on illness. This day I have spent on 'might-have-beens', along with my aches and pains from a strange bed, is drawing to a close. Maybe we all need something to rise above.

I live a blessed life and I know it. I'm thankful most of all for the spiritual riches that our parents and my dear sister passed on to me and for their love and the love that pours over me from our children. I will continue to minister to those who are ill, especially with something chronic, and learn to be even more grateful for the times when I have to wait for myself. While I'm being philosophical, a big "Thanks be to God" for my dear husband, who waits beside me. I love you very much and I'll try to keep it lighter next time. **JL Wheeler**

MAYBE WE ALL NEED SOMETHING TO RISE ABOVE

Home Health versus Nursing Home versus Retirement Home

When the time comes to seek additional assistance, it appears that little information is available to caregivers and their patients. As a Stage V patient now in a veterans retirement facility I have elected to offer my views on this difficult choice.

To establish my credentials, readers should know that my care has included family care, home health care, skilled nursing home care and retirement home care.

HOME CARE

Family care was provided when my symptoms included difficulties with basic hygiene, dressing and undressing, eating meals and balance and gait problems.

My cancer-surviving spouse experienced great difficulties with those tasks on a round-the-clock basis. To ease her burden we included a home health care facility offering aid on a daily basis. This proved to be more than satisfactory.

Properly credentialed certified nurse's assistants came daily to assist me from my bed, shave and shower me and dress me for breakfast. Blood pressure, pulse and oxygen levels were also checked. My family caregiver was responsible for meal preparation, serving and assistance as required.

At that time I was ambulatory and had a walker and wheelchair at my disposal. To assist me with gait and balance conditioning a licensed physical therapist visited three times a week.

Finally, home healthcare service provided a registered nurse on a weekly basis to check vital signs, check my general condition and consult with my caregiver. All were covered under Medicare part B, supplemental health insurance and nominal co-pay.

Following a fall, I occupied a hospital bed for two and a half weeks before being assigned to a skilled nursing facility. Many nursing homes are certified for skilled nursing facilities as are most retirement homes.

SKILLED NURSING CARE

Skilled nursing care includes rehabilitation and various medical and nursing procedures. Written policies and protocols are formulated with appropriate professional consultation. Law requires that these policies designate which level of caregiver is responsible for implementation of each policy, that the care of every patient be under the supervision of a physician, that a physician be available on an emergency basis, that records of the condition and care of every patient be maintained, that nursing service be available 24 hours a day and at least one full-time registered nurse be employed.

Other criteria stipulate that the facility have appropriate capacity for storing and dispensing drugs and a use review plan; that all licensing requirements of the state in which it is located be met; and that the overall budget be maintained.

As must be apparent, the choice of a skilled nursing home is of paramount importance. A review of facilities in your area (well in advance of the need) is advised. We were fortunate to have several skilled nursing facilities available. One in particular included extensive rehabilitation facilities, prompting my caregiver to transfer me. For those readers who are computer literate, I recommend searching for skilled nursing facilities in your locale. My state, Texas, offers a detailed analysis. Similar information may be available in your state.

For PwP, I strongly recommend enrolling in a rehabilitation program. The value of exercise cannot be overstated. I was unable to walk after my injury. Initial rehabilitation was basic with rudimentary arm and leg exercises. Within a week I was bicycling 20 minutes daily. I graduated to a walker and after several more weeks was able to do 100 yards using the walker.

The nursing home facility operated more like a hospital then a nursing home. Staff included a resident physician, registered nurses, vocational nurses and nurse aides. Patient care was adequate but far from outstanding. The message here is clear; "research, investigate and choose wisely".

Following my stay at the skilled nursing facility we decided to return to home healthcare. Unfortunately,

Stage V PwP require round-the-clock care and it was difficult to recruit people to work overnight. This is a drawback to the use of home care providers. Another alternative was available. The state of Texas sponsors a retirement home for veterans. After a short wait, I was admitted to this skilled nursing retirement home. I have been a resident for 4 months. What follows is based on my limited experiences there. I hope this will provide a little information to help those seeking retirement facilities in making their choice.

RESEARCH YOUR OPTIONS
AND MAKE A VISIT

Before making a visit to nursing homes and retirement facilities I recommend using a computer search to find basic information. Following a statistical analysis that included starred ratings, my caretaker and I visited several places and after careful consideration decided on a veterans retirement facility located 35 miles from home.

Most retirement homes provide a standard list of amenities coupled with optional alternatives. Probably the most important consideration is that of privacy. Typically, semi-private rooms are abundant. I had to wait 3 weeks before obtaining the private room needed to help develop this book. Private rooms include a shower, unlike the community facility available to others. TV is available in rooms and in some dining and recreational areas.

The next most important consideration is FOOD. I capitalize the word because it is the topic most talked about in group conversations. With varying tastes, diets and medical conditions, one can only imagine the nature of the dialogue. Planning the weekly menu must be as daunting as the creation of the atomic bomb. The resident must be prepared to accept the best and worst culinary capabilities and limitations. In this home away from home, I was able to request favorite dishes, desserts and breakfast cereals.

Ranking close to the top of your list should be a discussion with administrators concerning the duties and responsibilities of people charged with care and comfort. In this facility, primary care is a responsibility of a nursing supervisor, registered nurse and licensed vocational nurse, with assistance provided by certified nurse assistants.

As you would expect, a nurse assistant job is labor-intensive, particularly in a retirement home. CNA positions require dedicated, caring and personable individuals. Unfortunately, lacking credentials, they are underpaid, overworked and misunderstood. Turnover rates are high and burnout is common. A hot topic at our 'town hall' meetings for residents, is call-light response time. Many residents expect the impossible.... immediate response. Most of the service staff here suggest 10 to 15 minutes is reasonable.

You should check out activities, recreational facilities and available services. Usually retirement homes include a recreation area, an activity center and conference facilities. Many have libraries, computer access, barber and beauty shops. Many include physical and occupational therapy units. In this one, contractors are employed, as required, for the special needs of residents.

If the resident is elderly, confined to bed, or handicapped in any way you should discuss what special assistance is available. Power chairs, wheelchairs, walkers etc., may be available as a part of your package, or on a rental basis.

Heating and air conditioning utilities can present special difficulties for residents. The age-old expression "different strokes for different folks" applies. Some residents seem to be dressed like Eskimos, while others appear in the dining hall in shorts!

Ask and investigate until all your questions are answered. **Robert Cummings**

The message here is clear; "research, investigate and choose wisely"

Editor's note: When looking for care facilities, seek opinions and reviews from many sources including your support group members, community friends and acquaintances and others. Be aware of whether the info is current or long past. If you are a family member helping with this from a distance or need help for any reason, there may be social workers in your area who are knowledgable and available through a local government service or on a fee basis.

SOME SELECTED PARAGRAPHS FROM 'SPIRITUALITY'

Lurkingforacure

I read somewhere that the difference between being religious and being spiritual is that religious people fear hell, while spiritual people have already lived through it. I have a lot of thoughts about spirituality, especially with the PD card we have been dealt, as I am sure many here do. No need to get into all of those, I just wanted to share this, because for some reason I cannot explain, this distinction between religion and spirituality gives me comfort.

One thing PD does, is to force you to focus your energy and attention on those things that are most important to you, which unfortunately also exposes a great many problems in this world that we previously may have been blissfully unaware of. I can't believe some of the things I used to think were important, now THAT was sick! I may be going out on a limb posting on this, but if anyone gets comfort from this distinction, it's worth it.

Jaye

A younger friend once suggested that if I didn't feel as if I had faith, I could be thankful I had other gifts of the Spirit, such as love and hospitality.

I have observed one way to get into spirituality is to learn to still the Self and permit the Presence to make itself known. It can take 15 minutes or 15 years of practice to get to the point of occasional bubbling joy in the wake of one of these experiences. PD speeds up the process, maybe.

What some Christians call Contemplative or Centering Prayer, or The Practice of the Presence of God and the experience of Buddhist Meditation as taught to me by a Theravada monk seem to be related to each other.

Silence is important, but it means silence of the mind   "Ask and it will be given to you" generally refers to spiritual things more than to a Mercedes Benz. Spiritual disciplines like the use of prayer beads or regular prayers read at certain hours from a book can be useful in leaving the Self/Ego behind and attending to the Divine.

Looking at my life in a spiritual way and trying to live it from that point of view is the only thing that keeps me sane. It's not a constant high by any stretch of the imagination, but it has lifted me out of a few ditches.

Shake 'Em Up

Lessons from my cat Sunny

As life becomes more difficult, I find I have to dig deeper into my inner resources to find those grains of hope. The other morning I realized that my cat Sunny was sharing his way with me: rest, breathe deeply, unclench my fists, let my heart sing and allow myself to feel the beauty in every moment.

I have a long way to go to get it, but I'm working on it. Aren't we all.

THROUGH THE LOOKING GLASS - ALL THE WAY!!

Borrowing from **Alice in Wonderland** we have stepped through the looking glass and presented topics largely from the patient's point of view.

I intend to step through the looking glass one more time - this time all the way!

First, I would like to tackle some perceptions concerning mental health issues.

It seems to me the prevailing public view of patients afflicted with Parkinson disease is that it is a mental disorder as evidenced by such things as tremors, dyskinesia and dystonia.

PwP frequently are faced with these perceptions as they attempt to live normal lives. Balance and gait symptoms tend to reinforce their views. Prominent public people with Parkinson are ridiculed as punch drunk or overacting. Terms like dopamine, substantia nigra, and essential tremors are not a part of the average person's vocabulary. They simply do not know. That is a part of our mission.

Next, we should deal with the double D's (depression and dementia).

Neurologists, psychologists and yes, even primary care physicians, often have a series of exercises or questions designed to help identify symptoms of either depression or dementia. One would think it does not take a proverbial rocket scientist to predict the probability of some form of depression with patients diagnosed with Parkinson disease.

When advised "there are no survivors" what would you expect of your patient if you were a medical professional? Dementia, on the other hand, is a distinctly definable mental disorder. Parkinson patients diagnosed early in life seldom if ever show signs of dementia. It's us older folks that trip the switch from short-term memory loss to more profound lapses that may be the onset of dementia. In our case it is not a mental disorder, but in our opinion as patients, just plain aging.

The next subject is more delicate and one which my collaborators seem to want to avoid.

However I scanned postings from a caregivers forum as well as NeuroTalk's postings and found many patient-related discussions on compulsive behaviors. Based on my reading, I'm inclined to believe that they are more than prevalent in Parkinson patients, especially among the elderly. Posts detail compulsive behaviors including alcoholism, gambling addiction, shopping addiction, compulsive sexual behavior, and other obsessive-compulsive behaviors.

A key issue tends to compound the controversy. Is it a symptom or a by product of treatment? Debate rages on.

Finally, and regretfully, let's now turn to the very delicate subject of suicide.*
Quite naturally PwP are not inclined to discuss this issue, particularly since most contemplating this rash act are already severely depressed. A recently published book dealing with suicide of a family member illustrated much of what needs to be discussed in forums offered to both caretakers and patients. It is titled Imperfect Endings, by Zoe Fitzgerald Carter and I recommend it.

Robert Cummings

* If you or anyone you know are dealing with any of the issues on this page seek help **immediately** from a qualified professional or call your local social service agency for a referral.

LOSING A FRIEND

I had just visited my friend, who was in the final stages of Parkinson disease. My mental picture of her kept flashing in my mind. She had been unable to swallow since Tuesday; today was Friday. As I entered her room I saw an NG tube attached to her bottle of milky nourishment. Her frail body was covered to the waist by a sheet and her bare arms formed the top border. Her mouth was open to allow breathing, as the tube obstructed one of her nostrils.

I took her bony hand, warm from a slight fever and looked into her searching eyes. She was glad to see me. She had not been able to eat normally for four days. A swallowing test had revealed she was aspirating food into her lungs. Though she had been unable to speak for years, she could point to the letters on her 'communication board' and by trial and error she was able to tell me that a feeding tube had been refused. I wondered if she really knew what this meant.

We two were in our own little world, which was not unusual. I was doing well, I was being strong for her. Then she asked me to pray. I did so . . . from the heart. Quietly, under my breath, I asked God to not let her suffer any more. The nurses sat her up in a chair. She didn't open her eyes, but squeezed my hand to acknowledge my presence. Again I secretly prayed for God to not let her suffer much longer. The nourishment drip had been stopped.

I returned to the familiar room where I had spent the last 3 years attempting to create hope in a person whose desire to live was great, though the disease that ravaged her body was greater. Her husband gently placed her frail body back on her bed. I could see that her face was extremely pale and her once rigid body was now limp. I could see she had gone.

The nurse said she had checked her a few minutes earlier and had found a pulse and asked us if the family wanted her to perform CPR. After a moment's silence her husband looked to me - not so much for an answer, but a validation that the only answer possible was 'No'.

I retell this story for two reasons: 1) everyone should have a living will, and 2) we must do ALL within our power to find a cure for this and other neurological diseases.

When my friend passed from this life, her death certificate didn't say 'Parkinson disease' it said 'Pneumonia'. She only lived 6 years from diagnosis, and I only knew her for the final three. She had a rapidly-progressing type of Parkinson, never definitively diagnosed, possibly one of the Parkinson-Plus syndromes. I stayed with her weekly, often more than that. Within 2 years of diagnosis she had lost her voice, began to have extreme trouble with walking and rising from a sitting position and then started to fall often. Her final month saw her totally immobile, unable to swallow - and only able to open one eye. She died of aspiration pneumonia and kidney failure.

Some time later her husband and I visited her grave. I remembered my friend. She had loved nice clothes, make-up, jewelry, things she thought made her beautiful. When she was unable to move, trapped in a body that was skin and bones and all those things were taken away, she was still beautiful. I noticed a strong breeze blowing from SW to NE, the same way it blew here the year before. I reminded her husband of this, and said, "Do you remember that the wind blew this way last year? The balloons we released blew over the horizon just like this and nearly everyone standing here said together, 'She's free at last.'"

After a few moments of silence, we made our way back to our cars and drove away. We may be able to walk away from a gravesite, but we cannot walk away from death.

Peggy Willocks

Death isn't so bad.
But missing her will be.

Spiritual support in PD:

An instant messaging conversation in the night, between two people who have met in person only once or twice.

M: PLEASE SAY A PRAYER FOR ME
J: Anything in particular?
or I think I can put one together.

M: PEACE

M: BREATH
J: Dear intimate friend God our lover, who heals microscopically and rules universally, we love your healing ways and the whole-ness you bring to our lives, our hearts, our bodies. Your servant M lies in distress, loving you and yearning for your healing touch.

Send her, Lord, all comfort, peace and rightness of body, mind and spirit, as only you can give. Let her feel your touch. Let her snuggle as a child in your arms.

M: LOVELY
J: Let her body be aligned with your will.

M: AMEN
J: Let her heart be given to all others, to return to you and be given back to her again in her quiet rest. In the name of that holiness which gives us the gift of healing. Amen

M: AMEN and for my spiritual partner here with me, the same healing infusion of your love. AMEN

J: Amen

M: SLEEP

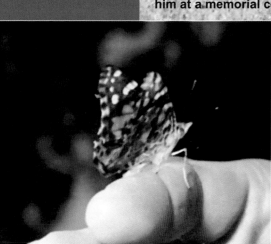

Butterfly

It was a long journey, twenty-two years of Parkinson disease with clinical trials, advocacy, pain. My partner had endured all of this until his death at age 68. He held on waiting for a cure, none came. He had accepted this disease without complaint, but with patience and class. He never gave up until the end and his last contribution to the disease was to donate his brain to research. I was invited to pay tribute to him at a memorial celebration, which I was thrilled to do. I wanted others to know him as I did. While we were seated, listening to a lovely guitarist, a beautiful large black and orange butterfly landed on the stage in front of us.

My friend and I glanced at each other, with questioning looks. It did not move, even as people went by. There was to be a butterfly release at the end of the tribute; however, this was an adult and when it did not move from the stage, so close to the performer, we were concerned. I had only seen butterflies fly, never stay in one spot for an extended period of time. My thoughts were, perhaps it was waiting for the rest of the program. I went to the podium to give my thoughts, the butterfly stayed there until the end. I knew this was my partner; he had passed away one month before and I had waited for some sign from him.

Here it was; he had promised me something. I silently said, "I love you. Good-bye."

We were in awe of this experience and I will remember it forever.
Gerry Haines

199

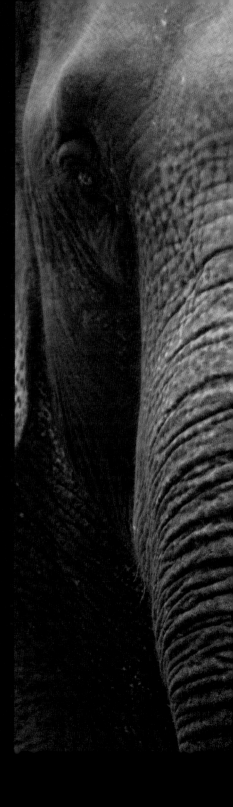

THE THINGS WE FEAR MOST

The things important to us are dependent on any number of factors. These factors are as varied as the people to whom they apply. For People with Parkinson disease quality of life is often measured by neurologists based on how well our motor symptoms are being controlled. Psychosocial issues involved with this disease are often mistakenly thought to be less important or to have a lesser affect on the way we perceive life than the physical symptoms, but more often than not, the psychosocial problems are the ones that make the difference between living and living.

When those of us with PD are asked what concerns us most, motor symptoms like tremor, rigidity and balance come in a distant second to the non-motor symptoms of depression, sexual dysfunction, memory loss, decreased cognition, loss of executive function and dementia. They are the conditions that most profoundly determine the level of satisfaction with our lives. From the perspective of a Movement Disorders Specialist or any neurologist, the first priority is to control motor symptoms. After all, that is their training. That is where they are best able to affect change. Considering how Parkinson disease is diagnosed and treated today, it is not surprising that the non-motor symptoms take a back seat to the impediments to smooth movement. The losses we suffer as a result of ever worsening motor symptoms seem almost insignificant when compared to the losses entailed in worsening psychosocial symptoms like memory loss and depression.

Being so depressed that we are unable to carry out the activities of daily living or having memory loss so severe that we are unable to recognize friends or family members represent the kind of reduction in the quality of life that causes the idea of being in a wheelchair to pale by comparison. Seeing a marriage dissolve as a result of sexual dysfunction or a promising career disappear due to the loss of executive function are things we don't want to think about or talk about even with those closest to us.

COGNITIVE DETERIORATION

Money will not be directed to discovering remedies for these quality of life issues until the ones in charge of funding research realize that it is not dying we are afraid of, it is dying badly.

Of course the six hundred pound gorilla that is always in the room is that most dreaded non-motor symptom, dementia. Dementia is defined as cognitive and intellectual deterioration, but that doesn't begin to cover the emotional horror that the word conjures. The prospect of dementia is a specter that hangs over each of us from the time of our diagnosis until the day we die, because only then are we certain we will not fall prey to this horrid condition.

Cognitive deterioration can rob us of our families, our friends, our pride, our dignity, our talents, our passions and our hopes. It can leave us unable to communicate and unable to care for ourselves in even the most basic way. Dementia eventually robs us of our capacity for joy and leaves us with a live body and a dead soul. It is evidence of the truth in the statement "there are worse things than being dead."

These are the things that many PwP fear most, the things we want the research to concentrate on and the things we want cured. These are the things we want to be assured are not being caused by the medication prescribed to control the tremors, rigidity and balance problems. Many of us are willing to give up smooth motor function if it means we can maintain those cognitive functions that largely determine the quality of our lives. Each and every one of us can participate in altering the priorities of the research.

Through personal advocacy we can contribute to a change in the way Parkinson disease is defined, diagnosed and treated. The method can be as simple as telling our neurologist about changes in any of the areas of psychosocial functioning and making sure they are aware of our apprehensions about them. Until the medical community becomes collectively informed of the importance of these issues to us, the emphasis of the research will remain the same that it has been for forty years. Money will not be directed to discovering remedies for these fundamental life issues until the ones in charge of funding research realize that it is not dying we are afraid of, it is dying badly. Pam Kell

Finding a collective voice for shared concerns

She found that was still able to do many things but was not able to work all day. She needed to time medicine for maximum effectiveness. She needed real breaks to 'recharge' her battery. In spite of that, she wanted to wear out and not rust out. She wanted to use time well, to belong and contribute.

She joined a support group. She went to an awareness event. She'll always remember the feeling of belonging when she saw many PwP and their supporters. There was information about about many different groups.

When she returned home, she checked further and chose the PD organization whose mission closely echoed her own philosophy. She got involved and raised her voice for the cause and felt better - tired but alive and still needed. She told her less mobile friends of her work and helped them write letters in support - it got them all involved.

In this chapter you will find a brief history of how some PwP connected, organised using the internet, and launched advocacy campaigns that helped start a world wide movement.

If you're as strong as those living with PD, read on.

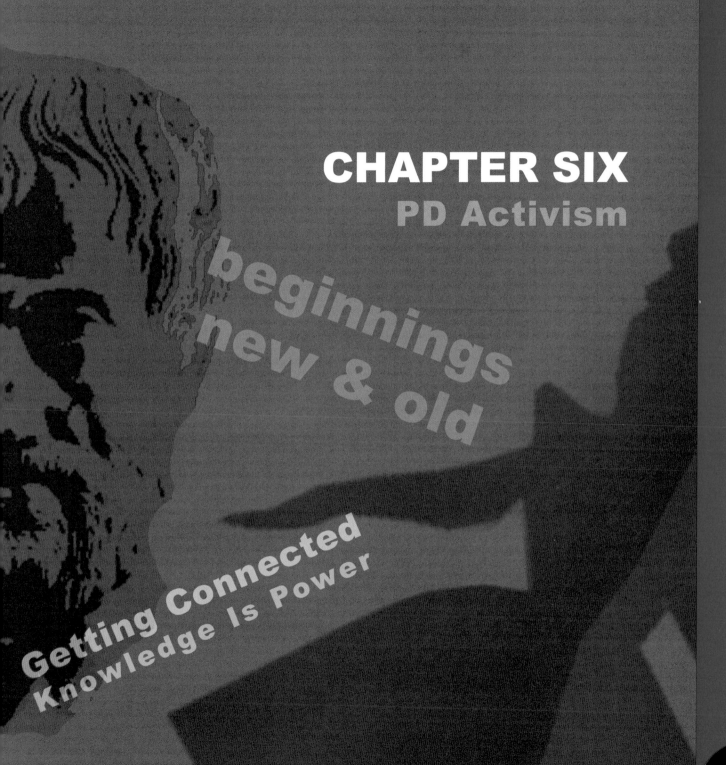

CHAPTER SIX
PD Activism

beginnings
new & old

Getting Connected
Knowledge Is Power

A WORLD PARKINSON COMMUNITY IS BORN!

In the autumn of 2010, in the grey and rather overcast city of Glasgow, Scotland, over 3000 people gathered for a medical conference. Nothing remarkable, you might think, but among the doctors and health workers who had assembled from around the world were another group, PwP, brought together by a remarkable chain of events that spanned the previous 15 years.

At first, it seemed as though this was to be another standard medical conference but with the 'novelty' of patients' presence. That is, until a quiet, kilted man, resplendent in Northern Irish tartan, rose to his feet and delivered a speech that reached the hearts of everyone. For each PwP, it resonated with feelings and issues that many had worked tirelessly toward for years.

After he finished, a hush fell over the crowd while his simple earnest words registered. Then thundering applause began spontaneously from all sections of the auditorium and the audience, to a person, stood in support of his extolling the "fierce urgency of now." That night, Bryn Williams became the voice of a new phase in Parkinson activism.

With the Congress and this speech, we became a true global community, working to raise the profile of this complex, long-lasting, debilitating, and currently incurable condition - the sense of community was exciting.

KNOWLEDGE IS POWER

Today, people recall that inaugural speech. It continues to inspire patients, carers, friends and families to action. We reprint it here and hope the words, the standing ovation and the sense of urgency will motivate ALL members of the Parkinson Community:

All of us arrive at this Congress with a common goal.

To improve the lives of people with Parkinson's disease.

Everybody in this room has something to contribute.

The clinicians and researchers bring extraordinary science and potential therapies to be discussed and dissected.

But this is not just a science meeting.
This is a Congress.

This is a gathering of the whole Parkinson's community and the patients and carers bring an extraordinary contribution too.

We bring the experience, we bring the knowledge, and we bring the passion that comes from living with this disease.

The value of this experience, knowledge and passion should not be underestimated.

The patients and carers bring something else to this Congress.

Something that only a person who lives with this disease, day in, day out, can truly understand.

Urgency

What Martin Luther King referred to as the fierce urgency of now.

I've only been diagnosed a few short years and already I have had enough.

My wife and my two little girls have had enough.

My friends who have been walking miles, running miles, and swimming miles to raise awareness have seriously had enough.

Their aching limbs and cramped feet long for a cure almost as much as mine do.

A cure that's been sitting tantalizingly below the horizon since before I was diagnosed.

A sunrise waiting to happen.

Every day I ask myself what can I do?

As a group of patients and carers what can we do?

What can we offer to advance the work of you, the clinicians and researchers?

We can offer you commitment, we can offer you cooperation and we can offer you collaboration. Clinicians and researchers we can be your Advocates.

As Advocates we can dispel the myths of Parkinson's.

The outside world believes this is a disease of elderly. We know it isn't. The outside world believes there are drugs that will see you serenely through your life. We know there aren't.

The outside world believes the cure is five years away. We know people who were told that 30 years ago.

As Advocates we can mobilise ourselves to deliver volunteers for clinical trials more quickly.
As Advocates we can become positive nuisances, pestering politicians, badgering budget holders and nagging decision-makers.

As Advocates we can express ourselves and the concerns of our community in a way which will deliver results.

As a community of Parkinson's Advocates we can be a resource for you the clinicians & researchers.

But to be effective we need your commitment, we need your cooperation and we need your collaboration.

We need your support and your encouragement to bring the value of our experience, knowledge and passion to bear.

We need your guidance to plan our journey, to point us in the right direction, and to propel us to the destination all of us here want to reach.

A partnership of equals.

This Congress is not just for the scientists to demonstrate what they hope to do for the patients, it is also an opportunity for us the patients to demonstrate what we can do to eradicate Parkinson's.

If the delegates whose life's work is Parkinson's, collaborate with those who live with Parkinson's, together we can deliver a future without Parkinson's.

But the road must start here. The opportunity exists this week. In this city. At this Congress.

Urgency. Ladies and gentlemen, Urgency.

The fierce urgency of now.

Now is the time to realise the promises of science.

Now is the time to bring our urgency to bear and deliver a future of hope for the victims of this disease.

Now is the time for a steady hand, a strong voice and a keen sense of smell for the opportunities that await us.

A steady hand.

A strong voice.

A keen sense of smell.

I had them once.

I want them back.

Bryn D. Williams
© 2010

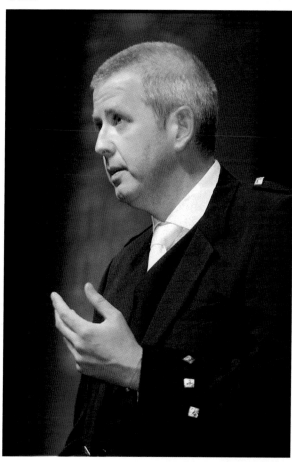

So how did this community of people with Parkinson begin to come together, and when?

What were the things that drew these people together, and what exactly motivated them?

Timing played a huge part. The new accessible Internet drew thousands of people to the most dynamic and forward looking patient-oriented sites, inspired by the ability to access information that until then was little known outside the medical community.

For the first time medical information was freely available to all, and PwP wasted no time in researching their condition, and finding others like themselves.

A host of groups generated a new dialogue about Parkinson, forming a rich interconnected community of people dedicated to helping each other, and finding out how to live well with their

Parkinson community tree....

MICHAEL J. FOX FOUNDATION

CURE PARKINSONS TRUST

SHAKE RATTLE & ROLL

PARKINSONS MOVEMENT

PATIENTS LIKE ME

PD PLAN FOR LIFE

GDNF 4 US

NEUROTALK

CLOGNITION

PARKINSON PIPELINE PROJECT

GRASSROOTS CONNECTION

PARKINSON'S ACTION NETWORK

PLWP

BRAINTALK

MGH FORUMS

PIENO

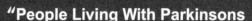

"People Living With Parkinsons
(PLWP) satisfied the social needs
for many displaced PwP diagnosed
with Young Onset Parkinson Disease
(YOPD), while BrainTalk filled the
need for intellectual stimulation, and
in a sense became our new 'job',
filling the void from early retirement.
But it was BrainTalk's roots, providing
an online meeting place, that
branched into numerous local events,
websites, activities and participation in
Parkinson national organizations."

Peggy Willocks

"We are in community each
time we find a place where we
belong....To belong is to know,
even in the middle of the night,
that I am among friends."

**Peter Block,
Community, The Structure of Belonging**

THE INTERNET PROVIDED AN ONLINE MEETING PLACE

JOAN SAMUELSON ADDRESSED THE PARKINSON'S UNITY WALK ON OCTOBER 15TH, 1995

You may wonder why an almost 20 year old speech is reprinted here. Joan's observations may be similar to your own experience with PD and unfortunately, many of the problems are still unresolved.

I don't know how many of you were in the same situation I was when I decided to come and people said are you going to walk and I said no I can't walk that far . . . because often I can't. And it was pretty nice for me personally to be with a lot of other people who I knew were probably in the same situation - others of you who probably didn't know if you could make it for sure the whole way. But the one thing I did know was that it would be O.K. if I didn't, which isn't always true in the world we live in.

We try to be equal to everyone else around us. We want to be normal. We want to be able to do all the things that we used to be able to do. And it's hard to give those up and it's real nice to walk up this way knowing that if at some point my foot started doing the crazy things it does or if I got tired that it would be OK. And that somehow somebody in this crowd would make sure that I got here by the end. So I just wanted to mention that.

The thing that really motivates me about this Unity Walk - the idea of it - and the symbolism of it is that it is symbolic of our strength but before I go any further I want to say that how deeply grateful I am to Margot Zobel and to Ken Aidekman because we in the PD community have a huge amount of strength that remains untapped and it's time to unleash it. I have a saying on the wall in my home from Freidrich Nietzsche, of all people, which states, "That which does not kill you will make you stronger." And I've been learning a little bit about that sort of philosophy in the 8 years that I've had PD.

I don't know what it was like for you but I'm sure your experience was very similar to mine. When I got that PD diagnosis the floor fell out from under me. Everything changed that day. I didn't know who I was going to be in the future. I didn't know if I would still be a lawyer. I didn't know if I would still have the dreams that I had held at that point. Many of those dreams have vanished because of PD.

And it was devastating. There's a picture in my home of Mt. St. Helens blowing up. And it was given to me as a bit of a joke, but it's symbolic of the day I got the PD diagnosis. It was the most terrifying day. It remains terrifying, those moments at 3 o'clock in the AM when I'm awake thinking what about the day when I can't cope anymore. It scares me to death.

Well, that ironically has given me strength that I never had. And I know that that's true of those of you who are standing here whether you're the person afflicted with PD or you are a loved one who's life turned into a complete tailspin the day you got that diagnosis in your family. What you have to do now is to make your family work to provide income because the person who was doing the work is now disabled. Just to make life go on.

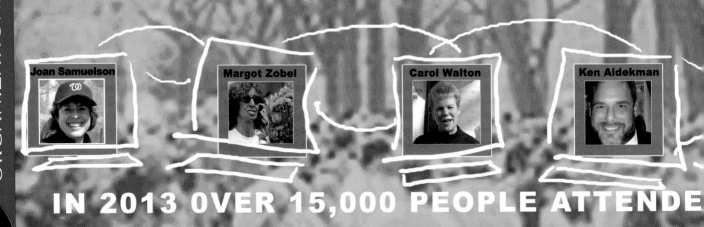

Joan Samuelson   Margot Zobel   Carol Walton   Ken Aidekman

IN 2013 OVER 15,000 PEOPLE ATTENDE

PWP ARE STILIL WAITING FOR BETTER TREATMENTS

A Unity Walk has been held annually in Central Park, New York. Since 2008 there has been a Unity Walk in Sydney, Australia and in 2013 Amsterdam hosted the European Unity Walk.

You're very, very strong people because you have to be. And we can be very proud of that.

What we have to do is tap that (strength) now in public action. But, unfortunately we have been very invisible - and for good reason. It's very hard to live with PD. There are lots of things that we have to do just to survive that everybody else in this country doesn't have to think about. Our lives are very hard. But we have to reach inside ourselves to find a little more time and energy to make ourselves public because we deserve a cure. We deserve attention in Washington and around the country. We deserve to have people in the US understand the affliction of PD.

When I started working with the PAN in Wash five years ago nobody knew what PD was. And if they thought they did, they were wrong. They thought, and many still think, and you know this, that it's a benign disorder. "Oh yeah, you have that drug, don't you? Oh, you're OK." And they see us in public when our Sinemet is working and so on. And they say, "I know somebody with PD and he looks fine." And they do that day or that particular ten-minute stretch. And some people think that they don't have to dig into their pockets for PD research. Or some Congressmen think that they don't have to support the Morris K. Udall Bill which would expand PD research in the Federal government. They think it's just not that important. They think it's not as important as curing AIDS or breast cancer or Alzheimer's.

Well they think that because people with AIDS and Alzheimer's and breast cancer have made it their business to get to Washington and to be in the public to talk about how hard it is to have that disorder, and it is, and get people talking about it and thinking about it and crying about it and worrying about it. And it produces results. Those diseases get far more money per patient from the Federal government and far more money from the private sector from peoples pockets and they're getting results with their medical research.

Well we're getting results because our science is so advanced. I'm sick of scientists coming up to me and telling me; "Don't worry, we've got tremendous potential . . . if we get the money for additional research." I want that money to be in their pockets so they can hire the additional people for their labs so that they can do the experiments.

We deserve that.   We need that.

We thank Joan and other early champions of PwP causes. They have shown us the way....

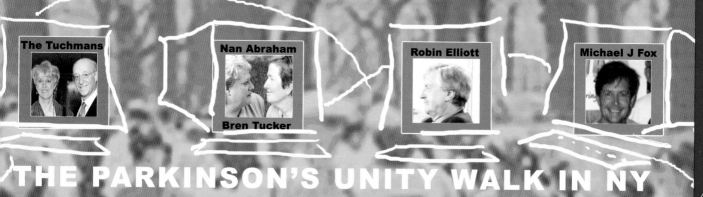

The Tuchmans | Nan Abraham | Robin Elliott | Michael J Fox
Bren Tucker

THE PARKINSON'S UNITY WALK IN NY

PARTICIPATORY MEDICINE:
What I've learned from e-patients.

Dan Hoch M.D. & Tom Ferguson, M.D.

In retrospect, the most important thing I have learned ... was that patients want to know about, and in most cases are perfectly capable of understanding and dealing with, everything their physician knows about their disease and its treatments.

I have also learned that an online group . . . is not only much smarter than any single patient, but is also smarter, or at least more comprehensive, than many physicians - even many medical specialists. While some posts do contain erroneous material, online groups of patients who share an illness engage in a continuous process of self-correction, challenging questionable statements and addressing misperceptions as they occur. And while no single resource, including physicians, should be considered the last word in medical knowledge, the consensus opinion arrived at by patient groups is usually quite excellent. And if more expert clinicians offered to consult informally with the online support groups devoted to their medical specialties - as I now do - we could help group members make information and opinion shared in these groups even better . . .

I had been taught to believe that patients could only be "empowered" by their clinicians. And while I do believe that clinicians can help in this regard by sharing their knowledge openly and by encouraging patient self-reliance, it now seems quite clear that growing numbers of patients are perfectly capable of empowering themselves, with or without their clinician's blessing. Physicians and other health professionals should do all they can to support them in this worthy effort . . .

Finally, I have concluded that few, if any, physicians could have created a system like BrainTalk Communities. As a tech-savvy non-physician intimately familiar with both the inner workings of medical care and the power of information technology systems to create effective online communities, John Lester was less proprietary than most physicians are about medicine's proper professional "turf." He was also less inhibited by professional biases regarding the potential value of the medical contributions that "unqualified" individuals might make. This is not an isolated occurrence. We suspect that the intensely professionally centered enculturation most physicians receive in their training and practice environments may render them, in the words of John Seely Brown and Paul Draguld, "blinkered if not blind" to the emergence of many promising new techno-cultural changes, which currently present new opportunities for health-care innovation [10]. Thus, physicians who seek to innovate in these areas might benefit greatly - as I have - from joining forces with web developers, net-savvy social scientists, experienced e-patients, and other colleagues unencumbered by the limiting belief systems that may result from our traditional medical training . . .

In light of their empowering social dynamics and volunteer economics, we suspect that patient-led online groups may prove to be a considerably more promising and sustainable health-care resource than professionally moderated therapy groups. And we are convinced that networked work teams linking patients, caregivers, and medical professionals will be an important model for future health-care innovation . . .

Hoch D, Ferguson T, 2005 What I've Learned from E-Patients.
PLoS Med 2(8): e206. doi:10.1371/journal.pmed.0020206

Online groups of patients who share an illness engage in a continuous process of self-correction, challenging questionable statements and addressing misperceptions as they occur.

And while no single resource, including physicians, should be considered the last word in medical knowledge, the consensus opinion arrived at by patient groups is usually quite excellent.

Massachusetts General Hospital & the Parkinson chat room

In 1998, after not feeling well for more than a decade and being diagnosed with Parkinson disease for six years, I finally typed the word 'Parkinson' into a search engine on my new computer and found the MGH Harvard neurological communities' Parkinson chat room. After reading the online chatters for awhile, it felt as if a hand was reaching out and pulling me in, ending almost 15 years of stressful isolation, denial, hiding, and my own ignorance about this illness.

The members of this community (one of the diverse neurological communities under the guidance of site owner John Lester, Ph.D., who believed in 'patients helping patients' and actively promoted strategies that worked) have never stopped connecting and building from these original MGH communities, which later became known as **BRAINTALK**.

Some years later, the BrainTalk site crashed catastrophically, leaving thousands of patients badly in need of each other. At this time, mid-2006, Dr. John Grohol of **PSYCH CENTRAL**, a large internet mental health and psychology forum, saw the need of stranded patients, and when it became evident that Braintalk's future was uncertain he offered its neurological patients a new online home for their forums.

THE BIRTH OF THE ONLINE Parkinson COMMUNITY

In the same year Dr. John Grohol replicated the lost communities and slowly people regrouped at the new forums. By patient consensus they became known as **NEUROTALK**.
Paula Wittekind

In the words of one member:

" **This whole site is a world of its own - huge collections of information, plus a constant buzz of many different conversations at once. This forum is a huge combination of I don't know what all - university, friendship, debate, fortress, battleground, fight for life, passion, comparison of drugs, advocacy, emotional rescue, free reading material, contacts around the world... You know this is new in the history of the world, this whole internet thing . . . and it has only just begun.** "

Bob Dawson

211

TWO ENDS OF THE TELESCOPE

Many of us with Parkinson, because of our physical and emotional reactions to our PD, grab the telescope by the wrong end, and totally distort the reality of what has happened, is happening and is going to happen with our disease.

A fellow Parkinson patient was at the end of his rope, and so I offered him a brief history of PD to demonstrate that if you look through the 'right' end of the telescope you will see that there is hope to be found.

It is almost certain that in a few years they are going to have this thing either completely curable or, at the least we will be beneficiaries of advances being made right now that will make our lives pretty much what they once were.

OK. This is what I re-read to myself every day now - my own words of wisdom (how egotistical, don't you think?), but they are helping.The most important thing to hold in my heart is the fact of the amazing telescoping of time lines in advances in the treatment of PD.

The first thing one of the best neurologists in the country said to me when he confirmed my diagnosis with a second opinion was: "If you had to get a progressive neurological disorder, this is by far the best one to get right now." I thought "Sure, pal, easy for you to say, you don't have it." After reading everything I could find on PD, however, I think that the neuro was right. Consider the facts, and remember the telescope.

1817   **Parkinson was first described in 1817**

1960   **It was not until 143 years later, in 1960 in Austria, that scientists discovered that levodopa could substantially relieve Parkinson symptoms, but at the cost of terrible nausea, because levodopa alone had a hard time passing the blood/brain barrier.**

1967   **As a result, use of levodopa was largely abandoned and only began to be revived as a treatment in about 1967, 150 years after the illness was first described.**

1975   **More importantly, it was only in 1975 that carbidopa was developed (the other active ingredient in Sinemet, which allows 90% of levodopa to pass the blood-brain barrier and greatly reduces nausea and other side effects). Did you know that "Sinemet" is of Latin derivation and means "without vomiting"? So widespread use of the most powerful drug in the PD arsenal, levadopa/carbidopa, only began 24 years ago, 159 years after the discovery of the disease.**

1983   **Then in 1983 came the "Case of the Frozen Addicts",** an event so important that it cannot be overemphasized – it literally revolutionized research into the cause and treatment of Parkinson. In short, a Stanford, USA, neurologist, William Langston, got a call from the police about six heroin addicts who seemed to have become literally frozen overnight. Langston and others discovered that all had taken a form of heroin that had been cooked up in a lab using a chemical called MPTP, which converted into MPP3 in the brain, and caused the destruction of the substantia nigra, where dopamine cells are located, producing almost instant full-blown Parkinson. Within a few years, and this is the important part, some bright soul realized that they had stumbled onto the biggest Parkinson research tool ever. Now they had a chemical which could induce Parkinsonism in humans in a matter of days, and these scientist concluded that it could also be used to induce it in lab animals for research. They were right, and the study of Parkinson disease took a QUANTUM LEAP forward.

1997   **In the years since that time many new drugs have been introduced that have prolonged the span during which a PD patient can expect to carry on daily activities with a substantial degree of freedom and independence. Selegiline was introduced as a result of experiments involving the frozen addicts. Mirapex and Requip hit the market in August 1997, and these dopamine agonists have been real improvements over the older agonists for most people.**

2001 - The present day Parkinson research is advancing on many fronts. A gene has been discovered for a hereditary form of Parkinson. The Parkinson's Institute announced a significant study of twins with Parkinson. There are new and greatly improved surgical techniques. Neuro-protective and neuro-restorative strategies are sprouting up all over the place now, and stem cell advances provide hope for the near future.

So that's the way I look at the FACTS through my telescope, not at pie-in-the-sky vague hopes. The snowball is speeding every larger and faster down the hill. As one Parkinson researcher put it, one day soon scientists all over the world are going to spring out of their chairs and shout "Eureka" as they read that someone has found the key that fits the lock to this disease.

So grab that telescope again for a quick summary. It took 43 years to find levodopa, which was combined for improved effectiveness with carbidopa in 1975, a mere span of 15 years. The frozen addicts case led to huge leaps in research potentials - a 10 year span.

Our futures looks eminently hopeful when we look through the right end of the telescope!

Greg Wasson

For people looking for answers to their own particular 'wear and tear' questions the internet has not just provided information. It has supplied something more - communication with people asking the same or similar questions, and the potential for these groups of people to come together and collect a powerful and informed body of knowledge themselves and to challenge the experts to prove themselves, their theories, and their solutions, in order to see a truer picture of the things that are shaping their lives. One such group of people is the international Parkinson Disease patient community, made up of people whose growing awareness that the view of their condition that was offered by the medical world was anodyne, incomplete and in some respects untrue. Some come together to bring about a better understanding of PD, to open up the burning issues that exist for people with a progressive condition, and to try to influence and bring about the solutions that they know are needed, not just for themselves, but for future generations.

They are out there, doing this, in many ways. This book is one of those ways, and has been brought to you with the hope that it will inspire you whether you are a patient, or family, carer or doctor, care home worker, physiotherapist, or part of the hierarchy of influence that exists to develop

products for us, from researcher and scientists, upward to decision makers across government, industry and finance. Like all disease, this one can touch anybody. Today it is me, tomorrow it could be you, your partner, parent, child or friend.

For those who came together in the infancy of on-line advocacy the years are passing, and their views and motivations have deepened and changed as their hopes of a treatment making it to the market in time for them have moved further away.

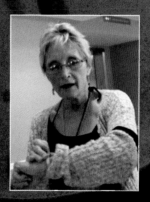

Some of us are reminded of this almost daily. In the tag of committed online advocate, PwP, and fellow contributor to this book, Paula Wittekind . . .

" Time is not neutral for those who have PD and for those who will get it. "

E ALL DISEASE, THIS ONE CAN TOUCH ANYBODY

PD
is the gift
that keeps
on taking

Michael J. Fox

Michael J. Fox and Mohammad Ali testifying at Congress in 2002. Ali's wife, Lonnie, described his fight with Parkinson. She said he "is facing an opponent unlike any he has ever fought.... Muhammad is battling a relentless, remorseless, insidious thief."

PWP TESTIFY IN WASHINGTON DC

Joan Samuelson, PAN's founder, created a strong grassroots PD network in the US. Through PAN, PwP learn about current issues and how to contact their legislators to keep them informed. At the DC PAN forum, the grassroots advocates network with each other and bring their message to Capitol Hill in person.

In 2002, the Parkinson Action Network patient forum was scheduled to coincide with Congressional testimony on the status of federal funding for Parkinson research. Patients were able to attend and quite an impressive list of PwP testified on the panel; among them Mike Fox, Mohammad Ali, Lonnie Ali, and patient advocate Tom Schneider. Science researchers were represented by Harvard's Dr. Ole Issacson, Founder Joan Samuelson represented PAN, and a National Institutes of Health representative rounded out the panel. This was a landmark event in advocacy and awareness and a catalyst for action.

At that time the principal concerns of patients and PD organizations were increased funding and stem cell research. In the press-filled room decisions were made that would affect PwP globally.

However, the real elephant in the room for PwP, was the illness itself. Millie Kondracke sat and watched with bent frame in a wheelchair, unable to speak. Lonnie Ali testifed on behalf of her husband Mohammad Ali, who was unable to speak. Even Michael J. Fox had difficulty (his dyskinesia steadily increased throughout his talk, leaving him breathless and not quite able to finish).

FLASHBACK:
ALL ARE ANONYMOUS IN CHAT ROOMS

One afternoon I was clicking through the TV channels and spotted Michael J. Fox on Rosie. There was a rumor circulating online that he had Parkinson Disease. Curious, I decided to watch him for any movement signs that would be familiar to another person with Parkinson.

I saw myself - things I did at school. Fidgeting throughout the interview, his movements were similar to my attempts to cover up other unwanted movements. When he swung his left arm over the back of the chair, I felt certain he did indeed have Parkinson.

Sitting on my porch that evening, my thoughts turned to Michael. It was hard to believe. I thought he'd probably enjoy the chat room. We were a bunch of clowns anyway . . .

It wasn't long before Michael did announce his illness and shortly afterward someone we thought may be him entered the chat room.

Mike's symptoms and length of time diagnosed were similar to some of us. We entered the chat several months ahead of him; he was a decade or more younger. He, as we all had, seemed to feel the relief that finally comes when we can be that person we are becoming . . . and from talking to others in the same predicament. He had just ended many years of denial and hiding his condition. He was far too young for this. The chat room was a haven for us, and we craved the opportunity to compare symptoms, experiences and knowledge.

Michael finally did disclose who he was to several of us, and the thoughts I had on the porch that night actually became a reality.
Paula Wittekind

Another forum member who was there wrote this about Michael's presence in the chat room.

"While on the surface I appeared to be accepting my diagnosis of Parkinson disease, deep down I felt like a misfit. In a culture that reveres youth, I was prematurely morphing into an old person while still in my early 40's. When I first discovered the Parkinson chat room, I was pleased to find a group of people engaged in the same struggle to retain their vitality, intelligence, creativity and humor as this 'dis-ease' steadily eroded the same. I was welcomed into this cyber world by a fellow teacher, and quickly became friends with other teachers, artists; representatives from all walks of life and corners of the globe. Humor, in particular, was our saving grace: laughing in the face of great loss.

I remember during one of these chats, we were joking with a teacher from Newfoundland about kayaking.

In typed banter, we tossed one liners like, "Be sure to bring enough drugs . . . in waterproof bags", though it seemed doubtful if any of our Parkie party could right a flipped kayak. Imagining this flotilla of stiff, weak, or even frozen kayakers careening aimlessly in the waters of the North Atlantic was our private joke.

So it was into this particular chat room conversation, that a new participant signed in. What caught my attention was his light touch and humor. I remember being delighted to have this guy along for the bigger journey that not one of us had volunteered for. I was later to find out that this was Michael J. Fox. His presence and spark added an energy that increased the levity and camaraderie. This saving grace was better than any medicine a doctor could give us."
Maureen Murphy

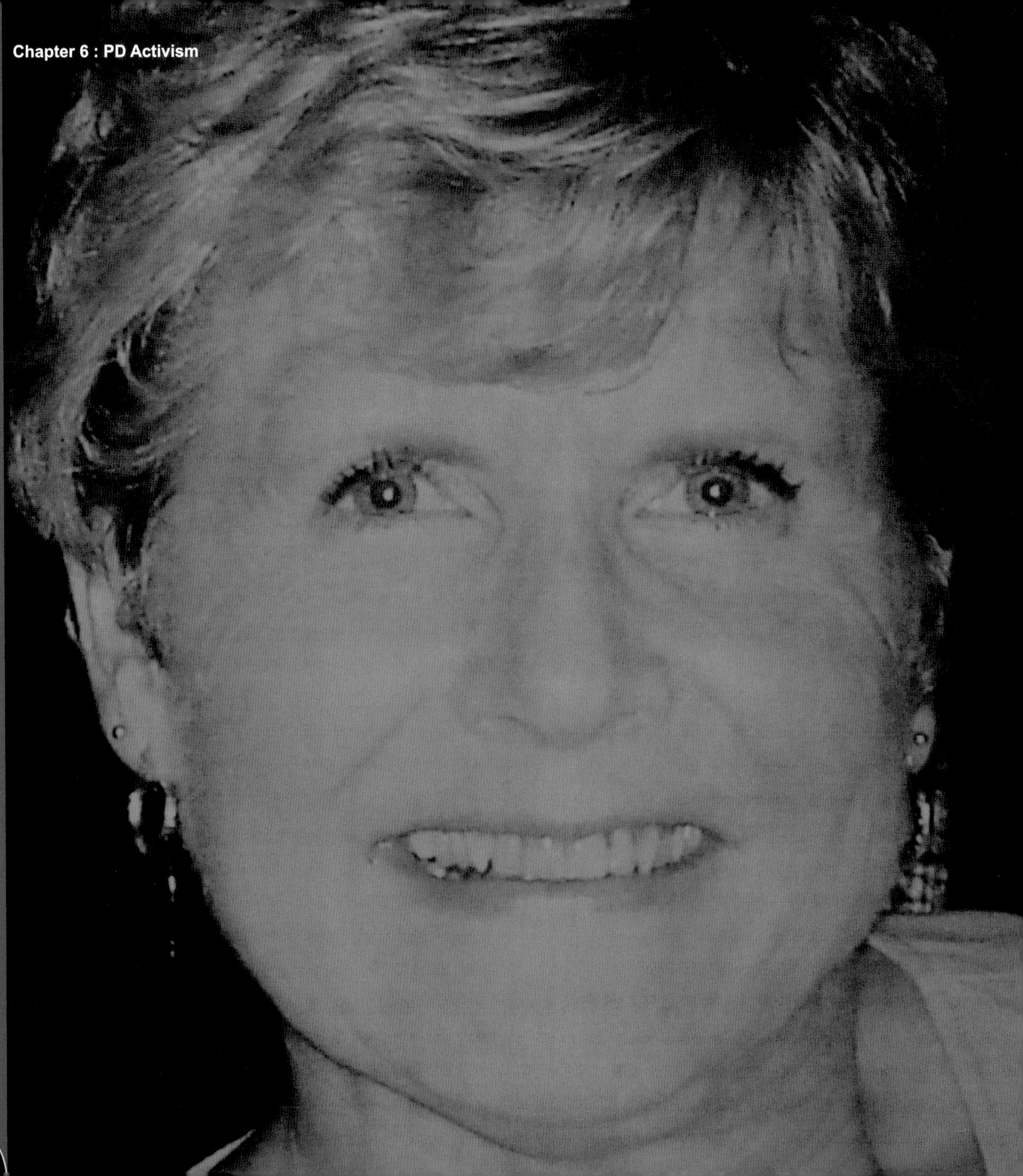

At age 44, I was diagnosed with Parkinson. I was at the height of my career, serving only eight years as an elementary principal. After a period of total devastation due to my early disability retirement, I began to reach out. I had survived what the doctor called a "Parkinson crisis." My need for understanding this illness began with searching the web. But there was a desire for more - something for my emotional needs. Then by chance I happened upon BrainTalk, hosted by Massachusetts General Hospital (MGH), a forum where information was shared intellectually and "virtual friendships" rapidly evolved.

John Lester, Technology Administrator at Harvard, was the creator of BrainTalk, and for some reason held a special interest in Parkinson patients. I met John face-to-face through an online support group called People Living With Parkinson's (PLWP).

PLWP satisfied social needs for many, especially those with young onset Parkinson.

BrainTalk filled the need for intellectual stimulation and in a sense became our new "job", to fill that void from early retirement. For the next five years, I journalled for PLWP and befriended many, even stumbling upon Michael J. Fox unknowingly, until he mentioned reading my posts from BrainTalk at a meeting in Washington, D.C.

For the last ten years I have played the role of patient advocate, volunteering for many non-profit orgs and pharmaceutical companies.

In a way, I am still teaching.

Peggy Willocks

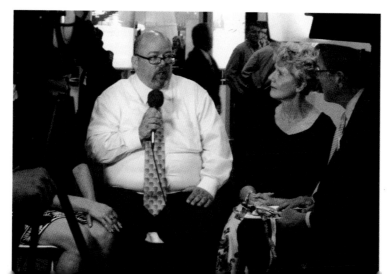

PwP representatives James Trussell (PAN) and Peggy Willocks (PD Trials) being interviewed at Biotechnology Org conference.

217

Parkinson's Outreach
"Hope for Tomorrow. Help for Today."

I came to terms with my diagnosis ten months after that fateful day in February 2007, when my neurologist told my wife and I that my MRI did not show any abnormalities, but that he felt that I had Parkinson disease because of the history that I had described to him, and my physical examination.

How does a seemingly healthy person just a few years earlier become one in need of constant medications to provide relief and live a normal life? This disease that moved into my life as an unwanted and uninvited burden soon came to be the best thing that could have happened to me. I had to look inward at who I truly was and then work out from there to helping those who couldn't help themselves.

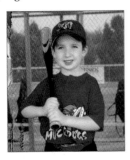 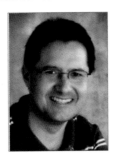

My motivating factor for becoming involved in advocacy work and wanting to help those less fortunate than myself came in the form a special little person named Landon Blake Mitchell, my grandson. He became my helper when the tremors started and would ask what color pill I needed to take at the time, often insisting on placing the pill in my mouth. When the days were long and the nights even longer during those first few months after my diagnosis, and I wanted to give up, my wife reminded me that Landon needed his Pop Pop to be there for him. It was then that I realized this disease was making me feel sorry for myself, and I needed to do what I could, while I still could, to make a difference. Many more people were out there who didn't have the love and support of a child like Landon, giving his unconditional love. This child would tell people, "If you shake, you need to go the doctor to get some medicine because you have "Parkins disease" like my Pop Pop".

I thought of providing financial support to national organizations doing so much for the cause of finding a cure for this devastating disease. At the same time, I kept hearing of people having to do without their medications because they were without insurance coverage, and meeting several people with severe tremors who had never been seen by a doctor because they couldn't afford the fees.

With the help of my wife, Chris, and several others, we decided to raise funds to start a foundation dedicated to helping people with Parkinson disease offset medication costs and physician's fees.

We took a leap of faith and had a Parkinson disease Awareness and Education Dinner/Fundraiser. All proceeds from the event went toward setting up the foundation as a non-profit organization, which has been a slow process, but a necessary one, in order to have the ability to seek tax-deductible donations.

Parkinson's Outreach is the name of our foundation. It is a 501(c)(3) organization. "Hope for Tomorrow" is intended to show that we look to the future and keep the hope of finding a cure. "Help for Today" indicates the need for providing assistance to those that need our help now.

I've often used the analogy of setting up a foundation to that of opening a store. You've done the background work to get it started because you know there is a need, but until people know what you can provide, the wait to get started and know if it will be a success can be excruciating.

What I have found most interesting about some of the calls that we receive is that people are seeking information about the disease and want to talk about what they are going through with PD. The chance to talk to another person who shares the same disease often seems good enough for them. When asked if they need help with prescription costs or physician's fees, many will say that they are doing well financially now but will keep us in mind if they ever need our help.

My daughter Ashley once wrote in an essay, "This disease wasn't meant to ail us, rather, put into our lives so that we would be so blessed as to help others." That pretty much sums up what our mission will be as we head forward.

We will keep spreading the word about the help we make available for persons with Parkinson disease in the West Texas area, knowing that we are helping to improve their quality of life.

Johann Wolfgang Von Goethe is quoted as saying, "Knowing is not enough, we must apply. Willing is not enough, we must do."

One thing is for certain as we seek a cure for this disease. We will continue to do our part in serving people locally and offering financial support for research on the national level, and by our involvement in clinical trials. We need to get more people involved in this because they can't find a cure without PwP as partners in the process.

Israel Robledo
Parkinson's Outreach
info@parkinsonsoutreach.org

ADVOCACY SPEECH

Peggy Willocks

This was originally presented at the UDALL awards dinner in 2005;
with slight alterations for inclusion in this book, it is still timely.

A • **AWARENESS:** Advocacy is NOT just about dealing with legislative issues. Advocacy is about getting the word out about our disease - whether it be as simple as wearing a PD themed tee-shirt when you go to the grocery store, or as elaborate as being a part of a major fundraising project for a foundation that funds PD research.

D • **DONATIONS:** I am not talking about just monetary donations (which are absolutely essential to continue the work of our Parkinson organizations). I mean the contribution you can make - donations of your time, your skills, your personal stories and your prayers. Or you might even donate your brain to science.

V • **VOLUNTEERS:** We need people who will dedicate their lives to fight Parkinson disease. We need to help recruit patients for research as well as patients to volunteer to be a part of clinical trials - because without volunteers we cannot have new treatments nor will we find a cure.

O • **ORGANIZATIONS:** We need the national and international organizations - APDA, NPF, PDF, Parkinson Alliance, the Fox Foundation, the Parkinson's Institute, The Cure Parkinson's Trust, Parkinson's Movement, World Parkinson Coalition, European Parkinson's Disease Association and the many more Parkinson organizations from around the world. We need the national Unity Walks in the USA and Australia, the conferences and congresses which bring these organizations and their research focus together and we need the people who organize these very successful events. For me, 'organizations' also include those pharmaceutical companies who genuinely care about the patient.

C • **CONGRESS:** Lobbying Congress (or any other governmental policy makers) is a necessary task we must do in order to get the most funding for our research and programs. We must visit our legislative leaders and recruit as many constituents as we can to help us receive our fair share for Parkinson disease research.

A • **ACTION:** We sometimes just can't wait for a good idea to develop. To borrow a phrase from Nike, we have to "Just do it!" We don't need to wait for someone else to write that letter to the editor, or call a congressman, or let someone else start that support group for the newly diagnosed. "Just do it!" "Just do it."

C • **CAREPARTNERS:** Let's not ignore the job of this irreplaceable group. I could not be here were it not for my husband, who has stood by my side through my sickness from day one and my kids who support me in my advocacy efforts. I watch carepartners interact with their loved ones knowing how difficult it is for all of us.

Y • **YOU:** Last, but certainly not least, we need YOU - EACH and EVERY ONE of YOU! And it takes all of us in a united effort to give of our most precious commodity - TIME.

GLOBAL ISSUES AND VISIONS

While they/we can see that globally uncounted billions of research currency have been spent, they/we can also see that on the ground, depending where that ground is, life can be precarious. In some developed countries the personal cost of medication, long term care, hospitalization etc., can be staggering, Healthcare plans both private and public have their shortcomings, and where these are felt is inevitably in the daily life of the patient. In less developed countries the picture is, as with all health issues, much more grim. Around the world many thousands of people never even get a diagnosis, let alone treatment, and the ones that do are often subject to paternalistic and outmoded models of healthcare that do not nearly meet their needs. For patients in developed and undeveloped countries the research currencies have yielded few benefits: a tablet that lasts slightly longer, an old drug delivered in a high tech way . . . and a lot of promises.

What patients are increasingly saying is that while they are waiting for a cure, there are other considerations, other needs to be met. These include being better informed about their condition, about having multi-skilled teams of health professionals to help them with maintaining the health they have, while optimizing existing treatments to their individual needs; and when and if they need it, hospital and care provision that understands those needs, and will tailor their care appropriately. All of these things require a quantum shift of vision, to one in which the patient is central to their health provision. Where compassion, care, and empowerment are not secondary to profit, corporate development, and political expediency. They would like to see it happen now, in their lifetime, for all.

Linda Ashford

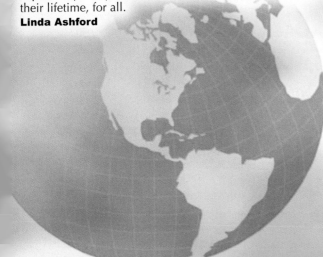

TRENDS IN U.S. HEALTH POLICY AND COMMUNITY ORGANIZATION

Trends in health care policy have a big effect on PD research and the ability of science and medicine to deliver the long promised cure. Fortunately, the current trends are starting to align behind our most powerful weapon against PD, the empowered activated PwP. This patient centered approach to medical research and health care is not only the ethical thing to do, but also is necessary to sustain healing to a point where PwP can ease our suffering and maintain our dignity sufficiently to make life worth living.

Over the past 20 years, the emphasis of PD advocacy in the US has been on NIH research funding, but in recent years this focus has widened along the continuum of medical research from bench to bedside - from basic science (great emphasis on "stem cell" research) to translational research (still mainly at NIH), to clinical research evaluation and regulatory review of new therapies, and then to actual delivery of patient care and management of quality. As the last frontier for medical science, the emphasis of medical research on the brain and central nervous system has been on basic scientific knowledge. Most disease-focused Institutes support a full continuum of research. The neurology institute (NINDS - leader for PD) has been slow to adopt activities such as epidemiological or population studies and quality management, so PD is disadvantaged compared with Alzheimer (NIA) and mental health (NIMH) in our understanding of the issues and the effects of the reality of service delivery on PD care (e.g. >50% of PwP are treated by primary care physicians and <10% see a movement specialist).

In recent years the PD community has started to branch out and become more unified. PAN has increased its activity with respect to FDA regulation. NPF has launched an extensive quality management effort in its centers of excellence and is collaborating on creation of the information technology needed to support patient decision making and to manage continuous quality improvement. Collaboration has been initiated between clinical researchers in the PSG and activist PwP in the Parkinson Pipeline Project and elsewhere on the creation of comprehensive information technology to provide mobile access to data collection on observations of daily living, as the key component of a personal health record (PHR) to better monitor symptoms.

Paired with the doctor-focused electronic medical record (EMR) in the quality project, shared decision-making will improve. MJFF has launched Fox Trial Finder to enhance the recruitment of PwP to clinical trials, and in the process established a community-wide coalition that we hope will be the basis for collaboration on the use of PHR/ EMR practice data for a variety of purposes.

Perry Cohen

SUCCESSES IN ADVOCACY

**Can patient advocates make
a difference in the fight
against Parkinson disease?**

The answer is emphatically "yes".

Look at what PwP have already done.

Patient advocates have helped legalize and fund embryonic stem cell research in several states, established patient advisory roles in government offices, put forward and passed legislation creating registries of the Parkinson disease population, worked with the medical community to inform and train staff, and held industry partners accountable for more responsible and transparent clinical trials. They have helped pass legislation, giving veterans exposed to Agent Orange a conclusive presumption that the exposure caused their PD, making them eligible for VA benefits.

As the voice of the patient has increased, doctors and scientists are proposing new theories about our disease that may overturn paradigms that have governed research into Parkinson for 100 years.

The most dramatic and obvious is the Braak staging scheme. Braak and his colleagues have proposed that far from being a simple movement disorder, what we call PD is a systemic disease originating in the brainstem. They argue that the involvement of non-dopaminergic structures long precedes involvement of the substantia nigra and the appearance of motor problems. This staging scheme has already had a profound influence on current thinking about PD. Questions are also being asked by both patients and scientists about the value of traditional models for clinical trials, including animal modeling.

These new directions in Parkinson research are not a step backward. On the contrary, they represent great strides forward, a Renaissance, if you will, in our understanding of Parkinson disease. The road to a cure has turned out to be longer than we thought it would be in 1999, but its new course promises to be straighter and more true. It appears that the road may be quite a bit shorter than we had supposed even six months ago.

Why does it take approximately 6½ years for cardiac medicines to get from bench to bedside, while it takes an average of 15 years for Parkinson medications to make that trip? The answer is that there are no biomarkers that can scientifically demonstrate the presence or progression of the disease.

Reliance for 200 years on clinical observation (eyeballing the disease) has greatly hindered the progress of scientific research. But now the Michael J. Fox Foundation for Parkinson Research has initiated an unprecedented $40 million quest to find biomarkers. To top it all off, after a great battle over the neurotrophic factor GDNF, largely fought by a patient coalition that included several members of this Forum, new GDNF trials are being organized after the corporation quietly licensed GDNF to a small group of doctors and researchers who believe in the great possibility of this treatment to halt and even reverse the progression of Parkinson.

Together, patient advocates, scientists, and industry are going back to re-chart the future in the fight against Parkinson disease. No small part of that future will be due to the past and ongoing efforts of so many of the members of this great place called Neurotalk.

Thank you so much.
See you at the Dance,
Greg Wasson

> **As the voice of the patient has increased, doctors and scientists are proposing new theories about our disease that may overturn paradigms that have governed research into Parkinson for 100 years.**

MAKING A DIFFERENCE

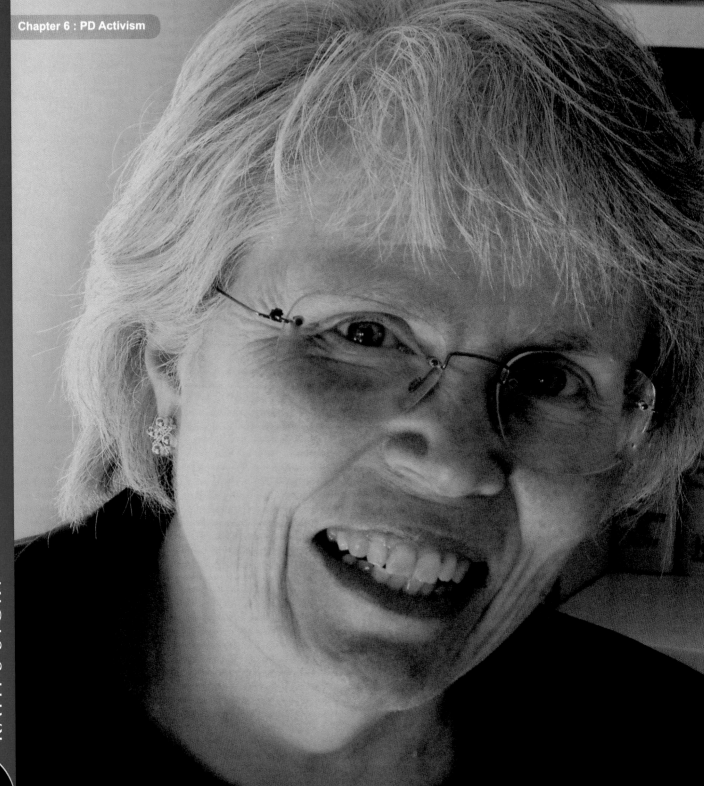

KATH'S STORY

HOW FAR BACK CAN I TRACE MY ADVOCATE'S VOICE?

Imagine a very young student who often asked "why?" and "why not?" and who never wanted to believe that things couldn't be changed. That was me in the 1950s - and I'm still asking the same questions.

When I decided to become an attorney, I thought that it was an appropriate role for an advocate. I didn't realize that attorneys must promote someone else's agenda and argue for things the attorney did not advise nor support. That role was not me.

In 2000, a year before my diagnosis with PD, I became a volunteer community organizer working for changes in U.S. gun laws. I was drafted to organize my city. I learned many specific skills and recruited thousands for the Million Mom March. Although the demonstration was huge and the lobbying continued, NOTHING changed. After that, I no longer believed that you could convince lawmakers and businesses to take a moral position by presenting persuasive, factual arguments and mobilizing large numbers of people. The key lesson for me was that only money and power were heard. I despaired and withdrew.

Strangely, my return to advocacy came through religion. Well, maybe it's not so strange since most people agree that all the great religious leaders were advocates. Two years ago, my activist pastor (who has been arrested and served time for civil disobedience) told the story about the widow who repeatedly petitioned her local, corrupt judge for her rights. He always rejected her pleas until finally he granted her petition -- but only because he wanted her to stop petitioning (Luke 18: 1-8). That helped me realize that you might get what you ask for, not because of the virtue of your cause, but because of your persistence, or some other reason you couldn't possibly imagine or influence. I learned from Buddhist writings that it's important to start the process, which might not be completed in one lifetime.

Since becoming a Person (not a patient, nor a subject, and never a patient subject) with Parkinson disease, I find it's important for me to use my advocate's voice for family members and myself. One example is when I ran my hand through my previously thick hair and noticed it was thinning and that large amounts fell out in my hand.

My internist just told me to: "Use Rogaine." My neurologist said, "It couldn't possibly be due to anything related to PD." I turned to the Internet, found that it could be a rare side effect of the dopamine agonist I was taking and brought a copy of the information to my dermatologist. Luckily, he was interested in research: he pulled together the few prior studies, ran tests to rule out other causes and then filed an adverse incident report with the drug company. I realized there was no way to establish that my hair loss was due to the drug without an unbiased trial. So on Halloween - an appropriate day - since I looked a fright - I stopped taking it. After a few tough months, the hair grew, though not to its former fullness. The dermatologist felt it was important to inform his peers, so he wrote a formal article including before and after photos of the top of my head. If I had followed my doctor's advice, I would have had an extensive collection of wigs or a very cold head.

Given that experience and many others, this is my sincere request to the entire medical community: First, please, see me as a Person; second, hear my statements (especially since PD exhibits symptoms and responds to treatments in many unique ways); and third, let's work together to find a cause(s) and cure for PD. (Unfortunately, I don't believe this will occur in my lifetime). Finally, and most importantly, treat me, as you'd like to be treated - with respect.

A side issue is that medical facilities need accessible exam tables so that people can use them without fear of falling. Imagine, adjustable height, dentist-style chairs or tables with adequate steps and handrails or any other solution, instead of the current tables which sometimes float like islands in the middle of the room with only a tiny pullout step.

For me, now, advocacy is speaking out, voicing my views, and trying to change some things in the world. I don't define success as achieving a goal. Success is using my voice. If I'm mute, "they" (whoever I'm up against) will have won because I've allowed them to silence me.

I will speak out as a model for my son and daughter. I will use my voice for causes and issues I care about and I won't let others silence me, either directly or through my own despair. I hope that I will be able to use my voice in advocacy till the end of my days.

Katherine Huseman

PATIENT ORGANIZATIONS & ORGANIZATIONS WORKING FOR CHANGE

We couldn't possibly list in this book all the groups working for change in the PD community. Throughout the book you will find some mentioned. A comprehensive list is is contained in the Parkinson's Disease Resource List. PDF listened when its PwP Advisory Council said such a list was needed. Thank you - it's an amazing help - every PwP should have one. You can view it at **www.pdf.org/en/resourcelink** or order a paper copy by calling **(800 457-6676)**. This publication highlights over 750 resources throughout the US and around the world that address many needs of a person living with Parkinson. It includes specific resources for early-onset Parkinson, the newly diagnosed, care partners and more. 114 Pages.

Resources listed include:
- **International, national and local Parkinson groups**
- **movement disorder centers**
- **financial, insurance and legal planning assistance**
- **clinical trials**
- **medical equipment**
- **caregiver-specific resources**

The Parkinson Pipeline Project

This patient led advocacy group is headed by Dr. Perry Cohen. It provides the patient perspective in evaluating new biomedical therapies and working on the issue of sham surgery. As a result of these grassroots efforts PwP are now participating in patient advisory committees and conferences. PD organizations around the world have adopted the Pipeline model.

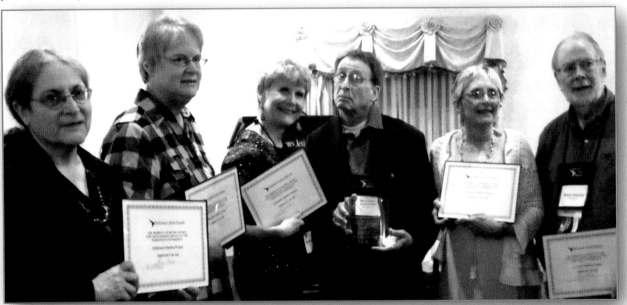

Pipeliners Linda Herman, Carolyn Stevenson, Peggy Willocks, Perry Cohen, Paula Wittekind and Tony Decamp receive The Murray Charters Award for their work together on The Parkinson Pipeline Project.

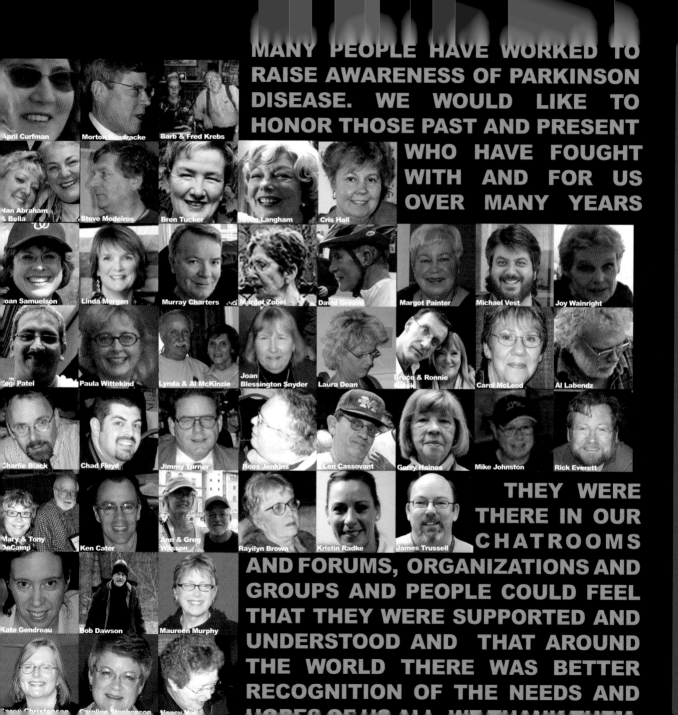

MANY PEOPLE HAVE WORKED TO RAISE AWARENESS OF PARKINSON DISEASE. WE WOULD LIKE TO HONOR THOSE PAST AND PRESENT WHO HAVE FOUGHT WITH AND FOR US OVER MANY YEARS

THEY WERE THERE IN OUR CHATROOMS AND FORUMS, ORGANIZATIONS AND GROUPS AND PEOPLE COULD FEEL THAT THEY WERE SUPPORTED AND UNDERSTOOD AND THAT AROUND THE WORLD THERE WAS BETTER RECOGNITION OF THE NEEDS AND

THANK PD ADVOCATES EVERYWHERE.

April Curfman
Morton Kondracke
Barb & Fred Krebs
Nan Abraham & Bella
Steve Medeiros
Bren Tucker
Kacee Langham
Cris Hall
Joan Samuelson
Linda Morgan
Murray Charters
Margot Zobel
David Greave
Margot Painter
Michael Vest
Joy Wainright
Yogi Patel
Paula Wittekind
Lynda & Al McKinzie
Joan Blessington Snyder
Laura Dean
Bruce & Ronnie
Carol McLeod
Al Labendz
Charlie Black
Chad Floyd
Jimmy Turner
Rees Jenkins
Len Cassovant
Gerry Haines
Mike Johnston
Rick Everett
Mary & Tony DeCamp
Ken Cater
Ann & Greg Wasson
Rayilyn Brown
Kristin Radke
James Trussell
Kate Gendreau
Bob Dawson
Maureen Murphy
Karen Christenson
Caroline Stephenson
Nancy Hall

PAN's Vision for the Future

Amy Comstock Rick, CEO
Parkinson's Action Network

PAN's vision for the future is that we are no longer in business. That would mean we had achieved our mission: we had advocated long and hard enough for federal biomedical research funding that led researchers to a cure. We would love nothing more than to close our doors and put Parkinson in the history books.

PAN's objective is serving as the unified voice for the Parkinson community, fighting for those currently living with the disease as well as future generations.

Federal funding of biomedical research - both basic research and translational science - is paramount to discovering better treatments and a cure for Parkinson disease. The federal government has a responsibility to invest in medical research that benefits taxpayers and fuels local economies.

PAN is the Parkinson community's advocacy voice for real change. The staff and grassroots advocates in all 50 states work with decision makers on policy initiatives supporting scientific research. PAN's grassroots advocates ensure that their voices are heard on critical issues in a substantive, results-driven way.

PAN advocates are the heart and soul of the Parkinson community's work. The work we do is fueled by our shared goals for collaborative scientific discovery and a future free of disease. There is a near-term vision for the future that I believe will get us closer to achieving our mission and it is all about using our voices to more effectively influence research and discovery.

All the interested parties have a responsibility to collaborate more effectively, including patients communicating closely with their doctors … doctors sharing information more broadly and systematically with the scientific community … and researchers working more collaboratively with patients through clinical trials and other venues. The focus on strengthening relationships and opening the channels of communication among these critical stakeholders must be a goal of all those who live with and care for people with Parkinson. No one can do it for us. With strength in numbers, we can set a new benchmark for how discoveries are made and get that much closer to achieving our community's goals.

This is PAN's vision for the future. But we wouldn't be PAN without sharing what our advocates hope and want. So, in closing, I'll leave you with two quotes from PAN advocates about their hope for the future:

"If I can bring some hope that future generations of Parkinson patients will have a cure, or a better quality of life, then it makes my work completely worthwhile."

Arthur Fitzmaurice, Ph.D., University of California, Los Angeles

"If you don't stand up for what you believe in, who will? Are you content to sit by and let nothing change? By advocating with others, you can, and will raise awareness and change things for the better."

the unified voice for the Parkinson community, fighting for those currently living with the disease as well as future

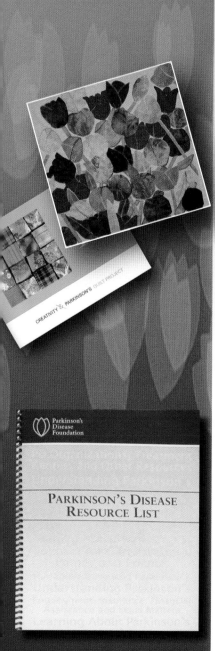

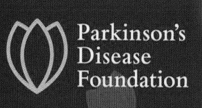

Parkinson's Disease Foundation

located in New York, trains patient advocates for clinical trial education and recruitment at their regional Parkinson's Advocates in Research (PAIR) Conferences.

What makes the **Parkinson's Disease Foundation (PDF)** hopeful about the future? To a large degree, this is a question about product - getting new and better treatments for Parkinson disease, faster and more effectively. But it is also a question about process - getting the right resources in place that will make the product possible. In the view of PDF, no resource is more important to this process than the people who live with Parkinson themselves.

Don't get us wrong; we are also hugely hopeful about the "product"- the exciting pathways that scientists are pursuing, the new therapies currently under investigation and the bright minds that are dedicating themselves to Parkinson research.

But truth be told, it is development of the process - centered on people living with Parkinson and informed by science - that gives us the greatest hope of all.

In our own work at PDF, we are driven by the same passion. It powers our People with Parkinson's Advisory Council (which incidentally includes several leaders and contributors to the Parkinsons Creative Collective). It is also demonstrated in our **Parkinson's Advocates in Research (PAIR) program**, which also includes leaders and contributors to the Collective. We created PAIR as a means to building a cadre of lay leaders who have the scientific knowledge and leadership skills they need to partner in research. Almost 200 PDF Research Advocates have completed our three-day trainings, along with hundreds of others who are in the process of completing our new online course. Other examples include the hundreds of people who write letters to the editor during Parkinson Awareness Month each April and share their artwork via the Creativity and Parkinson project.

Why do we feel so strongly about these and other patient-centered initiatives? Quite simply, because we truly believe our progress in Parkinson research, education and advocacy will only come when people with Parkinson and their families are recognized as equal partners in the process, along with scientists, companies and government.

The underlying point is that the role of people with Parkinson is indispensable to fulfilling our hope both for the long term (that is, defeating Parkinson for all time) and for the short term (that is, empowering people who live with the disease today to achieve and maintain the highest possible quality of life). And nowhere is this idea expressed more brilliantly than it is in the pages of this inspiring book by the Collective.

PDF proud to join hands and link arms with the leaders of the Collective, as true 'partners in hope.' We look forward to working closely with them in the twin causes of understanding Parkinson better and developing newer and better treatments to combat it more effectively.

Robin Elliott
Executive Director, PDF

23andMe

When Parkinson becomes personal, people become engaged. An outstanding example is the Parkinson's Research Community launched by leading personal genomics company 23andMe, whose cofounder Anne Wojcicki's husband discovered he carries the LRRK2 mutation known to be associated with Parkinson disease. He inherited the mutation from his mother, who has Parkinson disease and actively participates in research to help find its cause and possible cures.

The goal of **23andMe** is to analyze DNA from the saliva of 10,000 people who have been diagnosed with Parkinson. Facilitating a truly global research effort, **23andMe** has already enrolled people with Parkinson disease from 49 states and over 21 countries. In 2013 they met their goal but continue to need our help. Their research is expanding our genetic knowledge, encouraging scientists, with new areas of study, and patients with shortened timelines for new treatments to reach the market.

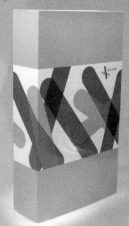

Overall, CEO Anne Wojcicki says, **"her scientists have one of the largest genetic databases in the world"** with more than 250,000 users who have supplied DNA samples to the company's lab. This makes it possible to do "a tremendous amount of discovery" about potential causes of many ailments, as well as to help customers learn to understand their own DNA, the genetic blueprint that determines everything.

New discoveries from the 23andMe GWAS study of people with Parkinson disease

In June 2011, the **23andMe** Research Team published their first scientific paper in a peer-reviewed, open-access online journal called PLoS Genetics (2). Besides confirming 20 known associations to Parkinson in the paper, scientists at **23andMe** have also discovered two novel genetic associations. The first novel association lies near the gene SCARB2, which is involved with known Parkinson disease pathways. The second lies near the genes SREBF1 and RAI1 and is of unknown function. The **23andMe** research team

also replicated twenty previously discovered genetic associations, providing support for the novel web-based design used in this study."

Existing genetic associations confirmed

- LRRK2
- GBA
- SNCA
- MAPT
- GAK

In spite of the rare chance of Parkinson developing from a genetic mutation, their analysis found that Anne's husband Sergey and his mother have the same LRRK2 mutation known as G2019S. Sergey shares his outlook in a 2008 blog entry:

"This leaves me in a rather unique position. I know early in my life something I am substantially predisposed to. I now have the opportunity to adjust my life to reduce those odds (e.g. there is evidence that exercise may be protective against Parkinson's). I also have the opportunity to perform and support research into this disease long before it may affect me. And, regardless of my own health it can help my family members as well as others."

Sergey and his family are doing their part to prevent the onset of Parkinson for everyone. Recently, scientists at Stanford University said they had been able to observe in the lab, for the first time, using cells from Sergey's mother, how neurons sicken and die in Parkinson patients.

Sergey is exercising and contributing to research, as Anne's company continues analyzing genetic blueprints. **23andme now offers their spit kits free of charge with prepaid postage to people diagnosed with Parkinson.** However, the study does not end with sending the DNA sample. **23andMe** has online surveys to complete that are very important to the study because Parkinson disease is suspected to be the result of both environmental factors and genetic predisposition. These surveys are critical to filling in the blanks between Parkinson, individuals' DNA, and their unique environments. **Paula Wittekind**

CALL TO ACTION

The rest is up to us. Our part for this study is simple and free of charge. Go to www.23andme.com and sign up for a spit kit. Fill out the online surveys at your own pace. If you happen to forget the URL, just Google '23andMe'.

References: (**1**) MercuryNews.com, Google-backed 23andMe hits major milestone: 100,000 users in DNA database, Peter Delevett, 6/11/11; (**2**) 23andMe Press Release, 6/29/2011, www.23andme.com/about/press/pd_discoveries_plos_62311; (**3**) Sergey Brin's blog post, September 18, 2008, http://too.blogspot.com/2008/09/lrrk2.html

23andMe

NATIONAL PARKINSON FOUNDATION

Recently, I have felt renewed hope for Parkinson research. The pieces of the research puzzle are being put together as never before. Researchers at Johns Hopkins have zeroed in on the exact protein in the LRRK2 pathway (LRRK2 being the genetic variation that has the highest chance of causing Parkinson). Drug companies are already developing plans to capitalize on this discovery. Plus, scientists at Columbia University and elsewhere have determined the fundamental mechanism that creates extra alpha synuclein clumps in neurons, leading to cell death. These two important discoveries are bringing together previously disparate scientific bodies of work as never before. As a result, I truly believe that within the decade, new classes of drugs aimed at slowing the disease at its source will be in clinical trials. Yes, I know, gene therapy and stem cells are what excite people. But they are invasive, not for everyone, and in the case of stem cells, light years away from the clinic - if ever.

Other progress also continues: formulations of existing drugs continue to be made better. Better absorption, extended effectiveness, better delivery - these don't sound sexy, but they can result in sound sleep, clearing thinking, fewer side effects, and improved ability to walk or get up from the wheelchair - all of which can make a substantial difference in people's lives. Just talk to anyone who has tried the pump, or undergone DBS.

So my message to patients is: stay healthy. Exercise, look for other ways to minimize your symptoms. Tweak your medications, use the new formulations, undergo DBS or try the pump if you're a candidate, but stay in the game, because there is likely to be a significant breakthrough down the road and you want to be there and be healthy for it.

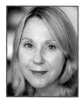

Joyce Oberdorf, President and Chief Executive Officer of the National Parkinson Foundation (NPF). Her aim is to transform NPF into a technology-enabled, 21st century foundation focused on the mission of improving care through research, education and outreach aimed at better treatments and better care now.

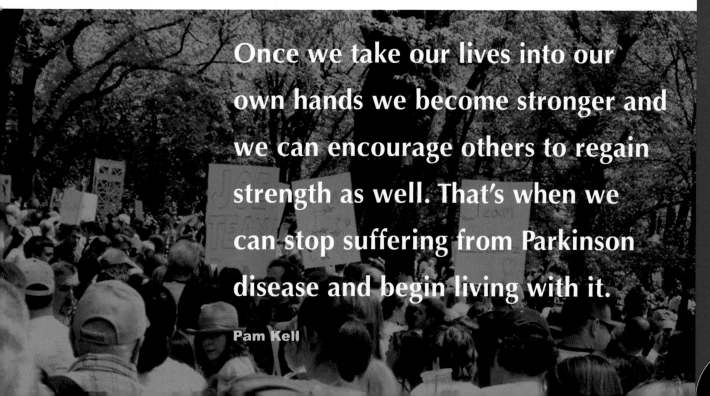

Once we take our lives into our own hands we become stronger and we can encourage others to regain strength as well. That's when we can stop suffering from Parkinson disease and begin living with it.

Pam Kell

PARKINSON'S MOVEMENT

Reaching out to connect people with Parkinson disease around the world . . . .

Parkinson's Movement aims to instill the relevance, urgency and more personalized approach necessary to ensure that those in charge of our healthcare sit up and listen.

Launched in August 2011, the Parkinson's Movement website has attracted visitors from more than 3,600 towns and cities throughout the world and is fast becoming a recognized portal for global patient advocacy activities.

Parkinson's Movement says that it will only consider itself successful when its members are present on every relevant drug advisory board, research grant-awarding authority panel and government policy advisory committee. It is currently building its membership from the 1,500 or so already committed followers who enthusiastically respond to a series of Parkinson's Movement polls, surveys and articles.The results are then disseminated to the wider Parkinson community via international conferences, articles in the scientific and wider press and through direct contact with its numerous stakeholder groups. At last, there is a platform for PwP to independently define the Parkinson agenda.

Together we will consolidate and communicate the opinions of the people who understand the reality of living with this condition so our priorities are represented in our quest for a better life with Parkinson and a treatment that is tailored inaccordance to our needs.

For more information, visit:
www.parkinsonsmovement.com

Parkinson's Movement, a patient-led, patient-inspired organisation, was founded by Jon Stamford, Sara Riggare and Tom Isaacs. Following Sara's departure to pursue other projects in 2013, Jon and Tom have given Israel Robledo, Steve DeWitte and Peggy Willocks higher profile roles in Parkinson's Movement.

"WAGING WAR....
as far as I'm concerned, a cure can't come a moment too soon. Every day that passes means another soldier lost in this fight. Make no mistake – this is a fight to the death.

But know one thing and know it clearly. This is a war our enemy cannot win. It's not a case of 'if' we win. It's when. And that is down to us. That's right - us. If we want this war to be won sooner rather than later, we have to make a personal commitment. It's not for others to win this fight our behalf. And if you think that, you're in the wrong place.

Because here we fight daily. We fight for every inch of the battleground for every minute of battle. We fight with every sinew of our being. For ourselves and for our brothers and sisters. We fight for those who can no longer fight. And we fight for those who do not yet know they will have to fight. If you haven't got the stomach for a fight, leave now. Because this is Parkinson's Movement!"

Jon Stamford, PhD

AMERICAN PARKINSON DISEASE ASSOCIATION

AMERICAN PARKINSON DISEASE ASSOCIATION

APDA is the largest US grassroots organization, serving Americans with PD and their families.

APDA's unique dual mission to '**Ease the Burden - Find the Cure**' offers both help for people affected by PD today and hope for tomorrow through research.

Ease the Burden - through a national network of chapters (volunteer organizations that raise awareness about the disease and funds to support research and patient programs), Information & Referral Centers (professionally-staffed resources for educational materials, community physician and services referrals, patient/caregiver programs), and more than 1,000 support groups, APDA means help and support now. In addition, three dedicated national centers (APDA National Young Onset, APDA National Veterans I&R Center, and the newest APDA National Resource for Rehabilitation that connects the caller to a licensed physical therapist to discuss all aspects of exercise) address the particular challenges and needs of specific populations.

In addition APDA's free educational publications, written by experts in the field, address all aspects of the disease and are available in hardcopy, online, and can be downloaded from the website www.apdaparkinson.org. A quarterly hardcopy and monthly e-newsletter are also available.

Find the Cure - as a funding partner in most of the major PD scientific breakthroughs in the past half century, APDA focuses on support research on all levels. APDA Centers for Advanced Research are located at nine prestigious academic and healthcare institutions and research grants are awarded to individual scientists both experienced and those entering the specialty. Summer internships in PD laboratories are offered to medical school students to introduce them and encourage them to consider research as a career path. All research grants are reviewed and recommended by APDA's Scientific Advisory Board composed of 15 recognized experts in specific areas of PD and chaired by David G. Standaert, MD, PhD., professor and neurology chair, University of Alabama - Birmingham.

**Leslie A. Chambers,
President & CEO, APDA
www.apdaparkinson.org**

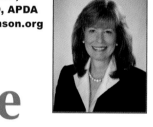

Ease the Burden Find the Cure

ADVOCACY 101 - or HOW TO GET STARTED.....

Now you've seen what others have done and may be wondering how to get started yourself.

The same question was asked on the NeuroTalk PD Forum and many forum members responded. Some of their advice on Advocacy 101 follows....
(http://neurotalk.psychcentral.com/showthread.php?t=136032)

AnnT2

I hate to sound stupid, but how exactly do you get involved in advocacy? Not how you did it, but how it would be done today at this stage? Where can we find a list of future conferences so we can at least attend those near our homes? I have volunteered for three studies, but I don't see anything but record-keeping coming from those studies. These may sound like silly questions, but I for one would love some Advocacy 101 exposure.

pkell

Those are excellent questions. I know it is frustrating to hear people extoll the wonders of involvement and yet leave no bread crumbs for others to follow. I am probably not the best to offer advice as I have mostly stumbled into the whole thing by accident and there are others who have taken a far more intentional path..... I honestly believe it (involvement in advocacy) is the best medicine we have available. It is completely restorative and I am personally certain, neuroprotective. On top of that it is great fun.

jeanb : Some ideas

I stumbled my way into advocacy, but here are some ideas. As Pam wrote, I hope others will share their experiences.

- Learn all you can about PD
- Join PAN (or any local PD organization)
- Contact them to see if they need volunteers; Ask how you can help them
- Join a support group
- Start a support group
- Talk to support groups
- Lobby your legislators about issues important to PwP
- Write letters to the editor
- Respond to newspaper or web articles or letters to the editor
- Write a blog / respond to blogs
- Write your story/ Tell your story / Share (publish) your story
- Create a poster for awareness
- Help the PD community by raising funds for:
    Research
    Awareness
    To help other PwP

GregW1 : Getting Started in Advocacy

We need to bring new people interested in advancing education and awareness and influence about Parkinson, both to increase the number of advocates out there and to replace those who have or will eventually reduce their commitment or retire from advocacy altogether as their disease progresses.......

To find out where and when conferences may be taking place in your area, the best resources are the websites for PAN, the Michael J. Fox Foundation, the Parkinson's Disease Foundation, the National Parkinson's Foundation, and the American Parkinson's Disease Association. Checking frequently with those sites will keep you abreast of any upcoming conferences in your area and will also provide important information as to issues currently being worked on in the Parkinson community. The NPF also sponsors support groups around the country. Contact them for a list of those in your area.

Large regional organizations also offer plenty of advocacy opportunities. Google for local and international PD groups.

pkell

One thing I would like to add. Advocacy may sound like altruism at its apex, but the truth is the rewards do not go to those you are advocating for, though that, of course, is a lucky by-product, but rather to you, the one advocating.

There is no feeling that compares to coming out of the darkness and standing side by side with other PwP, refusing to be silent. There is no substitute for the sense of power that comes from joining with others to make your voices heard. There is no joy like joining the communion of those who are striving to gain a seat at the table for the PwP and knowing that your participation, no matter how small, is still a part of the progress. There is such a regained sense of relevance that comes with grasping the genuine truth in:

**"TOGETHER WE ARE BETTER.
TOGETHER WE CANNOT BE STOPPED."**

violet green : Other ways to advocate

Folks have suggested joining support groups. That didn't work for me even though I love working in groups. So if any of the ideas given don't appeal, try another, or gather a group around you if that's your preferred style.

Another thing that I personally enjoyed was to join a local fund-raising event like a walk. Last spring I did my local one and also the Unity Walk in New York City. There's nothing like it - a sea of people all raising funds and awareness to fight PD - we are better together and you'll feel tired but high at the end of the day.

Ann, you've found this forum and I did too. It's been a great place for me to learn about PD from our experts, PwP and to connect with others perhaps more like-minded than those in your geographic area. Also, forum members post opportunities to participate in various campaigns and other actions here.

jeanb : good points ...

I'm not a member of a support group either....Like Katherine, I have made wonderful friends on line. That's how my buddy Sheryl and I met and started **pdplan4life**. Even though she is in Illinois and I am in Arizona, we work well together.

jeanb

One thing I can guarantee, you will feel good - feel better- after taking action in advocacy.

Debi Brooks wrote the following in another thread. They are good words.

> **"Get involved. Do something that fits you. Be part of the action. There are many things patients can do. Get educated about the disease. Get to a movement disorders specialist. Support research. Raise awareness. Volunteer for a clinical study/trial - by the way, not only are patients needed but healthy controls are needed too!"**

I can't think of a better way to start advocacy than supporting PPMI. It is searching for biomarkers for Parkinson. If scientists could identify biomarkers, it could lead to a cure.

The NeuroWriters message is:

JUST DO SOMETHING! TOGETHER WE CAN MAKE A DIFFERENCE....

My friend Jean Burns and I were 51 and 44 years old respectively when a twitching finger turned our worlds upside down. Diagnosed with young onset Parkinson, we set out to find a new purpose for our lives that would make the most of our skills - mine in writing and Jean's in art and design - and allow us to "give back" to the PD community for the support we have received on our own journeys with this disease.

The result is pdplan4life, our vehicle for sharing our daily challenges, triumphs, humorous moments, and coping strategies to empower others to live well with Parkinson by our example.

Collaborating on pdplan4life is a labor of love for Jean and me, and the most personally rewarding venture either of us has ever undertaken.

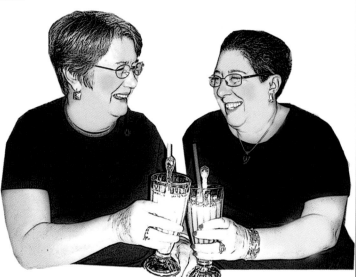

Jean Burns   Sheryl Jedlinski
www.pdplan4life.com

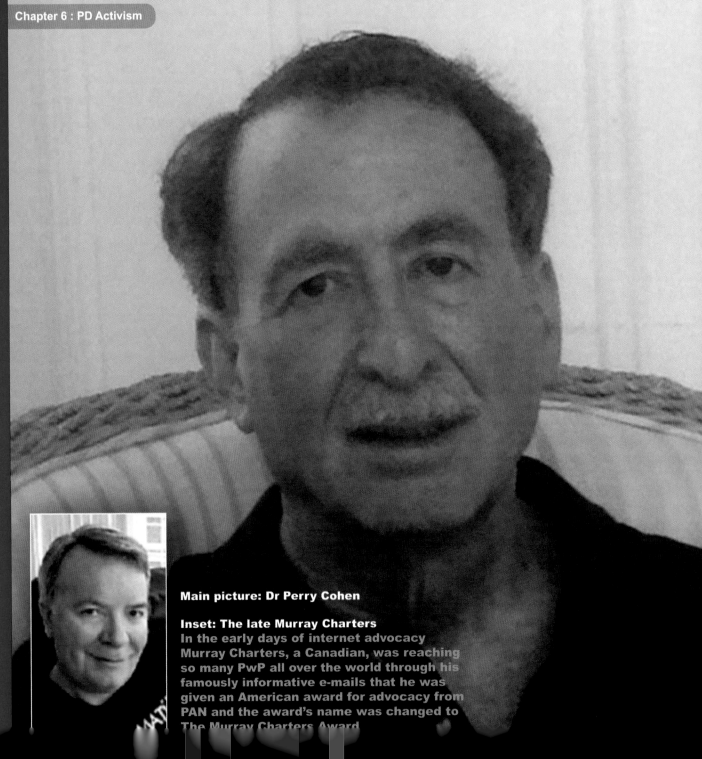

MURRAY CHARTERS / DR PERRY COHEN

Main picture: Dr Perry Cohen

Inset: The late Murray Charters
In the early days of internet advocacy
Murray Charters, a Canadian, was reaching
so many PwP all over the world through his
famously informative e-mails that he was
given an American award for advocacy from
PAN and the award's name was changed to
The Murray Charters Award

Perry Cohen, PhD: a collective tribute from the NeuroWriters Collective

Perry Cohen describes his first 50 years as "training for his most important role - to work with PD advocates and end PD as we know it."

We have not yet ended PD, but Perry has educated and inspired untold numbers of PwP with his belief that the voice of the patient is the missing element in the treatment development process and we must be heard. We must demand an equal seat at the table whenever PD is being discussed by researchers, pharmaceutical companies, doctors and other health care providers, or Parkinson organizations.

Before his PD diagnosis in 1996, Perry ran a successful health care consulting firm in Washington, DC. His knowledge of the health care and drug development system, pharmaceutical companies and his many personal contacts in government and industry have proved invaluable.

Several of the Neurowriters met Perry during the mid-1990s, on the Parkinsn email list. Perry was one of the leaders of a historic, mostly online, grassroots campaign to pass the Udall Bill to authorize and appropriate NIH funding specifically for PD research.

Perry is a true visionary, thinking about issues to be addressed next - usually years ahead of others in the PD community; pushing the envelope forward; focused on the prize - the end of Parkinson disease.

Long before terms like 'translational research' became buzzwords, he encouraged advocates to see that PD funding was "directed toward new knowledge and to translating knowledge into delivery of effective treatments to the population."

Perry was the first to advocate for PwP to lobby and work with the pharmaceutical industry to move drug development ahead more quickly. His goal (and that of the Parkinson Pipeline Project which he founded) (www.pdpipeline.org) was to develop a network of patient clinical research partners, industry advisors and FDA advisors to provide patients' perspectives in the drug development and approval process.

Perry's ideas were met with skepticism by some of the PD community. When first introduced, they might have seemed radical. Now, just a few years later, a number of these proposals have evolved and been adopted by Parkinson organizations. PAN is now tackling FDA and drug approval issues; PDF has instituted a Clinical Trials Learning Institute to train PD advocates to advise patients and encourage them to join clinical trials; four PwP have been appointed to an FDA Advisory Committee on new drug approvals. At Perry's urging, the NIH held the first international conference on the science and ethics of sham surgery.

(http://oba.od.nih.gov/rdna_rac/rac_sham_con.html)

In recognition of Perry's leadership and the impact of the 'Pipeliners', the Parkinson's Action Network awarded the 2011 "Murray Charters Award for Outstanding Service to the Parkinson Community" to the Parkinson Pipeline Project.

This award was especially meaningful because Murray was one of the original members of the group.

Linda Herman

The NeuroWriters of The Parkinsons Creative Collective would like to recognize the HUGE contribution Perry has made to the Parkinson community over the years.

We hope he can hear our heartfelt thanks and applause reverberating through cyberspace.

Note: In 2012, PCC was pleased and honored to welcome Perry to its Board of Directors.

Working for real change in science, medicine and health regulation

As her disease progressed and knowledge grew, she found herself exploring the science of PD more deeply through activism. She wanted to know what might help improve the chance for cure in her own lifetime.

She discovered that the research and drug approval process did not seem to accommodate the patient perspective. The patient should be the most important person in the whole process. Greater patient involvement could help create a real sense of urgency.

She heard about the rare practice of sham surgery that is used in certain PD trials She might volunteer for other clinical trials but was wary of anything involving sham surgery. There has to be a better and less dangerous way to show results.

In this chapter you will go deeper into the world of Parkinson: the science, possible system reforms, and the politics. Without a 'seat at the table', we feel like pawns in a game that has life and death consequences for us.

If you're as strong as those living with PD, read on.

CHAPTER SEVEN
Advocacy in action

A CURE ?

Research as partners in knowledge . . .

CONNECTING THE DOTS

CONNECTING THE DOTS
Girija Muralidhar, PhD

Though it seems like the Parkinson disease story is changing every other month, I believe it is coming together. PD scientific literature tells us that it is a neurological disease, influenced by the immune, endocrine and digestive systems as well as genetic factors. We hear about infections, inflammation and stress exacerbating PD, while exercise is beneficial. All these observations are like dots and the true identity emerges only when we begin to connect the dots. This is my perspective on what PD might be at the cellular level, based on current literature with a few hypotheses that are yet to be tested.

We often hear about genes (SNCA, Parkin, PINK1, UCHL-1 and LRRK-2), but how are they responsible for developing PD? Beginning with SNCA as an example, we connect a few dots to better understand the relationship and become familiar with some of the technical terms used in the literature.

Connecting the dots hypothesis 1
Gene mutations/modifications and PD
SNCA is alpha-synuclein (alpha-syn), a small protein present in the neurons. Though it is considered to be a chaperone protein, its function in the brain is still unclear. Mutations in the SNCA gene and/or exposure to certain chemicals make alpha-syn polymerize and form clumps.

In normal healthy neurons, if alpha-syn gets tangled and/or fails to perform, it is immediately removed from the job. It gets marked by another protein as inefficient or useless. This tagged alpha-syn is sent to a cell compartment where it is recycled. The process (called autophagy), involves many proteins that work together. Parkin and UCHL-1 are part of this system that keeps 'bad' proteins at bay.

Now imagine a scenario where mutations (whether inherited or environmental) make alpha-syn sticky and tangled. It can no longer chaperone other important proteins into the cell. Cell functions are disrupted and it is necessary to eliminate the tangled alpha-syn from the neuron. The system that recognizes this as a bad protein is already compromised in the genes of some people with Parkinson disease (those genes are Parkin and UCHL1).

Cells also recycle old and dysfunctional mitochondria, the generators in cells that supply power for the cellular processes. Mutations in genes, PINK-1 (seen among early onset PD patients), and LRRK-2 affect mitochondria by reducing its capacity to generate energy, thereby increasing the need for mitochondrial recycling (autophagy). At this stage there is a problem. If one bad mutation is present but not the others, it is possible for the cell to compensate, but with multiple mutations present proper clearing is prevented and tangled alpha-syn accumulates.

Connecting the dots hypothesis 2
Accumulation of Alpha-syn
Tangled alpha-syn is toxic to neurons. Dead or dying neurons release the toxins into the brain where they do not belong. Microglial cells (that police the brain for foreign material) take in the tangled alpha-syn as if it were a pathogen (virus or bacteria). As a consequence, cells begin to produce pro inflammatory cytokines, leading to neuro-inflammation. Inflammatory cytokines attract immune cells to the brain. These immune cells perceive tangled alpha-syn as the result of infection rather than a normal component of the body and they work hard to get rid of it. During that process, they produce more cytokines and neuro-inflammation increases, creating a spiral affect - toxicity causes neuro-inflammation and neuro-inflammation increases toxicity.

Connecting the dots hypothesis 3
PD and auto immunity
Tangled alpha-syn and/or fragments generated from it get into the blood stream and circulate in the body. The immune system is alarmed and assumes that tangled alpha-syn belongs to a pathogen that has infected the brain. The immune system dispatches T cells that are specifically designed to attack and eliminate 'infected cells', but in this case the immune system has made a huge mistake as there is no infection, just the body's own neurons making aberrant, tangled alpha-syn. The 'killer' T cells in the circulation are attracted to the cytokine signals coming from the brain and cross over blood brain barrier. (The blood brain barrier of people with Parkinson may already be compromised due to neuro-inflammation.) The T cells target neurons that have tangled alpha-syn and kill them.

Connecting the dots hypothesis 4
PD and infection
The immune system is designed not to attack its own body but to selectively eliminate invading pathogens. A variety of pathogens take advantage of this property and make proteins that camouflage as the body's own proteins. It is called molecular mimicry. For example, during influenza infection, some of the immune cells generated not only kill virus-infected cells but also the body's own cells that might seem like infected cells. Immune cells quite possibly confuse the body's own neurons with the virally infected cells and kill them too, thus initiating Parkinson disease.

As you can see, we are connecting the nervous system with the immune system. There are many more similar interactions within the nervous system, with the endocrine system and among the neurotransmitters and hormones that can fit into the Parkinson disease paradigm. There are many dots to connect because.....

PD IS A COMPLEX DISORDER.

"There is no one cause. There is no one cure. But multiple lines of damage provide multiple lines of opportunity to slow, halt, even cure. It's not a bug, it's a feature!" Rick Everett

If you look at this diagram and are confused, you're not alone. PD is complicated and progress in identifying the cause(s) and developing a cure for PD is slow in coming.

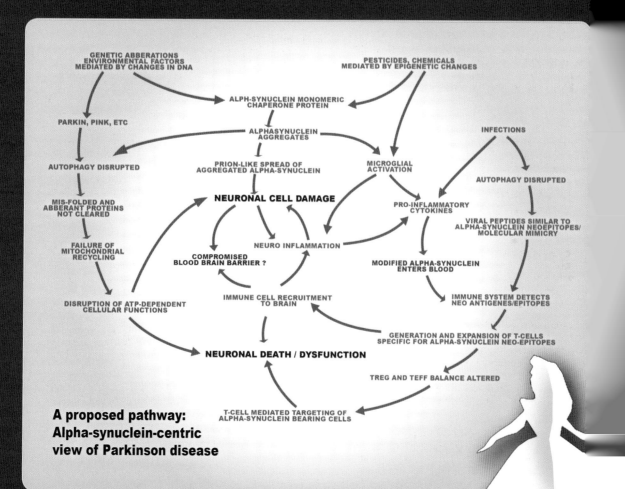

A proposed pathway:
Alpha-synuclein-centric
view of Parkinson disease

THE GULF OF MISUNDERSTANDING

Bridging the gulf between physicians, researchers and people experienced with Parkinson disease

Katherine Huseman

Another factor which impedes progress in unraveling the mysteries of PD is a lack of communication, especially between physicians and patients. In order to listen to people with different perspectives we must stay flexible and be willing to entertain new ideas as possibilities. Perhaps we can build this bridge together?

Too often, people don't really communicate - and that may be a special problem in an area as complex as Parkinson disease. How can we build a communication bridge across that gulf of misunderstanding? One possibility follows.

First, as with any physical bridge, we need a strong foundation of respect - mutual respect. Doctors and researchers may have survived medical or graduate school rigors, but people with Parkinson disease survive the challenge and progression of Parkinson disease, every day. We have different perspectives - all are valuable.

Second, most roads carry two-way traffic. Similarly, the roadway of listening on our metaphorical bridge requires travel in both directions. Let's attentively listen to each other; we may be surprised by what we hear.

Third, using the information we learn on the listening road requires us to suspend our fixed beliefs. People who think they have all the answers often dismiss viable, alternative theories. Just as a suspension bridge has strong but flexible cables, our minds and positions need to be like the cables - capable of movement to accommodate the winds of new ideas. If our positions are fixed, just like the cables, they can break under stress, cutting off other possibilities and discoveries.

We are all people; the only way to bridge the gulf between us is through respectful listening, coupled with curiosity and flexibility, so that we may explore the unknown together.

Perhaps we can build this bridge together

BUILDING BRIDGES

240

THOUGHTS OF A 'PATIENT THEORIST'

"After being online for several years and realizing that they wouldn't be cured in the five or ten years their doctors mentioned, some patients began to express their thoughts and ideas about the condition. They began to search for information about this movement disorder. This led to the development of a series of intensely debated theories.

The first to become a 'patient theorist' at Brain Talk was Michael7737". Paula Wittekind

Here is a statement he made about his research in 2001:

"Parkinson disease (disorder) is both complicated and simple at the same time.

Evidence leads us to believe that in many cases more internal environment is involved in causing the symptoms that identify what we call Parkinson disease. These include environmental toxins (the list is growing quickly), physical trauma, genetic mutation, certain medications, and emotional stress. The route taken by these stressors might vary, affecting several systems and causing a variety of symptoms along the way, but the final area of destruction is found in the dopamine producing neurons in a region of the brain called the substantia nigra. Within these cells, the mitochondria, tiny manufacturing plants which work with assembly line-like efficiency to produce substances necessary for our body to function, are deprived of substances required for their manufacture. In the end, the cell lacks energy and water enough to function and either becomes dormant or dies".

Michael 7737

241

THE NEED FOR NATIONAL REGISTRIES FOR PARKINSON DISEASE

W hat we still need is our grassroots, patient-driven data base and a web platform for taking patient surveys.

W hat we lack in money and fame we can make up in sheer numbers!

Carey Christensen

Why does the U.S. need a Parkinson registry?

For years the number of people with PD has been estimated at 1 million, but we don't know if this number is accurate. Better data on disease incidence and prevalence, geographic distribution, ethnicity, race, age, risk factors, and other epidemiologic information would help identify environmental triggers, advance understanding and treatment development and help identify needed patient services. It would also illustrate the immense burden of PD on the nation's heath care system and the economy.

What is the status of a PD Registry in the U.S.?

Bills HR1362 and S1273 were introduced in Congress in 2009. The bills were to establish a national "data surveillance system" for MS and PD, administered by the CDC (Centers for Disease Control). Data sources would include Medicare, Medicaid, VA, hospital and pharmacy records and state registries (although as of 2011, only one state - Nebraska - actually had a functioning PD registry).

With the efforts of grassroots advocates, PAN, and the MS Society, HR1362 was passed unanimously in the House in 2010.

The bill was expanded by the Senate to include all neurological disorders, (and placate Republicans insisting on "no earmarks" - although the bill wasn't really an earmark) and the title was changed to the "National Neurological Diseases Surveillance System Act."

Unfortunately, none of the Senators was willing to bring the bill to a vote before Congress adjoined in September 2010 and thus the bill "died" in the lame-duck Senate.

At the date of publication of this book, no registry bill has been approved by Congress and advocates continue to work on this issue.

So we still can't answer the question "How many people in the U.S. have PD?" **NeuroWriters**

SWEDEN IS SET TO BECOME THE FIRST COUNTRY IN THE WORLD TO HAVE A NATIONAL DISEASE REGISTRY FOR PARKINSON'S DISEASE.

The initiative is a collaborative effort between Lund University, Skåne University Hospital and Karolinska Institute, and tests of the database are scheduled to begin this spring.

"The register will really have an effect within two different areas. On the one hand, the immediate conditions for improvements in healthcare – doctors gain direct access to information of relevance to the patient; on the other hand, the research possibilities - being able to use the register to look at the impact of different treatments in larger population groups over a longer time period", Lund University professor Per Odin said in a statement.

Vivian Tse
Swedish breakthrough could slow Parkinson's
Published: 19 Jan 2011

I n Western Europe's five most populous nations (Germany, France, the United Kingdom, Italy, and Spain) and the world's ten most populous nations (China, India, United States, Indonesia, Brazil, Pakistan, Bangla Desh, Russia, Nigeria, and Japan), a conservative estimate of the number of individuals with PD over age 50 was between 4.1 - 4.6 million (Dorsey et al, 2007).

B y 2030, this number is expected, at a minimum, to double to between 8.7 and 9.3 million people with PD.

N otably, expected changes in the global population suggest that most cases of PD will be outside the Western world.

A Global View, Parkinson Report, Spring 2008.
Caroline M Tanner, Melanie Brandabur & E. Ray Dorsey

PATIENT REGISTRIES

HAVE WE MISSED PIECES OF THE PUZZLE?

Maria L. De Leon, MD

Ever since I was a young neurologist in training, I had the impression that we were missing a part of the picture when dealing with Parkinson disease. The books have always maintained that Parkinson disease primarily affects slightly more men than women, with most people over the age of 55, although a small percentage, (less than 15%) under the age of 45. As Parkinson patients, care-partners or experts in the field, when we attend various Parkinson related events we find that there isn't the same diversity present as there is in the general population. Why? We don't know and we don't know who is highest at risk among various ethnic and racial groups. Until we are able to get accurate numbers through national surveys (such as Sweden's) we may not be sure if the picture we are getting is the true and correct one.

Given my experience, I wonder if the face of Parkinson is changing or have we missed a piece of the puzzle all along by not including and analyzing ethnic and racial backgrounds in our research studies. My first recollection of a Parkinson patient was a young Hispanic woman of 40 who had had the illness for over 10 years. At that time, I thought she was the exception. During my 12 years of practice I encountered many similar patients. (I, myself a young Hispanic woman, developed Parkinson Disease in my late 30's.) We need to unravel the truth about the etiology and epidemiology of Parkinson disease.

However, while we are discovering the true numbers, we must make sure that ALL PwP receive best practice treatments and services regardless of their ethnic or racial background.

References: Incidence of Parkinson's Disease: Variation by Age, Gender, and Race/Ethnicity, Stephen K. Van Den Eeden et al, Am. J. Epidemiol. (2003) 157 (11): 1015-1022 ; Study Suggests Parkinson's More Common in Hispanics: Martin F. Downs, Reuters, 6/5/2003.

Israel Robledo

Outreach to those who have PD can be difficult, especially to those of different ethnic and racial backgrounds. For me, diversity did not play a role in my becoming an advocate. From the time of my diagnosis, I knew that I needed to seek the best medical care possible, to have the best quality of life possible and reach out to those who could not speak for themselves to help make their quality of life the best that it can be, regardless of who they were.

It was a few months later that I realized that there were very few advocates of Hispanic heritage that I could relate to on my journey. What I try to do is make personal contact and encourage all, regardless of ethnic and racial backgrounds, to seek the best medical care possible and encourage staying active and not giving in to PD. I help refer people to specialists and help in any way possible, (including through our foundation, Parkinson's Outreach, which pays for physician's fees and prescriptions for people with PD in our area).

One thing that I am most proud of is that my global 'Parkinson family' includes all, regardless of race, ethnicity, social status and any other differences. I'll continue to search for ways to increase the diversity represented in our family and I'm certain that I won't be alone in breaking down barriers for equal medical access and care for all.

CITIZEN SCIENTISTS

Personal experiences of living with PD and discovering that many of us have the same expertise on a particular aspect of PD gave us the confidence to project a bigger picture of PD. We discussed how PD is more than a movement disorder, how PD manifests in other organs. We contemplated the possible interactions of digestive, endocrine, immune and neural systems in developing PD.

These discussions were often based on specific observations, cause-effect correlations, on the experiments of curious "white rats" (a term coined by a group of self experimenting PwP), on alternative treatments that worked, and were many times backed by current scientific literature.

Awareness of these things - observations, analyses and hypotheses - got passed around the forum, and the ideas were leveled and solidified by active, at times tense and heated discussions. In the end the wilder aspects usually got weeded out and the core idea stayed on. Some of these are very feasible hypotheses, as in exercise and the non-motor aspects of PD, while others may appear speculative at this point of time.

NeuroWriters

So we offer some of these ideas in that spirit - as nobody knows what people will believe or accept as true in the future, or what will be proven to be useful.

We also reflect on patient involvement in health care.

Patients individually taking ideas to their doctors (i.e. communicating), is the way that doctors learn from their patients - the understanding of PD is a two way street...

CITIZEN SCIENTISTS AND RESEARCHERS:
A UNIQUE COLLABORATION

Summit4StemCell is working to advance a NON-embryonic stem cell treatment for Parkinson's disease. They are funding a new treatment that takes a patient's own skin cells and transforms them into dopaminergic neurons. Initially the reprogrammed cells will be tested in a rat model. Ultimately the transformed neurons, which will be an exact DNA match, will be injected into the patient's own brain, producing a personalized treatment.

To learn more visit www.summit4stemcell.org

CITIZEN SCIENTISTS

SCIENCE AND US
Rick Everett

White Rats

Rick is a PwP and experimentalist who views PD as a disorder encompassing neuronal, hormonal, immunological as well as digestive systems. He has been posting his hypotheses/theories on Neurotalk since around 2004.

The relationship between the medical community and a patient dealing with Parkinson disease can be an uneasy one. It isn't simply that medical science has yet to find a cure. It is, rather, that very little is known about the disease at all. **Despite two hundred years of effort, we do not know the cause, the course, nor the cure.** In fact, if the truth be told, the only thing we truly know is that levodopa helps with the motor symptoms for a while. It is like a jigsaw puzzle where one has managed to assemble a small section, but where the table is littered with pieces that do not yet make sense.

As a result of this state of affairs, the relationship between patient and doctor can be strained. A busy neurologist cannot be expected to feel joy at the sight of a patient waiting with a stack of printouts from the Internet. The patient cannot be expected to accept the ignorance that surrounds the disease that is stealing his life. Returning to the puzzle analogy, while the experienced may struggle with the pieces before them, a child may reach out and fit two together simply because she lacks preconceptions. Many PwP tend to be intelligent and well-educated self-starters. With the information offered by the Internet and the support of fellow patients, it would be absurd to expect them to idly wait as five years becomes ten, then fifteen.

On the map of the knowledge of PD there are vast areas labeled "Here there be Dragons", and most doctors lack the time and motivation to explore them. Ironically enough, time and motivation is precisely what the patient does have. It is true that they are self-educated, but that can be an advantage at times as in the case of the child and the puzzle.

There is an opportunity for a healing partnership and mutual education to relieve the ignorance of both parties. The doctor is accustomed to educating the patient, but may have some difficulty with the role of student. This is particularly so when the subject is unconventional, such as alternative approaches.

Many individuals facing a chronic, degenerative disease for which no cure is available are going to try alternative means sooner or later. It is totally unrealistic to assume otherwise. Sometimes they will find success. Things are out there and patients are going to look for them.

In closing, PD is no ordinary disease and it requires extraordinary approaches at all levels. One of the most important is the establishment of a true partnership with the scientific community and, if not acceptance, then at least mutual respect.

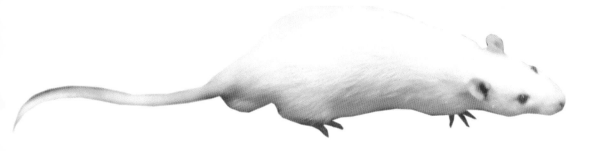

NASAL DELIVERY OF DOPA

Ron Hutton, a chemist by profession and PwP, comments on why DOPA could possibly be delivered directly to the location where it is needed (brain) via the nose. His observations date back to 2004. Despite his efforts to interest pharmaceutical companies, his approach was not validated by use until 2012.

I spent a lot of time studying this route (nasal) of drug delivery. I corresponded with several companies to try and persuade them to carry out research on the method.

It is recognized that the nasal passage goes directly into the brain. The advantage is that the nasal passage by-passes the BBB. This means you can get dopamine itself into the brain and it is instantly available. Having got there, it is 'locked in', since it cannot cross the BBB. So long as the dose is not excessive, presumably very little would pass into the bloodstream via the lungs. Most would get attracted to the receptors.

It is my understanding that the gut also produces dopamine - so I wonder if it could be 'harvested' with stimulation to produce more, attach it to a carrier to bypass BBB and have the body balance out your dopamine needs.

I have written to researchers to ask "Since dopamine is produced outside the brain as a body hormone by the same synthetic route as used in the brain, it means levodopa is also produced in the body. Levodopa CAN pass the BBB, so why doesn't the brain get a contribution of levodopa from the blood stream, and if it does, can it be increased?"

I never got a straight answer.

Ron Hutton, PhD

Editor's note: On January 6, 2012, a privately-held pharmaceutical company announced that it that is working on an inhaled formulation of levodopa (L-dopa) for the rapid relief from motor fluctuations associated with Parkinson disease.

Civitas Therapeutics,Inc. announces Positive Results from Clinical Study of CVT-301, an Inhaled L-dopa for Parkinson's Disease, Pharmacokinetic Profile in Phase 1 Study Supports use of CVT-301 in Managing Motor Fluctuations Associated with Parkinson's Disease Chelsea, MA - January 6, 2012

SURVEYS COLLECT DATA ABOUT DBS

In 2000, there was no comparative information about DBS. Margaret Tuchman corrected that. DBS is now recommended to early - onset PwP as one of the only treatments to buy time. There is still not enough information about it, how and exactly why it works, etc. A new generation seeks answers.

Imagine that you wanted to find organized, statistical data about DBS before 2001. When Margaret Tuchman looked for it she couldn't find any because each facility maintained its own records and didn't always publish its results. She discovered "that there was no collective repository of information about the types of surgery, the selection criteria of the patients, a description of the patients' condition before, during and after surgery, and [the surgical team's] protocol."

After her own bilateral DBS she developed a survey, a website and an organization, DBS-STN.org. (She is also the President of The Parkinson Alliance.) Now, many years and surveys later their research has been expanded to:

1. obtain a better understanding about the experience and well-being of individuals with PD who have received DBS, and

2. compare individuals with and without DBS in the context of both motor and non-motor symptoms related to PD.

They use standardized scales and intricate statistical methods to obtain sound results... investigating the experience of PwP as it relates to such topics as quality of life, depression and anxiety, sleep disturbance, speech disturbance, coping with PD, balance, pain, and fatigue and apathy.

Thank you, Margaret.
http://www.dbs-stn.org

DO CERTAIN DRUGS ALTER THE BALANCE OF OUR NEUROTRANSMITTERS?

It seems that another unknown is the interaction of certain drugs on the balance of our brain's neurotransmitters.

Is it the same for all with PD?
Do we know how to identify who will benefit from certain drug therapies?

Paula Wittekind, already a 'patient researcher' recounts a serious event which raises questions for researchers and physicians. She was given medications that may have altered the balance of neurotransmitters and caused problems.

Her experience supports the theory that PD is a problem of cell communication. Maybe researchers will delve into this area and find an answer. At the very least, it's a cautionary tale for all of us: Be very careful - note and report all changes in your body when you add a new substance to your daily medications. Trust your body's reaction - one size does not fit all.

Although I knew there are other neurotransmitters besides dopamine, I had never studied their relationship to each other or to our symptoms and general functioning. An experience with an Alzheimer drug a few years ago changed my outlook on Parkinson disease permanently. I believe what happened occurred because the neurotransmitters got too far out of balance.

"At that time, I was having great difficulty with weakness in my legs. It was impossible to ignore - I was wrapping my legs with Ace bandages just to walk. I asked my doctor to prescribe a drug I had taken successfully for similar symptoms. My doctor suggested as an alternative that I try a drug that is typically prescribed for Alzheimer. I went into 'good patient mode' and accepted it, but left the office thinking this outcome just wasn't right.

It didn't take long to learn that the new Alzheimer drug wasn't for me even though it is approved for use with Parkinson disease. In just a few days my legs were not the only part of my body that was weak. I became weak all over and my heart just didn't feel "right". I became so weak that I couldn't pick up my cell phone. Needless to say, I contacted my doctor and the medications were changed.

The Alzheimer drug they prescribed increases the neurotransmitter acetylcholine, which is said to be lacking in those with Alzheimer. This shortage is not a hallmark of Parkinson disease. Acetylcholine is toxic in large quantities. It can weaken and paralyze heart muscles.

In contrast, the drug I had originally asked for boosts norepinephrine; it is prescribed for depression and is a nerve painkiller with anticholinergic properties. I am still taking it successfully.

This experience has left me with several troubling, unanswered questions.
Was it acetylcholine that made me so weak?
It was obviously something in the Alzheimer drug.

- **How well do doctors know their neurotransmitters and illnesses' response to them?**
- **Could the drug have raised acetylcholine to an unsafe level?**
- **Are late-stage PwP being given Alzheimer drugs with the assumption that dementia is the same in both illnesses?**
- **Does the pharmaceutical industry, anticipating benefits of joining the research of Parkinson disease and Alzheimer, assume they can use the same drugs for both sets of patients?**
- **Should scientists be paying more attention to the interaction of neurotransmitters?"**

Paula Wittekind

THE DRUG DEVELOPMENT PROCESS AND CLINICAL TRIALS

CLINICAL TRIALS

Clinical trials, conducted in phases, are designed to determine the safety and effectiveness of a new drug or procedure in people. Each phase, with some overlap, has a primary objective with an ultimate goal of approval of the drug for general use.

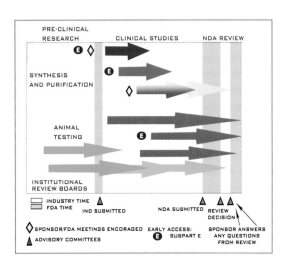

We have presented only a few examples of the challenges inherent in working on and living with PD. Now we turn to the challenges PD researchers and pharmaceutical companies must surmount to develop new drugs for PD.

Why is an over 40 year old drug still the best choice for treating PD?

PD is complicated & research takes time and money. The U.S. drug regulatory process is lengthy and is not uniform world-wide. This means that drug developers must repeat testing in multiple locations if they want to distribute widely. Many say it is difficult to recruit patients for clinical trials. Patients are reluctant for various reasons, including the need to travel to a test site, the level of participation necessary or the fact that some trials have ended suddenly leaving patients without a useful drug, or the reason why. Finally, unlike most diseases, (diabetes, heart disease) there is no objective test to determine diagnosis nor biomarkers to assess progression of the illness. The recently adopted concept of PD as a syndrome with multiple, different presentations is an additional challenge. A drug might succeed with patients in one disease profile but fail if the test group contains patients from many profiles.

Will this lead to more personalized medicine? Another unknown.

Peggy Willocks

PHASE I - Is the treatment safe?

These trials involve a small number of patients to test safety in humans and determine the correct dose of a drug.

PHASE II - Does the treatment work?

Once the experimental drug proves to be safe for human volunteers, Phase II studies test for effectiveness - does the treatment work? Since a larger number of people are studied, further information is gained on safety during Phase II trials.

PHASE III - Does the new treatment work better than the standard treatment?

Phase III trials test the new drug or treatment on hundreds of individuals. These studies are often 'double-blind' trials, meaning neither the patient nor the investigator knows which treatment is being used. They are designed to answer the question of whether or not the new treatment works better, or has fewer side effects, than the standard treatment.

PHASE IV - Is the treatment safe over time?

Phase IV trials are less common and serve to answer questions after the FDA has already approved a drug for general use. This can address questions such as long-term safety of a drug.

Also note that the approval processes in the U.S. and in other countries are not identical. Often the same treatment must be approved in many different countries at the same high cost before all patients worldwide can use it.

Girija Muralidhar, PhD

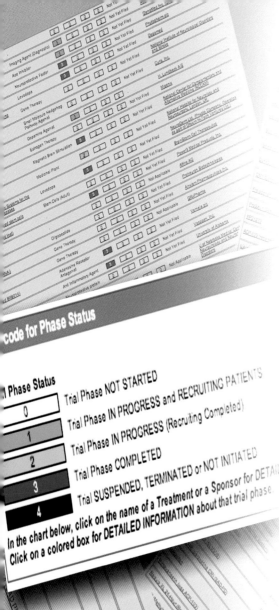

code for Phase Status

Phase Status	
0	Trial Phase NOT STARTED
1	Trial Phase IN PROGRESS and RECRUITING PATIENTS
2	Trial Phase IN PROGRESS (Recruiting Completed)
3	Trial Phase COMPLETED
4	Trial SUSPENDED, TERMINATED or NOT INITIATED

In the chart below, click on the name of a Treatment or a Sponsor for DETAILS.
Click on a colored box for DETAILED INFORMATION about that trial phase.

BRAIN TO BENCH TO BEDSIDE: AKA THE SAGA OF DRUG DEVELOPMENT

Why does the research you hear about in your morning news take so long to get to patients?

The process of developing new drugs - 'Brain to Bench to Bedside' is.a complex as well as complicated journey. It takes you to universities, biotech and pharmaceutical companies and government organizations. It requires a team of scientists, clinicians, financiers and patients. It brings out many ethical issues about laboratory animals, human volunteers and of course time, money and most importantly the lives and hopes of PwP.

Drug development: Brain to Bench to Bedside:

What is the cost?

(Adapted, with permission, from Debi Brooks' Neurotalk Post)

"If you were to visualize the path of an 'aha' idea by a brilliant basic science lab through all the necessary steps and expert hands before ultimately landing as an approved drug or procedure for patients, you would expect the journey to take 20 to 30 years and estimate the total cost to be one billion dollars."

Brain to Bench

Why is that? Well, to start, biology is hard and many ideas take decades to tease apart and to determine their relevance. Ideas can take one step forward and then, after additional results, take three steps back. Additionally, the path requires work from scores of highly specialized experts. U.S. Government money ~ $28 billion annually (chiefly through NIH) goes to academic researchers in labs at esteemed institutions to fund basic science across all diseases (~$175 million for PD). These taxpayer dollars fund 'discovery' and likely drive innovation.

Bench to Bedside

At the other end is 'industry' which takes discoveries to therapeutics. The gap between the basic research and the finished product is huge, requiring time, money and more importantly human participation. This area is commonly referred to as the translational 'valley of death'… The investments required are staggering…these are rough numbers but a Phase I trial for PD (open label safety in 10 patients) $2 - 5 million and 1 to 2 years. If successful, you go to Phase II ($15 - 40 million and another 2 years) - so, now cumulative investment (including your preclinical investments) is probably at least $50 million and you don't yet know if you have a decent candidate for a Phase III trial… Sorting out which targets will go into the clinic is data driven.

In addition to high cost, there are leaps of faith.Can success in an animal model predict success in humans? Can success in open label trials predict success in double-blind, placebo-controlled trials?

We are still seeking answers to such questions.

All these years I was on the other side of fence, wondered why patients complain, hesitate to take part in clinical trials and appear to be in a rush all the time. Now I know, I tell you, it is a lot easier to be the researcher working in a lab than be a patient waiting for the research to benefit me.

GIRIJA'S STORY

THE GRASS IS NOT GREENER ON THE OTHER SIDE...

All these years I was on the other side of the fence. I wondered why patients complained, hesitated to take part in clinical trials and appeared to be in a rush all the time. Now I know. I tell you, it is a lot easier to be the researcher working in a lab than to be a patient waiting for the research to benefit me.

As a kid growing up in India, my goals were clear and my path was straight - leading me to research in Biology. I marveled at the power of a tiny cell to accomplish so much with so few errors and enjoyed the challenges I faced in research. I sincerely believed that science had answers to curing the incurable diseases. I chose research projects that had direct connections to human diseases and hoped someday my work would be useful. When I received queries from patients about my findings and their relevance to real life, I always had the same answer: a few more experiments and only a few more years before it gets to the FDA . . .

From my point of view it was just a question of time and I had plenty of it. I never understood their urgency. I was living blissfully in my own little world of research . . .

I clearly remember the day when a colleague of mine asked me if I had injured my leg while exercising. She had noticed that I was 'dragging' my foot. With a project deadline due the next day, I joked with her while waiting for my cup of coffee, that it was obvious why I was dragging my feet. Little did I know what was in store for me! I was too busy with life. My precious little girl was just 18 months old and my career as a researcher was on the right track. I had a new home and family and there was no room for something like PD in my life. PD was already there, quite well established in all its manifestations and about to change my life.

It has been 10 years since the first symptom of PD appeared and I have now been on medications for seven years. I have to admit that I went through a couple of years of emotional roller coasters, the 'why me' phase, but I eventually accepted PD as my unwanted companion. The only time I forget about PD is when I am in the lab completely focused on an experiment I am doing, or interpreting data. Science is still an escape from reality and so I decided to try to use my escape mechanism as a move towards a better reality. I switched my research towards PD diagnostics and therapeutics, though I know it may be a long journey to reach my goal. Now that I am a PwP I understand the value of time, the urgency to find a cure, the anxiety about the future and the hope that science will come through with a miracle so that the next generation will never have to live with PD... I understand the human face of the disease, now I feel the same pain, anxiety and frustration as the millions of people behind the words 'People with Parkinson'. I hope this new 'me' can become a better person/scientist and hope to add my two cents worth to the world of PD.

Girija Muralidhar, PhD

Parkinson disease is complex and the drug regulatory process is lengthy. Further complicating matters, there is NO test which can identify PwP nor is there any lab test to measure the progression of the disease. These interesting, different approaches include the MJFF Biomarker Project, the Fox Trial Finder and mathematician Max Little's voice analysis phone call test.

THE PARKINSON DISEASE BIOMARKER:

A Critical Missing Link for Understanding PD, Currently Under Investigation by The Michael J. Fox Foundation

One of the greatest hurdles to developing new treatments for Parkinson disease – particularly therapies that prevent, slow or reverse the progression of the disease – is the lack of clear and reliable PD biomarkers. From 2002 to 2010, The Michael J. Fox Foundation (MJFF) invested over $28 million in biomarker discovery and development, setting the stage for a comprehensive study to validate promising biomarkers of Parkinson disease. In 2010, MJFF – in collaboration with industry partners and generous funders – launched the Parkinson's Progression Markers Initiative (PPMI), a $45-million landmark study to definitively verify biomarkers of Parkinson disease.

So what is a biomarker? In general, a biomarker is defined as a substance, process or characteristic in the human body that can be correlated with the risk or presence of a disease, or that changes over time, in a way that can be linked to disease progression. For example, blood pressure can be objectively and easily measured and serves as a biomarker of both normal cardiovascular function and (when high) of potential cardiovascular disease.

Parkinson disease is a complex neurodegenerative disorder with many underlying causes that may differ among individuals. For this reason, identifying a biomarker - or set of biomarkers - for PD requires sophisticated methods of measurement targeted at various aspects of the disease. PPMI uses advanced imaging, biologic sampling and clinical and behavioral assessments to evaluate a cohort of 400 recently diagnosed Parkinson patients who are not yet on medication and 200 control participants who do not have a close relative with PD.

Identifying biomarkers will be transformative to the PD community, allowing scientists to objectively diagnose, monitor and predict the disease. Currently, there is no way

to definitively diagnose Parkinson disease in a living person. Instead, a diagnosis is based on the presence of clinical symptoms including resting tremor, rigidity and bradykinesia (slow movement).

In addition to aiding diagnosis, PD biomarkers are critical to developing long-awaited disease-modifying treatments for PD, enabling researchers to concretely determine whether a candidate therapy is, or is not, impacting disease course in PD patients. Furthermore, a biomarker that can identify people with PD - or those at risk - could make it possible to intervene with protective and preventative therapies (once available) before significant dopamine neuron loss has occurred.

PPMI is the first clinical study to assemble a population of sufficient size and collect biologic samples and clinical information, draw meaningful scientific conclusions over time and try to develop better ways to measure the progression of PD. All biosamples and clinical data acquired from the study's participants will be made available to qualified researchers around the world in a comprehensive Parkinson database. By fostering such collaboration within the scientific community, PPMI will help increase the pace of biomarker validation and clinical testing as well as accelerate the pace of discovery.

PPMI is currently under way in 19 sites across the United States and Europe. Two additional European sites are set to launch in fall 2011, and the Foundation is exploring the possibility of bringing PPMI to Australia by 2012, making it a truly global study. PPMI is an opportunity to be part of a new model focused on collaboration and knowledge sharing - with a goal of creating the tools that will enable the development of transformational therapies and ultimately, a cure for Parkinson.

If you would like to help knowledge grow by participating in a clinical trial, the Fox Trial Finder makes it easier to make a good match.

FOX TRIAL FINDER
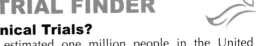

Why Clinical Trials?

Today, an estimated one million people in the United States and more than five million worldwide are living with Parkinson disease (PD). PD affects one in 100 people over the age of 60, though some people are diagnosed as young as their 20s or 30s. In the United States, 60,000 new PD cases will emerge this year alone. As the U.S. population ages, this number will only grow. According to a recent Wall Street Journal opinion piece by Nobel laureate Stanley Prusiner and former Secretary of State George Shultz, three out of five Americans will suffer from a nervous-system disease such as Parkinson or Alzheimer.

Clearly, the need for high-impact investment in research has never been more urgent. While financial investment is critical, dollars alone will not take us across the finish line in pursuit of therapeutic breakthroughs. The active involvement of Parkinson patients and their loved ones in clinical research is vital to finding the cure.

Clinical trials and studies play a critical role in the development of new and better medicines. In Parkinson and across many diseases, there is a significant opportunity to streamline and increase the flow of willing volunteers into these studies.

Under-enrollment in trials slows research progress and deters potential funders from investing in research - and we all pay the price for higher costs and longer time horizons to therapeutic breakthroughs. Currently, 80 percent of clinical trials finish late due to difficulties enrolling participants. Even more alarming, nearly one-third of trials fail to recruit a single subject and cannot ever begin.

According to a 2005 Harris Poll survey commissioned by The Michael J. Fox Foundation, only one in 10 people with PD takes part in trials. At MJFF, we understand that real-world issues, including work, distance and finances, can prevent even the most motivated volunteers from taking part in a trial. We also realize that simply identifying appropriate nearby trials can in itself be a hurdle to getting started. Yet in spite of the challenges, we know that this low participation rate belies the Parkinson community's significant interest in stepping up.

For patients and their loved ones alike, the reasons to participate in a trial are numerous. Recent research conducted at the University of Lisbon in Portugal identified the prevailing factors that motivate people with PD, the most prevalent of which was a desire to help the advance of science. The study also highlighted participants' overwhelmingly positive response toward clinical trials: approximately 67 percent reported that they would participate in the same trial again and that they were willing to participate in a future trial.

The dedicated engagement of the PD community - both people with and without PD - will make progress toward a cure come more swiftly. You can be an agent of change. Take a more active role in your own health care. Contribute to the understanding of Parkinson disease. Volunteer for a clinical trial and you could be the key that helps us unlock a cure to Parkinson.

You can create a profile on Fox Trial Finder

AND NOW FOR SOMETHING COMPLETELY DIFFERENT:

Max Little, PhD from MIT Media Lab, is trying to develop a new way of evaluating Parkinson symptoms that is inexpensive and objective. If you live in the US, Canada, UK, Brazil, Mexico, Spain or Argentina you can help, see below!

To introduce myself, I'm a scientist at MIT working on Parkinson (www.maxlittle.net). My aim is to help patients and their carers help themselves by creating low-cost, noninvasive, symptom monitoring technologies. In particular, I have a method for quantifying symptom severity on the Unified Parkinson's Disease Rating Scale using voice recordings alone. This could be very useful, because then it would take only about 30 seconds to get an objective symptom score, which would enable daily, or even more frequent, symptom tracking. I am hoping that you will be interested in exploring the use of this technology in managing your own symptoms on a day-to-day basis. To help in improving the quality of this technology, we launched the Parkinson's Voice Initiative (PVI) at the TEDGlobal 2012 conference in Edinburgh. We have telephone numbers set up in several countries, people can call in and leave a voice recording. We've had an extraordinarily positive response so far; more than 3,500 people from across the world, have contributed, totally exceeding our expectations. We have now reached our 10,000 and we'd be very happy if you want to follow our research, at **www.parkinsonsvoice.org**

Max Little

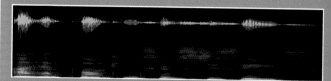

John Turner in the UK was the first to post information about PVI on Neurotalk. He added this update and comment:

As of 16th August, 2012, PVI had received 11,217 calls (US, 6601; UK, 2097; France 1337; Canada, etc.) In my view this is an exciting initiative. It's getting huge numbers of people taking part. With these numbers its benefits should go way beyond diagnosis. As I understand it, when fully developed, the technique should be able to give a Parkinson score. This should allow very rapid clinical trials, e.g. ring in to give a baseline, take curcumin for a week, ring in an end-point call, a day later have the results.

John Turner

THE ROUTE TO CURES, A PATIENT CENTERED MODEL

Perry D. Cohen, PhD

My vision of the "cure" for Parkinson (PD) is derived from my lay person's understanding of neuro-scientific knowledge and my own educated understanding of human systems, as well as my 16 years living with PD. There is a paradigm shift underway toward patient-centered models that takes into account a strong psychological component in the effective treatment for all chronic diseases.

In the patient-centered model the importance of activation and engagement of patients and their spirits, hopes and expectations are paramount. A PwP's own evaluation of the risks and benefits of therapies will be the operational objectives for each individual who will profit from becoming a full partner with medical professionals, who take roles as experts to assist in the interpretation of scientific evidence and the specification of alternative choices for treatment decisions.

What does this patient-centered paradigm mean for patients, doctors, medical research, healthcare delivery and what tools do we need to implement patient-centered health?

We need a better understanding of what motivates and what inhibits PwP from becoming more activated and engaged in their own care. We know that there are effective actions, such as regular exercise, that we can take to help our symptoms. Everyone can do more to self-activate. How can we reinforce and support self-activation, including participation in clinical research?

We need information technology to provide personalized information support for health decisions and to facilitate communications between doctors and PwP, such as a diary with a standardized method to collect individual data on observations of daily living (ODL). We also need a standardized data set and electronic health records (EHR) to provide a rich source of observational data for tasks such as monitoring safety of therapies throughout their life-cycle.

We need PD community wide support for **patients as true partners in medical research and healthcare, not merely research subjects or customers for medical products.** We also need greater consideration of the patient perspectives in regulatory decisions, especially where they differ from the scientists' views, including 1) TIME DELAYS; the balance between safety for patients versus time delay for additional preliminary studies or reviews, 2) ERROR TOLERANCE: the balance between the likelihood of acceptance of false positives (statistical model default) versus acceptance of false negatives (patient preference) in clinical trial design, and 3) BIAS CONTROL: the characterization of psychological response to context of a study (i.e. placebo response) as bias versus part of the treatment.

Unanswered questions in CLINICAL STUDY DESIGN:

• Why do many phase II placebo controlled trials fail?

• Is a placebo control group always needed?

• In surgical trials, is sham surgery always necessary?

• Is sham surgery ethical?

• Does the selection criteria for volunteers reflect the variability of PD?

• Should gene profiling be used to tailor treatments and trials to specific populations?

• How can patients' observations be integrated into the study data?

• Are the end points realistic and measurable?

NEW DRUG ACCESSIBILITY:

• Should sponsors continue to make a study drug available to the trial participants once the study is concluded?

• Should new treatments be made available to patients facing debilitating or life threatening disease before they receive full FDA approval?

HUMAN SUBJECT PROTECTION:

• Are federal guidelines for the protection of human subjects sufficient or do we need a stronger Declaration of Rights for clinical trials?

• How can patient input be recognized and accepted at every level of new treatment development?

Linda Herman and Girija Muralidhar, PhD

TRANSLATIONAL MEDICINE:
KEY TO PROGRESS OR BRIDGE TO NOWHERE?

"Drug safety would continue to be ensured by the U.S. Food and Drug Administration. While safety-focused Phase I trials would continue under their jurisdiction, establishing efficacy would no longer be under their purview. Once safety is proven, patients could access the medicine in question through qualified physicians. Patients' responses to a drug would be stored in a database, along with their medical histories. Patient identity would be protected by biometric identifiers and the database would be open to qualified medical researchers as a "commons." The response of any patient or group of patients to a drug or treatment would be tracked and compared to those of others in the database who were treated in a different manner or not at all. These comparisons would provide insights into the factors that determine real-life efficacy: how individuals or subgroups respond to the drug. This would liberate drugs from the tyranny of the averages that characterize trial information today."

Dr. Andy Grove, Science 23 September 2011: Vol. 333 no. 6050 p. 1679

Girija Muralidhar, PwP, attended the Stem Cell Summit in Pasadena in October 2011. Her notes and responses follow -- this is her interpretation of Dr. Grove's recommendations to improve the drug approval process.

At the Stem Cell Summit he stated the following:

Drug Development: In the traditional path of drug development, academic and research labs do the basic research. Then pharmaceutical or small biotech companies do the translational work and manufacture the drugs. The average time for drug development is almost 14 years, cost is close to 1.4 billion dollars. Less than 1% of tested therapeutics reach the market. For anyone with PD, these are frustrating and utterly discouraging facts.

Dr. Grove recommends that we encourage medical centers to become more goal-oriented, provided with scientists dedicated and funds targeted to assure timely and efficient transition of basic research to translational research.

Patents and Intellectual Property(IP): While Intellectual Property and patents are valuable in converting an idea to a product or therapeutics, [sometimes] these issues keep key products off the market. Trivial and obvious inventions choke up the system and hinder innovation. We need to limit the number of patents, recognize exceptional IP as well as protect the patent rights of inventors.

Reorganization of regulatory processes: Dr. Grove reported that FDA's role in drug development changed from monitoring the safety of new therapeutics (1930) to determining the efficacy (1980s) and much more (2010). The FDA's additional tasks have not kept pace with technology which makes it difficult to utilize the vast information on drugs that are stored by the FDA.

Dr. Grove suggests that FDA should store all the data in digital format and provide easy access to all the stakeholders--for patients' benefit. He continued with the often-quoted (see above) concept of returning the FDA to its earlier mission of ensuring safety and leaving proof of efficacy for post approval. This would significantly shorten bench-to-bedside time for a new drug.

Describing such a scenario, truly exceptional drugs or inventions would rapidly move on to translational research, go through Phase I and II clinical studies to establish the safety of new products in humans as per FDA standards. Once safety is established, the product would be available to patients as an experimental drug while the Phase III efficacy studies and FDA reviews for marketing are moving in parallel tracks.

If a drug is safe for human use, I would have a choice to use it or wait till the FDA approves it. That is my idea of Participatory medicine. **Girija Muralidhar, PhD**

ANDREW S. GROVE, PhD
Dr. Grove served as President, CEO and Chairman of Intel Corporation. He is a prostate cancer survivor and PwP, author of papers and books, including Only the Paranoid Survive. As a Patient Advocate at the University of California San Francisco, he helped to develop a program leading to a Masters Degree in Translational Medicine. He is an advisor to the Michael J. Fox Foundation and the International Rescue Committee.

ARE WE RISKING ALL BY RISKING NOTHING?

Opinion by Tom Isaacs
Summer 2012 | EPDAPLUS | 9

In the world of Parkinson, risk affects everyone - from people living with the condition to international corporations. Tom Isaacs discusses how the communication of different attitudes to risk has a critical role to play in the speed of development of new Parkinson treatments.

Parkinson can often impair people's capacity to make large strides forward at speed.

In my case, when my medication stops working, every step forward involves a shift of balance and momentum for which I have to take a calculated gamble as to whether my feet will follow my body at sufficient speed to prevent my falling over. Having lived with Parkinson for the last 17 years, I have grown accustomed to the fact that this condition is a risky business - a never-ending game of chance and a constant battle for consistency and control. Yet as people with Parkinson (PwP) wrestle with this reality, I wonder whether we are sacrificing our ability to contribute to the wider issue of risk assessment in the context of scientific progress. It is surely no accident that medical advances in Parkinson over the past 45 years have made about as much tangible impact on PwP's lives as my subscription to Advanced Knitting magazine has had on mine.

Having said that, there have, of course, been huge scientific advances in the last few years – involving growth factors, calcium channel blockers, gut hormones, gene therapy, stem cells and small molecules – so do they suggest that we have something to get excited about at long last? (I also know from the funding applications we receive at The Cure Parkinson's Trust that these and other relatively new approaches are vying to become the first undisputed disease-modifying therapy in Parkinson.)

THE BLAME GAME

The speed of translating this new science to the actual delivery of treatments is largely beholden to the complexities of the regulatory system – an 'entity' that has become the single biggest obstacle in the quest for improved therapies.

While it is easy to apportion blame to a faceless group that we call 'the regulators', the truth is we are all equally responsible for this state of affairs.

Together the stakeholders in the clinical trial process - industry, healthcare providers, PwPs, scientists, payers and regulators - have conspired to render the regulation, clinical trials and outcome measurement systems to a state in which they are, quite simply, not fit for purpose. For me, there is one critical and all-encompassing factor that stems the flow of progress across European healthcare: the control of risk. You only have to look at the phrase "contains nuts" on a packet of peanuts or the words "contents hot" on a takeaway coffee to know that the grounds on which consumers are currently litigating are bordering on the absurd.

It is precisely the same situation with innovation in healthcare. Industry, regulators and scientists alike are so intent on looking over their shoulders that they have little incentive or motivation to innovate or pioneer. Because of this, the system that aims to promote scientific advancement is pushing its own self-destruct button. Regulation is being heaped on regulation and the inevitable result is that nothing ever happens. To break this cycle, risk needs to be effectively communicated and then responsibility shared between consumer (patient), administrator (clinician), regulator (government) and manufacturer (industry). A team approach to risk is an essential component if scientific advancement in the field of medicine is to be achieved.

The race is certainly on but the reality is that scientific breakthroughs have not yet been translated into anything meaningful for PwP.

After all, how can someone without the condition make an informed judgment on the risks - namely, the pros and cons of a potential treatment - without first seeking opinion from patients?

I cannot understand why - when health is the most important aspect of our lives - we must hand over all responsibility and control to others. There is simply no reason for the natural autonomy that we have over our own destinies to be subjugated to government controls when we suffer ill health. Of course, the damaging consequence of our risk being managed exclusively by other agencies is not just restricted to increased litigation: it also adversely affects people's freedom of choice and the industry's ability to innovate; prolongs clinical trial timescales; prevents the prioritization of potentially high-impact medicines; and suppresses the ability to tackle the important issues of disease specificity and personalization.

A PARTNERSHIP OF EQUALS

There are solutions available to us. Healthcare is at its best when it is conducted as a partnership of equals and patients, such as myself, are far more likely to share in the responsibility of our own health if we understand all the issues. Therefore, healthcare professionals must give their patients a better understanding of the risks involved in the proper management of their health. What we need is proper representation – a voice to communicate the respective levels of risk and benefit that we think are appropriate and which better reflect our first-hand experience of Parkinson. After all, how can someone without the condition make an informed judgment on the risks - namely, the pros and cons of a potential treatment - without first seeking opinion from patients? Without better, more experience-based input into regulatory procedures, there is a real danger that the demands of the system will suffocate the translation of highly promising science and, instead, encourage the development of treatments that are either inconsequential modifications of existing therapies or have little relevance to a patient's needs.

As PwP we must look beyond our own circumstances if we are to help change the emphasis in the management of the disease from care to cure and from degeneration to regeneration.

Tom Isaacs is president and co-founder of the Cure Parkinson's Trust (www.cureparkinsons.org.uk) and a co-founder of Parkinson's Movement He has lived with Parkinson for 17 years.

Patient concerns about Clinical Trials and
SUGGESTED REFORMS

Clinical trials are necessary and useful to develop safe and effective treatments. Patient advocates are concerned that trials can take a very long time before yielding results, put patients at risk and there is inadequate communication.

Additional issues are a lack of trust among different stakeholders and a lack of transparency of data.

When clinical trials are suddenly terminated without explanation to trial participants it can and has caused suspicion and mistrust among researchers, sponsors and patients.

Many potential participants believe that involving patients in all phases of the design of the trial along with transparent and complete reporting of all trial results would reduce fears and increase participation.

It is interesting that our last few writers stress patient involvement in the regulatory process including patient risk analysis for new treatments. NeuroWriters

Many of the questions above affect others with chronic diseases. Let's work together to advocate for change.

SUGGESTED REFORM • INCREASING TRIAL PARTICIPATION

257

Funding Groups

People with
Parkinson's

Doctors

Organizations

Regulators

Drug Companies

Researchers

Families &
Care Partners

PATIENTS ARE STAKEHOLDERS

PATIENTS BELONG AT THE TABLE FOR EVERY STEP IN THE EVALUATION OF NEW THERAPIES!

Without patient advocates sitting at the table during the drug regulatory and approval process - those who are included make decisions for their own reasons, without patients' sense of urgency and perspective.

We believe that if patient advocates participated in trial design, trials would cost less, succeed more often and have increased patient participation. The GDNF case (next page) provides a good example of what can happen without patient involvement.

Trends in medicine today are moving toward greater 'patient centered' research and care. We observe that other groups (e.g. clinical researchers, industry sponsors, regulators, advocacy organizations) involved in the evaluation of new therapies claim to speak on behalf of the patients' interests, but are really speaking for their own interests that may overlap with patients' interests.

PwP activists contend that actual PD patients are the best qualified to speak for the patients.

Our bottom line is very simple: we want no decision about us, without us. **NeuroWriters**

No decision about us, without us.

Quilt square was PCC's contribution to the WPC 2010 quilt exhibit.

QUESTIONS TO ASK

Anyone interested in participating in a clinical study should know as much as possible about the study and feel comfortable asking the research team questions about the study, the related procedures, and any expenses. The following questions might be helpful during such a discussion. Answers to some of these questions are provided in the informed consent document. Many of these questions are specific to clinical trials, but some also apply to observational studies.

- What is being studied?
- Why do researchers believe the intervention being tested might be effective? Why might it not be effective? Has it been tested before?
- What are the possible interventions that I might receive during the trial?
- How will it be determined which interventions I receive (for example, by chance)?
- Who will know which intervention I receive during the trial? Will I know? Will members of the research team know?
- How do the possible risks, side effects, and benefits of this trial compare with those of my current treatment?
- What will I have to do?
- What tests and procedures are involved?
- How often will I have to visit the hospital or clinic?
- Will hospitalization be required?
- How long will the study last?
- Who will pay for my participation?
- Will I be reimbursed for other expenses?
- What type of long-term follow-up care is part of this trial?
- If I benefit from the intervention, will I be allowed to continue receiving it after the trial ends?
- Will results of the study be provided to me?
- Who will oversee my medical care while I am in the trial?
- What are my options if I am injured during the study?

From USNIH Clinical Trials information at:
http://clinicaltrials.gov/ct2/info/understand#Questions

GDNF

You've now explored some of the issues in clinical trials. The patient who is central to the process is rarely involved in decisions nor are patient voices heard when assessing risk. The GDNF trial brought these issues to the PD community and it responded by organizing protests to reverse the corporate decision to halt an ongoing trial. The story of GDNF is important for PwP because it illustrates many of the problems in the current drug approval process.

A new era of PD advocacy began when a biotech company halted all clinical trials in its patented synthetic Glial-cell Derived Neurotrophic Factor (GDNF) one of the most promising Parkinson treatments to emerge in many years. GDNF is a large molecule protein found in the brain and used to repair damaged neurons.

In 2003, two open label Phase I trials were completed. GDNF infusions brought significant improvements to many trial participants. Some were able to return to work after years of disability. GDNF was considered a 'miracle drug' and the best chance for a cure. Six months into the Phase II trial, interim statistics did not support what some patients were experiencing. (The statistics were based on rating scales but did not incorporate performance of daily living tasks.) Citing a 'lack of efficacy' and safety concerns the trials were abruptly halted. Trial doctors were instructed to stop the infusions immediately and remove the pumps. Some disagreed with the decision and, in defiance, kept their patients' pumps operating with a saline solution in the hopes that GDNF infusions would be resumed.

Several trial doctors spoke out on behalf of the GDNF patients and argued against the company's decision. Trial participants were devastated physically and emotionally by the withdrawal of GDNF. They pleaded with the company to reinstate the treatments, offering to sign waivers, absolving them of responsibility for any adverse effects. The company refused to change the decision or to speak directly to any of the participants.

The Internet was the perfect vehicle for GDNF trial participants, doctors and advocates to connect and collaborate. Advocates began a campaign to support the rights of trial participants and lawsuits were filed. The court decided in favor of the drug company.

The British medical journal, The Lancet, in an editorial commented: "The fact that the case has ended up in the courts highlights the lack of a suitable mechanism through which evidence from individuals can be taken into account in decision-making about experimental treatments. The case also shows that although patient choice has become a mantra for health services, when it comes to setting the research agenda, patients have barely any involvement at all."

Lancet Editorial: Patient Choice in Clinical Trials, The Lancet; 6/11/2005, Vol. 365 Issue 9476, 1984.

A generation of PwP lost their best chance for a normal life.

Revival of GDNF

In 2008, a new company obtained the license for GDNF. The NIH is planning a 2013 gene therapy clinical trial. In the UK, supported by the Cure Parkinson's Trust and Parkinsons UK, a new Phase II study will begin with GDNF infusions using a newly designed delivery system.

In the prior study the improvement of trial participants' symptoms was attributed to the 'Placebo' effect. For PwP, who benefited from the treatment and some of the physicians who had witnessed their recovery, three years of placebo effect was difficult to believe.

Besides GDNF, two other trials of significant importance and potential benefit to PwP ended similarly. The first was, **Spheramine** (retinal pigmented epithelial cell transplantation to restore dopamine production) and the second, CERE 120 (gene therapy with Neurturin, a growth factor similar to GDNF). Significantly, both involved neurosurgery and sham surgery for some trial participants as controls. Researchers gave the same reasons and used the same words as reasons for failing to continue with trials: 'the placebo effect', 'unmet endpoints' and 'failed clinical trials'. Most of these trials did not hear or heed patients' reports of substantial improvement in daily living activities.

In a partial reversal of the halting of the CERE 120 trial Ceregene with the Fox Foundation (MJFF), is conducting a Phase II B study with modifications in location of delivery and dosage.

Neurowriters

GDNF:
LESSONS LEARNED

The struggle was a seminal event for PD advocacy because:

- It was the first time such a large number of PwP advocates rallied behind a single objective.
- It was the first large scale attempt of patient advocates to lobby industry.
- It was the first attempt to ask a big corporation to justify its actions and consult with patients regarding decisions made on their behalf.
- It enlarged the role of patient advocates.

Advocates meet in 2004:
In 2013 we are still awaiting results of trials for GDNF

What are reasonable expectations for people with Parkinson regarding treatments and quality of life? We weren't sure after the GDNF experience.

"FAILED" CLINICAL TRIAL:

A participating PwP view

While waiting on a list for a DBS clinical trial, I found out about the Spheramine trial and enrolled immediately. The Spheramine surgery involved transplanting retinal cells from a donor eye into my brain.

The first six patients in Phase I had open label surgery - we knew we were getting the real thing. After forty-eight months, a presentation at the Annual American Academy of Neurology reported that the average improvement of these six people was a significant 49%. I was observably "better." Four years after this promising beginning, on July 8, 2008, the Phase II statistics were in and "my" miracle trial was dropped.

Seventy-two people participated in the Phase II Spheramine trial. In this phase half the participants received sham surgery, an invasive procedure where holes are drilled in the skull and nothing is infused.

Of the seventy-two participants in the Phase II trial no one knew who received the genuine retinal cells and who did not. Based on observations the trial was still showing moderately good results, but after the statistics were analyzed the trial results did not meet projected endpoints and the trial was halted. The obvious improvement of so many of the participants was credited to the placebo effect.

Now, twelve years since the first hole was drilled into the first man's head, one of the first six was deemed to have been misdiagnosed and three of the remaining five in my trial have had Deep Brain Stimulation. Is it possible the placebo effect is still responsible for my being better after twelve years and with only a little more medication than I took then?

I haven't made my mind up yet to have DBS, but I am 12 years older than I was when I had my first experimental surgery and I have been living with Parkinson for nearly eighteen years so I won't be on the surgical schedule until I have explored ALL the options.

Peggy Willocks

SHAM BRAIN SURGERY IS NO SUGAR PILL

Perry Cohen & Neurowriters

You probably know about double-blind, placebo controlled clinical trials by now. Neurosurgical trials involve drilling holes in the patient's head and inserting a substance or device that is intended to treat PD. If the researchers are trying to determine whether the treatment works, in the US, FDA policy would require some of the patients to have the holes drilled but no substance or device would be inserted. Those patients would serve as a control for the placebo* response to brain surgery. The total procedure is called sham surgery.

For moral and ethical reasons, sham surgery is rarely, if ever, used in Europe, nor anywhere else in the world. Patient activists think that sham surgery should be prohibited because the research volunteer is at a relatively high risk for adverse events from brain surgery and psychological stress from blinding/unblinding. In addition, the entire premise is based on a giant deception. (Wittekind 2012)

In an attempt to limit the use of sham control groups in US neurosurgical trials, patient activists in the US and UK have identified scientific rationale to explain why sham surgery trials fail so often, and have presented the patients' position to industry and the government.

Note: *A Placebo response or effect has traditionally been seen as a patient's response to the administration of an inert substance, such as a sugar pill, or simulated procedure, such as sham surgery, that does not actually deliver the treatment substance. The patient expects to improve. This creates a totally psychological but real effect that releases dopamine and lights up MRIs and PET scans in the lab.

PATIENT ADVOCATES CONTRIBUTIONS TO THE SHAM SURGERY DEBATE:

1. As patient advocates, the Parkinson Pipeline Project had ethical concerns about sham neurosurgical control groups. See their article on ethics in clinical neuroscience. (Cohen 2007).
2. Then, after the third (GDNF, Neurturin, Spheramine) consecutive "failure to meet primary end points" in a pivotal trial, followed closely by the publication of the successful DBS study (Weaver 2009) which did not include a sham control group, Pipeliners examined the characteristics of the study designs and conduct in light of the recent research on placebo response. Their analysis was presented at the ASENT (2009) Annual Conference. (Cohen 2009)

3. All of this work was the catalyst for the NIH Recombinant DNA Advisory Committee's sponsoring the 2010 NIH conference on Sham Surgery. Dr. Perry Cohen helped plan the conference and was invited to present the patient activists' view.
4. Pipeliners identified differences in vantage point and assumptions of scientists vs. PwP (ASENT 2011). They concluded that from the patients' viewpoint the strong placebo response to brain surgery was not bias to be eliminated but rather part of the treatment, and that prolonged blinding not only distorts and dilutes the treatment (and the validity of the trial), but also potentially harms PwP. (Cohen 2011)
5. A report from the NIH conference was published in The Lancet Neurology (Galpern 2012). It included 13 authors with no patient participation. Pipeliners with Cure Parkinson's Trust and Parkinson's Movement responded with a letter to the editor stating that patient activist views were not adequately represented in the report. Quoting the letter:

"Patients, as the ultimate stake-holders, are in many ways best positioned to discuss the ethical issues surrounding sham surgery and how the interface of risk, benefit, and development of techniques can be best assessed, in relation not only to science, but also to their lives." (Cohen 2012)

ALTERNATIVE APPROACHES

So how should you respond if a researcher or physician says sham surgery is necessary in clinical trials? Perry Cohen provides us with some answers:

Researchers could use single-blind, randomized controlled trials comparing the new treatment against the best medical treatment available. (This was done for the evaluation of DBS.) Also providing a follow-up time long enough to assess results after the placebo effects have worn off. Other advantages are that doctors could use the information directly in their practice, and safety data from the experimental treatment would be grounded and more useful.

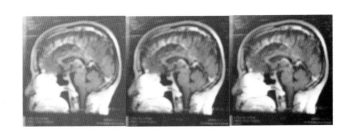

In addition, a patient-centered design would blind and centralize the clinical outcome raters to control for most of the evaluation bias and to reduce noise from variable raters.

A patient-centered design would NOT arbitrarily modify and dilute the treatment with purposeful deception and prolonged uncertainty for the sake of comparison.

Perry Cohen believes: "[A]s the medical miracles from research based on a science-centered model have waned in the first decade of this century, adoption of a patient-centered paradigm that emphasizes collaboration with activated patients will be necessary to conquer chronic diseases."

A FEW ADDITIONAL COMMENTS

Currently requirements for double-blind placebo-based tests increase the cost of clinical trials (sham surgery trials are very expensive and difficult to conduct.) Also, since it is not required in other countries, this delays introduction of potentially useful treatments and is an additional hurdle to pass before it is introduced in the US (for example, at the date of publication, Duodopa is still not available in the US after more than a decade of use in Europe and more than 4 years beyond the initial meetings with the FDA of sponsors who want to offer this therapy in the US.)

Many treatments currently in development involve surgical placement of substances or devices in the brain. Therefore under existing US policy more sham surgery trials and participants would be scheduled. (Note: US law does NOT require sham surgery-- it is only FDA common practice.) This is a critical issue for patient action now.

If you'd like to read more and see full arguments on both sides of this issue, they are well described in the article titled, "Why Fake It?" by Alla Katsnelson in Nature. (Katsnelson 2011)

WE LEAVE YOU WITH A DESCRIPTION OF WHAT HAS HAPPENED TO SOME PWP, A THANK YOU TO TRIAL VOLUNTEERS AND SOME QUESTIONS FOR YOU TO DECIDE.

Can you imagine being put under anesthesia, having holes drilled into your head, perhaps even penetrating the outer fabric of your brain. Then years later you find out you were in the control group and received no actual treatment. But it's not all bad - you already have the holes in your head so you can receive the real thing now. But that can only happen if the trial had positive results and the treatment was approved. If the trial was suspended or halted (which often has happened), you are left with holes in your head and most likely will be unable to qualify for any other trials.

Some brave and altruistic PwP do volunteer for these trials. We thank you!

WHAT DO YOU THINK?

• Do you think sham surgery is ethical?

• Do you think the benefit outweighs the harm?

• Would you enroll in a clinical trial where you might receive surgery but no potential treatment?
The majority of activist PwP in on-line surveys say "no".

"We should avoid institutionalizing the practice of drilling sham holes just because it has been the practice in the past."

Andrew Grove

(from Grove's article on trial design in this chapter)

ETHICS & ARGUMENTS

ENDNOTES:
Cohen PD et.al. (2012) Sham neurosurgical procedures: the patients' perspective. Lancet Neurology. 2012 Dec; 11(12):1022.

Cohen, PD (2011) Sham control groups for evaluation of neurosurgery delivered therapeutics: Patient activists views. Presented at The American Society for Experimental Neurotherapeutics (ASENT) Annual Meeting; 2011; Washington, DC.

Cohen, PD et. al. (2009) Examination of 'Failed' Clinical Trials Using Placebo Brain Surgery Controls - poster session presented at the American Society for Experimental Neurotherapeutics (ASENT) Annual Meeting; 2009; Washington DC. Available from http://www.pdpipeline.org/advocacy/2009%20poster_update.html

Cohen, PD et. al. (2007) Ethical Issues in Clinical Neuroscience Research: a Patient's Perspective. Neurotherapeutics. 2007 July: 537-44.

Galpern WR et.al. (2012) Sham neurosurgical procedures in clinical trials for neurodegenerative diseases: scientific and ethical considerations. Lancet Neurology. 2012 June; 11, 643-650.

Katsnelson A. (2011) Why Fake It? Nature. 2011 Aug. 11, 476; 359.

Weaver FM, et.al. (2009) Bilateral deep brain stimulation vs best medical therapy for patients with advanced Parkinson disease: a randomized controlled trial. JAMA. 2009 Jan 7; 301(1):63-73. Available from:http://www.ncbi.nlm.nih.gov/pmc/articles/PMC2814800/

Wittekind, P. (2012) Be here now. 2012 October 15. In: On the move newsletter, Autumn 2012, 2;21. United Kingdom: Parkinson's Movement. Available from: http://www.parkinsonsmovement.com/2012/10/

IS IT TIME TO RETHINK INFUSION TRIAL DESIGN?

By Andrew Grove, PhD

Former CEO & Chairman, Intel Corporation; PwP

Surgical Delivery of Therapeutics

After two decades of painstaking work, pressure-driven infusion is emerging as drug delivery method of choice for introducing substances with large molecules into the brain parenchyma. Some half a dozen trials involving infusion of Parkinson-related substances have taken place in the last few years with more being planned in the near future.

Some of these trials are safety trials; others are aimed at establishing efficacy. Following standard protocols, the efficacy trials are double blind and compare the infused substance with a placebo. Placebo in this case is a sham surgery in which holes are drilled into the skulls of trial participants without introducing any drugs.

I wonder how necessary this method is. Wouldn't one such placebo trial be sufficient to establish the extent to which a placebo effect takes place in all similar circumstances?

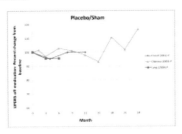

Figure 1 Outcome of sham surgeries

Figure 1 shows data from the sham surgeries of three different surgical trials. In two of these, burr holes were drilled in the patients' skulls without breaking through the dura. In the third, the holes were completed and a cannula was introduced but only saline solution was pumped into the patients' brains.

The three sham trials produced very similar outcomes. This should not be surprising: in all of these cases, the surgeries were similar and the patients had reason to hope for a good outcome.

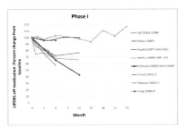

Figure 2 Outcome of Phase I infusion trials compared to the sham surgeries of Figure 1.

Figure 2 shows the outcomes of five different open label trials along with the placebo results of Figure 1. The open label trials had no controls. They were only intended to establish that the procedures and the substances in question were safe. Each of these trials followed extensive pre-clinical studies which gave reason for high expectations. The comparison of these open label trials to the sham results indeed suggests marked improvement.

Pressure-driven infusion, combined with accurate stereotaxic placement of cannulas, proper control of the flow of the infusate and confirmation with interoperative MRI may emerge in the near future as the standard method for delivering substances involving large molecules. Consequently, this may be a good time to think through how we can redesign such trials so they don't bring with them a corresponding explosion in the number of sham surgeries.

To be sure, we rely on the reproducibility of the results of the sham surgeries. Figure 1 supports this. (If the results of a sham surgery cannot be reproduced, why would infusions of the drug be reproducible?) Another issue is the natural optimism of the investigators which can cast doubt on the rating of clinical results. This can be addressed either by having the clinical rating be performed by third party clinicians and/or by the incorporation of objective measurement techniques which have been developed in the last few years, and may be ready for use.

As infusion enters mainstream use, we should avoid institutionalizing the practice of drilling sham holes just because it has been the practice in the past. Such a re-examination would also allow us to focus early on the question, which of the competing infused substances is most effective? It is an issue we have to deal with urgently, as suggested by Figure 2.

Reference: Christine CW, et al., Safety and tolerability of putaminal gene therapy for Parkinson's disease, Neurology, 2009 Nov 17;73(20):1662-9.

INFUSION TRIALS

WHAT "PATIENT CENTERED" MEANS TO ME:
A realization from Holland on the role of the patient in research

e-Patient Dave is a cancer survivor, blogger, keynote speaker and advocate for patient engagement. He is a board menber of the Society for Participatory Medicine. He discovered the Parkinson patient community in 2012 and became avidly interested in issues of how science uses the scientific method. As we were finishing this book he graciously granted us this excerpt of his blog article:

I'm sensing a number of things coming together, creating a new view of what's possible and what's changing in healthcare. It clarified my shifting view of the role of the patient in medical research - no small subject!

"Doing medical research without the cooperation of patients is like car-racing backwards blindfolded. The idea is to take away the blindfold and give the patient the role of **navigator**," says Lucien Engelen of the Radboud University Medical Center in the Netherlands. There they are using a patient participation model which includes patients from the beginning (see http://e-patients.net/archives/2012/12/the-patient-as-partner-in-medical-research-at-radboud-university.html.)

In my [Dave's] view,
• There should be an entire research agenda that's **patient-generated**, without any process of submitting ideas to a non-patient board. Not everything everyone wants can be done, but efficiency will improve if patients can declare an agenda with nobody's approval. So:

• **An unfiltered, unfettered list of what patients want** is a key component of any forward-thinking planning process. How else can we strive to create the most patient value for our research investment??

• As the Dutch article says, **the patient list is in addition to (not instead of)** what the establishment is working on. (It's just a mistake to say that all decisions should be made by well-meaning paternally protective proxies.)

• To get the most for our money - and to give patients what they value most - we need to let **them** say it, from the outset. Anything else can't possibly be as on-target.

And that brings us to:

RETHINKING WHO KNOWS WHAT'S BEST

In the Society for Participatory Medicine we say "patients shift from being mere passengers to responsible drivers of their care." In the past we've written about going beyond "compliance," to a vision of a future where patients design and create a safe, decent, patient-centered healthcare system. This takes it to whole different level: imagine patients directing the engineering agenda!

It reminds me of a talk by internet visionary Clay Shirky (Wikipedia) at the very first conference I ever attended, Connected Health 2008: "The patients on ACOR [Association of Cancer Online Resources] don't need our permission, and they don't need our help." Four years later, patient opinion is finally being expressed not just among patients, but in the domain of science itself.

LET PATIENTS HELP

It's no coincidence that this leads back to the closing line of my TED Talk: "Let Patients Help" heal healthcare. One route is to re-prioritize the research strategy - someday even the budget - around the ultimate stakeholder: the person and family whose lives are affected. And what I see in this initiative is a new pathway to allow organic growth of new research projects, in a new space, in addition to current methods.

e-Patient Dave
Dec. 29, 2012

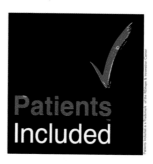

PATIENT-CENTRED HEALTHCARE

Looking Back...Looking Forward....Going Backwards

Many think stem cell therapy is one of the most promising potential treatments for Parkinson, yet federal funding of embryonic stem cell research (ESCR) was very limited by politics. Like many other patient advocates during 2000-2008, I devoted a good deal of my time and energy advocating for change in the federal policies set by the President. I firmly believe our futures depend on funding the most promising research and that those decisions should be based on science – not politics or religion.

Since my diagnosis I did what I could to advocate for increased funding for all types of PD research, including embryonic stem cell research. On the state level I was a patient representative to NYAMR – New Yorkers for the Advancement of Medical Research – a coalition of research institutions, medical schools, disease organizations, scientists and patients pushing for NYS funding of stem cell research (which became a reality in 2007 with the establishment of the Empire State Stem Cell Board and $100 million in funding over 11 years.

http://stemcell.ny.gov/about_nystem.html

NYAMR member Dr. Mark Noble is an internationally recognized stem cell researcher who also has great talent for explaining science to the lay public and for fostering consensus among people with opposing viewpoints. He often took part in state lobbying efforts and would start off the discussion with this "what if" story...

> "Imagine you are in a lab that houses hundreds of frozen embryos, all left over from fertility treatments and destined to be frozen indefinitely or discarded in the trash. Suppose a fast moving fire suddenly broke out in the lab. You notice a young child who was separated from her parents and unable to make her way to safety. You have only enough time to rescue either the hundreds of frozen embryos or the one child. What would you do?"

Dr. Noble said no one ever replied that the embryos should be saved over the child. By framing the controversy in such very human terms, he got people thinking and talking about embryonic stem cell research and clarifying their understanding of the science ... sometimes even changing minds and votes.

Our collective efforts, often led by grassroots advocates from the Parkinson's Action Network, paid off when President Obama signed an executive order in March 2010, lifting President Bush's limits on stem cell lines approved for federal funding. It seemed that finally after so many years, the research was poised to make significant progress.

While the heated debate on stem cell funding had been raging on, scientists were also studying ways to coax stem cells from adult cells, possibly eliminating the need to use embryos in the future. Induced pluripotent stem cells (iPSCs) are adult cells that have been genetically reprogrammed to an embryonic stem cell-like state by being forced to express genes and factors important for maintaining the defining properties of embryonic stem cells.

However, it is not known yet if iPSCs and embryonic stem cells differ in clinically significant ways. Researchers hope to develop iPSCs cells from the patients' own cells, thus eliminating problems with rejection and controversy on the use of ESCs. In addition to future clinical use, iPSCs are already useful tools for drug development and modeling of diseases.

And growing in a lab in Buffalo, NY - a line of my own stem cells are hopefully multiplying and creating new cells that will be used in PD research. How did this occur? I'm active in Internet discussion groups, such as Neurotalk. There I first learned from a posting about Dr. Feng, a researcher at a local university who is working with iPSC cells for PD. I suggested he might be an interesting speaker at our support group meeting. He was a hit! I think it might have been the first time he met and talked to PwP and the first time many of our group members had the chance to hear firsthand about research from a scientist. Dr. Feng announced he was looking for PwP and their relatives to donate skin cell samples for his research.

My husband Ed and I volunteered that night and a few weeks later were accepted. In June we underwent a punch biopsy to collect our skin cells. The samples were rushed from the doctor's office to Dr. Feng's lab by a graduate student, toting a soda pop cooler. Dr. Feng explained to us (many times) these cells will probably never be usable for treatment – the science isn't at that stage yet. It is enough to know they will be playing a role in moving the science along, and someday, custom-made stem cell treatments derived from patients' own cells may be available.

The icing on the cake is that Dr. Feng's research is funded by a NYS stem cell research grant, which we fought so hard for. It is one of those rare times in life when the stars seem to be in alignment.

If I was asked the 'burning lab' question... Of course I would save the child, but I'd also hope that someone else might be able to carry "my" stem cells to safety as well.

LEGAL AND POLITICAL ISSUES

Many advocates for ESCR felt they could rejoice and relax a little after President Obama's executive order making many new stem cell lines eligible for funding - both embryonic and adult - the scientists were finally unfettered and could concentrate their efforts on finding the promised cures. But on August 24,2010, we awoke to the shocking news that a federal judge had ordered an injunction preventing use of U.S. government funds for embryonic stem cell research. The injunction was the result of a lawsuit filed by 2 scientists who claimed the NIH was not funding their work with adult stem cells.

The legal actions threatened to close down ongoing federally funded research programs and withdraw future grants that had already been approved, sending ESCR in the U.S. into a tailspin, and denying PwP and their

'A line of my own stem cells are doing their thing by (hopefully) multiplying and creating new cells that will be used in PD research'

WHY STEM CELLS ARE IMPORTANT

Human stem cells are important because they can be used in research and in the clinic in the following ways:
- To better understand events that occur during human development.
- To learn more about the causes of diseases and how to treat them.
- To test new drugs
- To develop cell-based therapies, custom designed for each patient

families the very thing that has given us the strength to fight our battles with Parkinson - hope for a cure.

The government appealed the ruling. As the case moved through the appeals process from 2010 - 2012, scientists were unsure if their work would continue to be funded.

Finally in August 2012 the DC Circuit Court of Appeals ruled that federal funding of human embryonic stem cell research is not prohibited by federal law.

In January 2013 the Supreme Court refused to hear arguments against federal funding of ESCR.

However, funding is still vulnerable, because the Congressional supporters of ESCR failed to pass legislation that would protect funding from legal challenges in the future. When politics is considered to be more important than science, patients are the biggest losers.

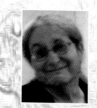

Linda Herman

A Vision of Beauty

Rick Everett is a PwP and an experimentalist. This is his homage to the elegant beauty of beings on a cellular level.

How does one convey the awesome beauty and incredible complexity of the informational flow that forms the center of a living thing, particularly one as amazing as a human? Viewing a living system as the movement of information is anything but fanciful. It is the reality. At any given instant, billions of tiny messengers scurry about our systems carrying instructions from one part to another. Not just in our brains, but in every tissue are found recipients awaiting those messengers. The information they convey ranges from "take a rest" to "commit suicide" to "send help."

Analogy is a useful tool if one keeps its limitations in mind. The portrayal of these messengers as keys that bump up against locks that open if the key is a proper fit is a good example of both analogy and its limitations. It provides a glimmer of understanding, but only a glimmer, as it sacrifices complex beauty in hopes of conveying understanding.

Beauty is a term that is not chosen lightly. Science takes a perverse pride in avoiding such words, but there are times when no others will do. When we confront something beyond our experience, our recourse is to compare it to the familiar by analogy.

Imagine you are floating far above a fantastic landscape of what seem to be diamonds the size of a fist. Hundreds of thousands in a wide range of colors lie below you. They seem to float upon a sea and are in motion as currents move them along. This dynamic and ever-changing surface below you is a single cell and the diamonds which float upon its surface are receptors, ports that receive information from the other cells in the body. Each receptor is "primed" to react when it encounters a particular molecule in its environment. These molecules, called ligands, come in many colors and both ligand and receptor must match in hue.

The receptors add further richness to the scene by not only moving about the cell surface in their hundreds of thousands, but also by shifting rapidly between configurations or shapes so that they, in effect, twinkle in the night. Their colorful twinkling in some unknown and

marvelous manner attracts ligands of a similar color and pulse - but only if they are present in the surrounding environment. If an appropriate ligand is, indeed, within range, it moves into position and gently bumps the receptor. Sometimes only once and it firmly locks into place in a "high affinity" relationship. Other times it bumps the receptor and backs away momentarily, then it repeats the action.

Each time the ligand activates the receptor, a message is passed through the cell membrane and a cascade of actions begins within the cell. What specific actions take place are dependent upon the "colors" or types of the pair. Cells not only "listen" via their army of receptors, they "speak" by producing ligands themselves.

If a macrophage encounters an invader, it sounds a warning by releasing a cloud of message bearing ligands which move rapidly through the bloodstream like tiny Paul Reveres. As these messengers wash past other components of the body and are drawn in by their receptors, they trigger defensive reactions such as the production of antibodies. Other macrophages follow the "smell" back upstream to assist. Still other cells respond in other ways and release their own messages.

This admittedly simplistic treatment of a truly wondrous interaction is but one of thousands occurring by the billions within our bodies every second. Ligands such as cytokines, hormones, and neurotransmitters are the way the body communicates with its various parts. Their division into groups relegated to the immune, endocrine, and nervous systems is an artificial one. Receptors are not necessarily limited to one specific ligand nor are ligands limited to one specific receptor. Our cells are in constant communication with one another as surely as the guests at a social function. How well that communication takes place determines our health and even our lives.

Once more, let us return to our position floating in the darkness high above the twinkling jewels of the single cell below us. Now that we know to look for them, we can see that we are floating in a cloud of dimly colored ligands like fireflies, each drawn to its individual destination below. Far away through this cloud we become aware of distant bejeweled planets and know that we are looking at other, nearby cells. Everywhere we look, information is being passed and the heavens glow with the force of life.

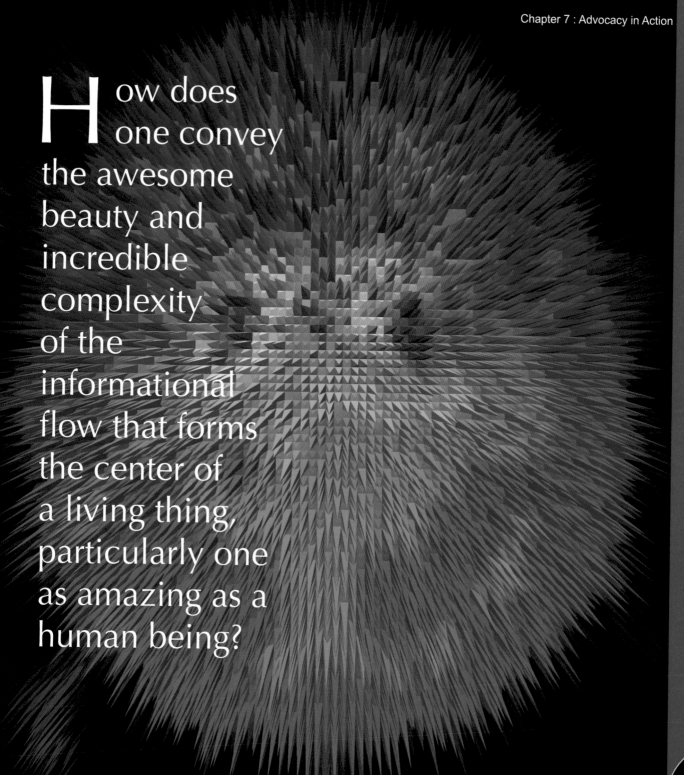

INCREDIBLE COMPLEXITY

How does one convey the awesome beauty and incredible complexity of the informational flow that forms the center of a living thing, particularly one as amazing as a human being?

PD activists speak

She continued to learn, becoming more interested in the wider world of Parkinson. She wrote to people in other parts of the world who had similar issues and concerns. Their common language was Parkinson, and they supported each other through many challenges in their lives. It was a wonderful way to move into the next stage of her Parkinson life journey.

In this chapter you will find a 'conversation' with fourteen PwP leaders and activists who live in Canada, Korea, New Zealand, Norway, Spain, Sweden, the UK and the US. We asked them to tell us about their experiences as PwP and advocates and to share their vision of the PwP community - past, present and future.

If you're as strong as those living with PD, read on.

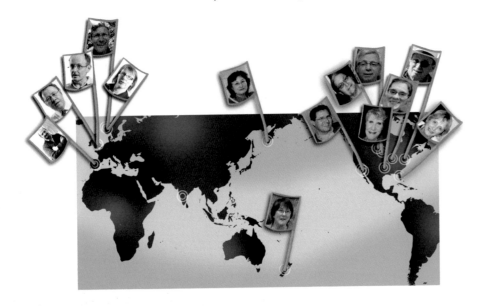

Note: This chapter was the special project of our editor-in-chief and designer. Although she was seriously out-numbered by us Yanks, she kept this whole book true to its goal of having international voices.

CHAPTER EIGHT
Going International

connecting globally

New Kids on the Global Block...
and some old hands...

Several of Parkinsons Creative Collective members are members of other Parkinson activist groups and include Pipeliners, PM Ambassadors, and more, as are many of our contributors, so what is it that makes Parkinsons Movement unique? Started in mid-2011 it has quickly become the holder of the hopes of the fledgling Parkinson international patient community.

Many of its newest members are new to this sense of community among PwP and are still at the stage of discussing their personal concerns. As they become aware of the potential to raise awareness they are raising the same questions as our seasoned advocates raised. After many years of campaigning this could feel disheartening, but we feel it is indicative that the message is spreading and this time it is happening on a much wider scale. As another World Parkinson Congress approaches we are thinking globally. We know the need to ensure that there is more awareness in the world about PD. The many efforts of PwP now need to connect up and reach the wider world.

We brought 14 advocates together for a virtual 'conversation' to talk about the next steps for global PD advocacy and asked them a few questions.........

Q1 Could you introduce yourself and say where you come from and how long you have had Parkinson disease......

Peggy This is Peggy Willocks, from Tennessee, USA. I was diagnosed in 1994 at age 44 and have had young onset PD for 18 years.

Paula My name is Paula Wittekind, Florida, USA and I have had PD for 25 years.

Bob My name is Bob Kuhn. I'm from Canada. I have lived with the adventure of Parkinson since 2006. . One of my favorite things to do is write, which I indulge through my blog "Positively Parkinson's".

Israel My name is Israel Robledo. I live in Midland, Texas, USA. I was diagnosed five years ago at the age of 42.

Linda I'm Linda Herman, I've lived with PD for seventeen years. I was diagnosed in 1995 when I was 45 years old. I live near Buffalo NY.

Sara
Sara Riggare, living in Sweden, engineer and co-founder of Parkinson's Movement. I had my first symptoms of PD in my early teens, was diagnosed with it until 2003, when I was 32 and my daughter was nine months old.

Jackie
My name is Jackie Hunt Christensen, from Minneapolis USA. I am an activist of 25 years working on health and environment issues . Since diagnosis in 1998 at age 34, I have focused on PD issues. I am the author of 2 books about my experiences with PD.

Jin
Hi, I am Jin Kyoung Choae. I am an activist for PD in Seoul, South Korea. I administer the webpages at 'facebook.com/groups/tulipfriends' and 'tulipfriends.org'. I have been suffering from PD for 7 yrs.

Perry
Perry Cohen, Washington DC, USA - diagnosed with PD in the spring of 1996.... that's right, more than 16 years.....

Jon
Dr Jon Stamford, UK, neuroscientist by training with a particular interest in PD. I was diagnosed in 2006, having researched the condition on and off for 26 years.

Tom
Tom Isaacs, UK, co-founder and President of The Cure Parkinson's Trust, living with PD for 18 years, diagnosed age 26.

Dilys
I am Dilys Parker from New Zealand and I was diagnosed with Parkinson in 2008 while living in the UK. My working life has been mainly community based nursing and I also spent some time working in allied health and social services.

Anders
Anders Leines. I am 49. I live in Oslo, Norway, with my wife Annika and children Leo and Isabel. I work as a videojournalist at Norwegian Broadcasting Corp. I have been in the TV business 23 years. I was diagnosed with PD in January 2010.

Fulvio
Fulvio Capitanio (Spain). I'm an economist and ITC manager. I was diagnosed with Parkinson in 2007 and retired in 2009. In January of 2008, with a group of PD friends I met over the Internet, I started an online organization called "Unidos contra el Parkinson" (Together against Parkinson disease).

Q2

For many of us there is a defining 'something' that brings us to advocacy. What burning issues, people or events brought you to the point of deciding to be an activist for PD, and how has it affected your life? Have you helped newer PwP get involved? What life lessons has it brought?

Peggy

I believe I came to advocacy as only three years after diagnosis I had to stop working and was forced into disability. I had identified myself with my work and my job was who I was. I went on-line seeking information when the internet was new to me and to most of the world. I found people in other similar situations, quickly befriended them. Many were close to me in proximity, and so I became an advocate face to face and personally. Initially I was trying to fill the void in my life from not working. Advocacy has become my life, and I feel a great sense of worthiness from helping other people like me, and together finding out that it is not a death sentence, but a life sentence.

Paula

Going online! Making many friends for support. Meeting Michael J. Fox. Believing that there would be a cure in 5 years. Getting involved in creating websites and attending PAN advocacy got me through it. Through PAN, PWLP and other online groups, you could bring new people into advocacy all the time, especially through the forums. Advocacy changed my life completely.

I met so many people, travelled to so many places I never thought I would go, published pieces, learned science. Things I would never have done before. It was like doing a Ph.D. in Neuroscience, I learned so much! The clinical trial process and all its shortcomings.....

We can make a difference. Patients can make a difference; we learned that. PD is a business for some, but not for us. I learned that PD organizations are mostly elementary in what they offer, they don't really get past the early stages of learning about PD, they are always teaching the newcomers.

Bob

This is cheating! There is more than one question. I realized fairly quickly after diagnosis that I could use the advocacy skills I learned as a lawyer to communicate with others about PD. My desire has been to remain positive, and to encourage others to do likewise. The response to my blog provided an impetus to do more, and led to me attending the WPC 2010 in Glasgow. Spending time with PwP. My view is that the biggest help to convey to other people with PD is to encourage them by whatever means necessary. I have tried to do this one-on-one locally, through my blog, and through my recent round the world trip. It is the individual that really matters, not the organization, Internet, or even the disease. In the end we share the struggle to make the most of the life we have been given, finding purpose in pain, finding wisdom in difficult circumstances.

PEOPLE COME TO ADVOCACY IN MANY DIFFERENT WAYS

Israel The defining 'something' for me was my experience with deep depression after having been diagnosed. I was suicidal for about nine months. Through prayer and a constant seeking for what I needed to do, I found that looking outward and away from my own problems of dealing with diagnosis, I could be of service to others that were less fortunate than I had been with the support of family and friends. In essence I had become the most vulnerable that I had ever been. There was no way out of my situation but to embrace the fact that this disease was going nowhere and it was I who had to adjust my way of thinking. I work as a school teacher but my life begins when I get home and work as an advocate for awareness, education, and clinical trial participation, and all that comes with seeking new treatments and a cure for PD.

Linda At that time in the US there was a bill in Congress that would increase funding for PD research, called the Udall Bill, in honor of Mo Udall, the congressman who also had PD. Pioneer activists such as Joan Samuelson, founder of PAN and Jim Cordy, used the Parkinsn list to recruit other activists and spread information about the Udall bill. This was an early use of social media, though we did not call it that at the time.

So I became active in this grassroots campaign and I found that doing something about Parkinson disease helped me deal with my diagnosis. It was on the Parkinsn list that I met Barbara Blake Krebs, who was also a young onset PwP.

At that time there was very little information about young onset Parkinson, so we decided to write a book composed mainly of postings from the Parkinsn list to help newly diagnosed patients and to educate the public about Parkinson. It was called 'When Parkinson Strikes Early'. Since its publication in 2001 more than 5000 copies have been sold worldwide.

Sara The very first time that I realized that I could actually do more about my situation with PD was at a course in Spain arranged by a company specializing in personalized rehabilitation for stroke and PD. The course gave me a lot of very useful state-of-the-art knowledge from very knowledgeable healthcare professionals. I was made to realize how much benefit there is in physical exercise. This was the first time in my entire life that I was able to push my body far beyond what I thought was possible by learning how to walk a tightrope. Absurd as it may seem that experience is what brought me to advocacy as well as changing my life. In fact, the 7 seconds it took me to cross the entire length of that tightrope for the first time, back in 2008, actually led up to me now being a doctoral student at the Karolinska Institutet in Stockholm. My research aims to encourage people to help themselves by exploring and providing structured ways for people with chronic diseases, such as PD, to use their personal health observations to improve their own health, but also potentially be useful for other patients as well as for healthcare and research.

LOOKING OUTWARD CAN HELP IN COMING TO TERMS WITH PD

275

Patient-supplied data adds to the knowledge of how people experience Parkinson Disease

Computers dramatically changed the way we communicate. Now they are providing new tools for PwP citizen scientists. They are helping PWP to research in new ways. From crowd-sourcing to online surveys and measurement tools via computers and smart phones - the democratization of medical research has begun.

You can participate in the search for a cure for PD!

Parkinson Measure

Wouldn't you like to have specific quantitative proof of your body's reaction to an intervention (i.e. a supplement, activity, medication etc.)? John Turner designed an online tool that measures your fine motor skills and reactions.

Recently he posted the results of one of his own trials on the NeuroTalk Forum. He tested whether there was a difference in his motor skills after taking medication. He checked his fine motor reactions over a period of time and charted the results. It showed when his medication had the maximum effect.

His site **Parkinsonmeasurement.org** features tools to help you start a similar project or analyze data already there. Don't worry - even though the data is open source, your privacy is important and won't be linked to the data. **Parkinson Measure's** goal is to speed the development of PD therapy!

PwP bring fresh eyes to medical knowledge

In the traditional model of science, PwP voices are rarely acknowledged, but often contribute fresh thinking. Examples of PwP observations preceding research include: anosmia (lack of sense of smell), identifying the non-motor effects of PD, the behavioral effects of agonists, and the shortfalls of trial design. On experiencing a change or symptom, they brought that information to others, including their peers and neurologists, and at times research supported their initial theory.

In this new model, PwP citizen scientists, using Participatory Medicine ("networked patients shift from being mere passengers to responsible drivers of their health" (see the Society for Participatory Medicine)) share their experience in their preferred online communities, such as Patients Like Me, Parkinsons Movement, NeuroTalk, and 23&Me. With luck and work, together they advance issues in science and treatment.

The availability of personal genetic information has opened new doors for PwP to pursue independent research. This permits citizen scientists to enroll in or even design genome studies. The era of personalized medicine is dawning. Beyond the world of PD, citizen scientists are active in a movement in the health community which advocates openness, sharing information from multiple sources and helping use it for the common good. We encourage its use in PD: bringing together people with different ideas and information to create new possibilities. *NeuroWriters*

HOW IS YOUR QUALITY OF LIFE AFFECTED BY MOTOR SYMPTOMS?

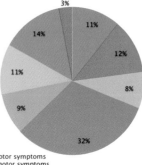

- Much better than expected from my motor symptoms
- Rather better than expected from my motor symptoms
- A bit better than expected from my motor symptoms
- Directly related to my motor symptoms
- A bit worse than expected from my motor symptoms
- Rather worse than expected from my motor symptoms
- Much worse than expected from my motor symptoms
- Other (please comment)

What was the FIRST key PD symptom you experienced?

- Tremor
- Rigidity
- Bradykinesia
- Balance problems

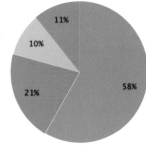

Poll Charts by kind permission of Dr Jon Stamford of Parkinson's Movement

Parkinson's Movement Polls

Parkinsons Movement regularly post polls on their site, encouraging PwP to respond with information that only a PwP would know. See the pie charts for results of recent PM polls.

If you'd like to contribute to the growing knowlege base, look for polls at **parkinsonsmovemnent.com** or other groups gathering info. Do read the site's privacy policy and learn whether any of your personal information will be collected, connected to the data or whether your info will be anonymous.

> "The process of scientific discovery - how we do science - will change more over the next 20 years than in the past 300 years."

Michael Nielsen, Reinventing Discovery: The New Era of Networked Science

Jackie

I have been an activist all of my adult life. If an issue is important to me, I cannot ignore it, even at times when it would be healthier for me to take a break! I see advocacy as working within the status quo, which needs to be done, and I can do some of that and help others find their passion for that. What I NEED to do is try to work outside the status quo, to push the boundaries and raise new issues that I believe are important. Two of my biggest issues have been helping fellow Parkies feel comfortable and worthy of speaking for themselves, even if they stammer, or take a long time, or seem to be devoid of emotion; and taking action to truly prevent environmentally-induced PD by keeping toxic chemicals out of our homes and workplaces. On the topic of speaking for ourselves for as long as we can, I have 'burned some bridges' with powerful people whose attitude is "How can you be so ungrateful? We've done so much for you!". I appreciate their work and we need it, but we also need to speak up about what we truly want and need.

Jin

At the 2nd World Parkinson Congress I got to know about the many support groups which are helping find a cure and fund-raise for PD research. The people I met at WPC, including Jean Burns, brought me to advocacy. It really affected my life. From a shy homemaker to an activist who organizes people with PD and their supporters! My doctor now introduces me to new patients when they want a support group. I'm happy I can help them. I realize the more open I am about my disease, the more I can support people.

Perry

The diagnosis of PD itself was a life changing event. I was dissatisfied with the way my work life was going and I quickly found a real need for my skills and contacts in health policy, and people ready to listen to my point of view. Thus, many things came easily to me, so much so that I would say that I "trained 50 years for the job". I just didn't know it until I saw it. I have an analytical mind fostered by a wonderful education, and try to extend my vision further into the future than most people. I was raised with charitable values and am able to campaign on issues of value to society and still live comfortably.

Jon

I regard myself as a slightly unusual advocate. Indeed I would not even describe myself as an advocate as such. I am someone who believes in acting for the benefit of the PD community, so perhaps I'm an advocate with a small A. As a patient I was struck by the degree of passivity of the Parkinson patients I met. They seemed to accept everything the condition had to throw it at them and every decision that their physicians took without question. Everything was accepted, nothing was challenged. As someone who has worked in Parkinson research, I was perhaps more aware than most that what is promulgated as the conventional wisdom is in fact often flawed. I was also aware of the knowledge gap between scientists/physicians and their patients. There was no common language. If I have helped to get newer patients involved it has been through the website, my blog and books.

OPENNESS ABOUT PD MAKES IT POSSIBLE TO SUPPORT OTHERS

ADVOCACY CAN HELP IMPROVE YOUR QUALITY OF LIFE

Tom

I was amazed by the support I received from doing sponsored events and it made me realize that with this kind of support one person could achieve a lot but as a group we really could make a difference. The burning issue for me has always been the fact that there is so much that we can do to contribute to progress in PD and the scope for this progress is so vast. Being an advocate has saved my life. It has given me a new perspective, a sense of fulfillment and has in many ways improved my quality of life. In terms of life lessons, Martha Washington's quote says it all:

"The greater part of our happiness or sadness, depends not on our circumstances but on our disposition."

Dilys

I haven't had anything that particularly stands out as the burning issue and defining moment, but I have met amazing people from the time I was first diagnosed. At first this was on line but soon I met many in person. I continue to meet inspirational people who are using their situation and talents to effect change. These are just ordinary people who are living their lives with Parkinsons in a way that says I am going to make something extra ordinary of this hand life has dealt me. These people were and are my inspiration and Parkinson's Movement provides a context and a supportive network. Advocacy affects life generally because it becomes an orientation and a way of responding to life. I know some people first get involved with advocacy after they are diagnosed but for others it is a continuation of how they have always engaged with the world. Personally I see it as an extension of my interests and work to date. I guess I have mostly worked with marginalised people. Now the marginalised group I have a passion and interest in working for and with are people like me with Parkinsons. I feel a strong commitment to raising public awareness generally and to challenging health professionals to be better informed.

I like being with people and building a sense of community. I see my work as connecting people to sources of knowledge and to each other. Hopefully this creates an environment where people can learn and grow confident in dealing with their condition. In this way they become their own advocates.

Anders

The event was that I made a Parkinsons Pledge video for WPC, which lead Eli Pollard to hook me up with several advocates. Soon after I went to Stockholm to meet Sara Riggare and her friends. All of a sudden I felt like I was near the center of a group of VERY competent people, with PD! I was then asked to be a PM ambassador. It has lead me to meet some very interesting neuroscientists, through the films we've made.

Being with optimistic and competent people like these people gives me hope and new insights on the disease. When it comes to advocacy I mostly do that through my films, which can be found on my Youtube Channel.

Fulvio As with many PwP I've been depressed for a period after being diagnosed. My "inflection point" was attending the Parkinson's Unity Walk in New York City. Being with thousands of people gathered together for the same reason made me realize that I was not alone. I saw crystal clear that if I was not happy with the situation I was in since PD entered into my life, the change should start from me and that there was no time to waste.

I believe that, first of all, people need to be informed.
Information gives you the tools to deal with the challenges of your daily life better.

It may seem that advocacy can be a tremendous job to only to bring one drop to the ocean. Nevertheless, the ocean would be less because of that missing drop, and even the ocean would dry out if all these drops would stop falling.

Q3 What are the changes/developments you personally hoped for; of these things, how much change have you personally seen?

Peggy I hoped for a better way to positively diagnose PD, because there is so much ambiguity in diagnosing. It is starting to evolve right now through the Fox trial finder, and lots of professionals are now starting to think differently about PD, that it is so much more that a tremor, or a motor condition alone.

Paula I personally hoped for more in the line of treatment if not a cure. We were very naive in the beginning. I hoped for more patient organization involvement and more involvement with research organizations. Things are getting better. Some orgs have now got patient councils and training programmes for advocates. They are paying more attention to us, and recognizing our value.

Bob To be honest, my hope is not in changes or developments. Yes, it would be great to find a cure, better medicines, a way to slow this beast of a disease down. Yes, there is a great deal happening out there. But I am not going to pin my hopes on some man-made miracle, finding a needle in a haystack, finding a magic wand or a silver bullet. Don't get me wrong. I will work diligently to pursue alleviation of disease, pain and suffering. But I also recognize the great strength that it can build in the process. We are a soft and undisciplined generation/culture that does not know the meaning of deferred gratification. We want a cure RIGHT NOW, as if we somehow deserve it. I guess the way I see it is that we are all called to serve people in different ways. For me, it is to live in such a way to encourage those who lack courage to face the demons, the disease, the devastation that so often marks living.

THERE IS STILL A LOT OF AMBIGUITY IN DIAGNOSIS

Israel

The change that I have personally hoped for is the inclusion of the patient in all aspects of the research process. I have seen some change in thinking among younger researchers who are more open to the patient as being an equal in the process. It won't be too long before the day that all researchers will value the patient perspective in PD research and include them as they strive to develop new treatments.

Linda

I hoped for more money for PD research, especially stem cell research - and that has increased over the years. Now I would like to see more patient-centred research and see patients involved in all aspects of research and clinical trials - and that is beginning to happen. It is starting, but we still have a long way to go.

Sara

I am hoping to be able to help PwP learn to help themselves by facilitating the process of individual empowerment. I have personally seen a lot of empowerment taking place in individuals, but in my view this aspect is not being recognized and acknowledged to a sufficient degree in the majority of healthcare settings and patient organizations.

Jackie

I have hoped for more awareness of PD's effects on communication and relationships and finally it is becoming a topic of articles and Parkie conference sessions. I am still working toward and hoping for it to be an integral part of medical/health care conferences and training for any medical or health personnel who deal with Parkies and our families.

On 'PD & environment' issues I am deeply frustrated. The weight of evidence (figuratively and literally) demonstrates that, at least for pesticides, we know there is a link to PD. It is time to DO something about it. Stop production and use of chemicals we know are linked to PD (and many other health problems). Educate people about pesticides and alternative pest management strategies. Require thorough neurotoxicity testing for new chemicals being considered for use.

Jin

I 'm hoping for a better public understanding of PD symptoms in Korea.
I'm just taking the first step towards tomorrow......

Perry

One of the main missions of my advocacy is the activation of people with PD. Everyone can do more than they are now doing, which not only helps the cause but also helps the individual. I make a point of explaining this to all the people who work with Pipeliners!

Jon

My personal mantra as always is the interaction between those living with the condition and physicians. This point of contact forms the basis for improved healthcare. Extending this to its logical conclusion is my view that patients should not only influence their own personal healthcare but should have a wider influence throughout the field of Parkinson medicine. In a nutshell, my view is that patients should be represented on every advisory board, every committee and every body that makes decisions related to current and future Parkinson treatment.

Tom

1. Better communication and transparency between scientists improving, particularly amongst Pharmas.
2. The recognition of the need for disease-modifying therapies. Management is not enough. We want it reversed - work in progress.
3. Parkinson is a whole body condition and a quality of life disorder, not simply a movement disorder - more work has been done in this area in the last two years than ever before.
4. Accurate measurement will allow personalized treatment of Parkinson and will bring more effective and more relevant results in clinical trials. This in turn will attract more investment into the area - one of the fastest growing areas of Parkinson research.

Dilys

Like many others, my hopes are that Parkinson becomes as known and generally understood by the public as is, for instance, cancer, heart disease or diabetes. This has been my personal hope from the early days of my diagnosis. I have not yet seen significant change in this area. There still is a lot of work to do.

Anders

I am hoping that PM will grow to be a real movement, but my experience is that it is struggling, due to a need for more financing and support.

Fulvio

The day of diagnosis the neurologist told me to have faith because there are people investigating on PD all over the world like never before and every day we get closer to find the cure or, more likely, to have much better drugs to treat PD.

One thing the neurologist couldn't tell me was "how far we are" from the finish line.

In five years the drugs available to treat PD remains the same and a cure for PD is still possible only in laboratory rats.

Q4 Do you think patient advocacy has been able to move the thinking of medicine, science and government and to what degree?

Peggy

Yes, and no. Yes the patient has now been recognized as playing a more important role in identifying the causes of PD, but no, they are still trying to hang onto the totally scientific approach and we are only just starting to recognize the importance of personalized medicine, which is patient-centric.

Paula

Yes, but not nearly to the degree it could have. We are still trying to get our own organizations to let us participate more instead of them speaking for us!

Bob

Yes. But we must be careful. We must define success in larger terms than our own community of people with Parkinson. I have seen many lawyers advocate for their client using every strategy and trick available to them. In the end, the system suffers and people become jaded and cynical. We must be careful to avoid advocacy becoming a turf war.

Israel

I think the early advocates such as Perry Cohen, Linda Herman, Paula Wittekind, and Peggy Willocks in the US, who fought so hard for so long to have the voice of the person with PD heard in all aspects of the process have paved the way for those of us whom have come to advocacy over the last five or so years to gain a more productive outcome. Newer movement disorder specialists have embraced PwP and are working towards making us true equal partners in the process. I will forever be grateful to these advocates for not giving up, and for allowing us to fight with them and share the torch of change as we start to advocate on a wider international level.

Linda

It is beginning to.

Sara

I think the process has been initiated, but there is still a long way to go. I also think that we all would benefit from working together with other diseases on different aspects of this process rather than to compete for the attention.

Jackie Yes, definitely. This past June in Minnesota, we (a team of Parkies and reps from PD orgs) put on a conference with an agenda chosen by PwP, and with Parkies and care partners speaking in most sessions. The awareness we raised about PD's effects on relationships and families was profound. One health professional who attended said "You know, this made me realize that I had never really thought about our patients' families." And this was coming from a person whom I know and consider to be a generally compassionate person!

Jin Patient advocacy, like trial participation, could move the thinking of medicine. It is now becoming a much bigger matter.

Perry Yes, over the past ten years I see a gradual progression now accelerating, like a snowball down a hill, toward patient-centered collaboration for research and care and away from doctor centered, expert treatment.

Jon I think there are a small number of enlightened pharmaceutical companies who acknowledge that patient advocates are pivotal to future drug development. It would be nice to see this attitude taken up by other pharma companies and governmental committees as well.

Tom Yes, in certain conditions such as AIDS and Breast Cancer, but not in Parkinson.

Dilys Yes, I think patient advocacy has power and does make a difference but we still have much to do. Recently PwP challenged members of the health profession to pay more attention to the side effects of agonist drugs. The possibility of compulsive behaviour with its devastating effects was not being acknowledged adequately. I have seen the positive effect this online lobbying by PwP has had and the resultant heightened awareness by health professionals. It is a very local example and when considered globally the effects may be seen as small, but they still give me hope.

THE EFFECT ON THE FAMILIES OF THOSE WITH PD IS PROFOUND

Anders I don´t have a lot of experience on this, but I´m sure that patients can add an emotional dimension through their stories that may inspire scientists and decision makers into working harder.

Also, as a critical voice, patients can contribute.

Fulvio Absolutely.
Especially in adapting the healthcare model to the real needs of PwP.

PARKINSON DISEASE NURSE SPECIALISTS

THE HEART OF THE MULTI-DISCIPLINARY TEAM
PDNS: who are they & what do they do?

- **What will the future of PD medical services look like?**

- **How will we cope with the scarcity of neurologists and motor disorder specialists?**

- **Who will staff telemedicine for PwP?**

The best answer to all three questions is the Parkinson Disease Nurse Specialist (PDNS)

In the UK, PDNS are very special people working to improve the quality of life for PwP. By training, they are nurses with advanced education and excellent inter-personal skills. They work in many different settings from rural areas to major PD centres. In most cases they perform some of the same tasks as other professionals but often have more time to devote to the patient and his/her carers. In addition, their role is flexible and the normally scheduled appointments may be supplemented with phone and email consultations with their PwP patients.

PDNS order medicine, treatment, tests and coordinate care with other specialists and directly support PwP who are using sub-cutaneous and jejunal infusion therapies. Good communication increases the chance to optimize the benefit of a PwP's treatment. PDNS provide targeted regular input, individual or group instruction such as, teaching and customizing the proper dosing and use of the PwP's medications plus conducting seminars on new research. Through all of these activities, PDNS improve the quality of PwP life.

PDNS, Anne Martin said, "I get the most enjoyment from my role when I see the PwP and families becoming the expert patient and family and feel empowered to cope with the diagnosis."

Why is the PDNS model important?
The Kings College Movement Disorders Unit in London, UK has had PDNS for over twenty years. With PDNS coordinating and customizing care for PwP, this model enhances care for more patients per physician, thereby making better use of existing resources.

In the US, specialist nurses have been working in similar ways and in a pilot program to expand the reach of neurologists caring for PwP in remote areas. In that program, a combination of telemedicine (via secure Skype) plus in-person nurse assessment (for cogwheeling, etc) will reduce PwP travel time and permit more PwP to 'see' specialists.

The UK model is time-tested; PDNS provide their excellent care, education and support there and in many other countries. It is now being adapted for world-wide implementation by an international collaboration of PDNS led by the UK's own Anne Martin, who is also Lead PDNS for Europe.

We thank the Parkinson Disease Nurse Specialists whose skills enhance our lives, providing the extra care we need and a potential solution to a shortage of motor disease specialists.
NeuroWriters

Parkinson's Disease Nurse Specialists and the King's College Hospital model of care, Anne Martin and Jane Mills, British Journal of Neuroscience Nursing, February/March 2013,Vol 9 No 1, 185-191

Can Free Video Consults Make Parkinson's Care Better? Nancy Shute http://www.npr.org/blogs/health/2013/03/12/174110032/

Q5 What is your view of the future for PwP, short and long term? Will there be a cure for PD, and how soon? What needs to be done to help bring a cure to patients? In the meantime what needs to be done to manage living with a chronic disease like PD? What is your view of your own future as contrasted with a newly diagnosed PwP?

Peggy

One of the biggest changes in my 18 years, is that most people were put on very strong doses, of dopamine replacements therapy early on in treatment, now we know that it is not the best way to treat PD because of long term use side effects.

I think a cure is just around the corner. When I say this, I mean not eradicating the disease but managing the symptoms. I have heard them say a cure will come in five years for two decades; it has now been 40 years since anything really new has been developed. The reason for that is not treating a patient holistically - I mean using alternative and complementary therapies, along with traditional western medicine, i.e. writing a prescription for western medicine, and then writing a prescription that will take care of the side effects of that pill. I think the cure is going to be relatively simple. I don't think it will require surgery in all cases, or viral vectors. I believe it will be a mild therapy along with a huge change in life style, and it will come within the next decade. I say that from my experience of my symptoms being exacerbated and enhanced by stress, lack of sleep, depression; we have got to look at that. Out of hundreds of people I have seen and known, there has always been some kind of psychological/psychiatric trauma that has preceded the disease which then manifests or evolves into very real physical and neurological symptoms. We need to treat the whole patient with a multi-disciplinary team approach.

Paula

I don't think there will be a cure anytime soon if ever. If anything, I think they are going to stop it with a vaccine. Maybe they will be able to prevent it, not cure it. The human body is too complex, too complicated for man to figure out. They figure it out in small doses, but how good are they at putting it all together to make the bigger picture? Money and use of more patients may help, but it is a big question, trying to bring a cure. I don't know the answer to that. Maybe more collaboration and sharing. They need to build disease specific facilities, with nurses who are skilled and trained in PD.

I like to hope a that a newly diagnosed PwP has it better than I did; that they get better treatment, access to more direct research results, and more effective clinical trials procedures.

Bob

Let me answer it this way. Sooner or later there will be a cure. It will stumble, even crawl, struggling to get to its feet long before it will run. And when it runs there may be a disastrous fall or two before it can truly be called a cure. My guess: 20 years. The biggest impediment: "turf wars". We need better coordination, cooperation, communication, built through better relationships. Since diagnosis I have begun to learn that living with a disease like PD is a game of inches, both mentally and physically, both won/lost. I have learned that my future is unlikely to be affected by any cure or major development in treatment. But that does not dissuade me one bit from doing what I can for the next generation, if that is how long we must wait for the system to work.

TREAT THE PATIENT WITH A MULTI-DISCIPLINARY APPROACH

WE HAVE SEEN TWO DECADES PROMISING A 'CURE IN FIVE YEARS"

Israel

The future for PwP is a bright one because the information that we are learning about PD is amazing. The best and the brightest from all parts of the world are doing their part. As for long term, finding at the very least a way to halt the progression of the disease will come, while the work to find a cure keeps going. Recently people were asked what a cure for PD meant to them and I was quite surprised to see how many people would be satisfied with stopping the disease progressing. I look back to when I was first diagnosed five years ago and see the newly diagnosed in a position to make a greater impact because of the opportunities for involvement that were not there just a few years ago. There is room for all to get involved in the advocacy process to the extent that they feel comfortable participating.

Linda

When I was first diagnosed, the doctor told me there would be a cure in 5-10 years, and then I learned that everyone since has been told the same thing. The cure has proved to be more elusive than was originally thought, so I think as of now there will be better treatments in the future, I don't think there will be a cure just yet. I don't think my generation of PwP will see a cure, but I think there will be better treatments to help us live better with the disease and there will be more discoveries of lifestyle changes like increasing exercise that will improve our quality of life. I think, especially, newly diagnosed people have a lot to be hopeful about.

Jin

I don't know when it will be. Who can tell the exact time that it will come, but some day, one day, I hope it will. A way that we as PwP, especially as newly diagnosed patients, can help this happen is to actively participate in clinical trials.

Jackie

I think that it is best that (at least in the U.S.), the PD orgs are focusing on supporting Parkies and our families as we cope with the disease, since those services are so necessary. I think there will be a cure but even if it were found today, it would not come to market for at least 10 years because the pharma companies have no interest in curing us -- not when they can make hundreds of millions of dollars off of the meds that we take. I believe that best way to find and expedite a cure would be to issue an international research challenge of, say, $5-10 million for a demonstrated (i.e., more than one study, randomized double-blind, etc.) cure that would then go into the public domain; there would be no intellectual property rights for pharma companies to inflate prices.

In order for folks who currently have PD to live well, we need MASSIVE public education efforts that also include health care providers; many more assisted-living facilities specifically for Parkies, especially those of us w/ young-onset; treatment for caregivers and family members, who are also impacted by disease; and subsidy (in the U.S.) for complementary therapies such as exercise, tai chi, yoga, etc.

Sara

To me personally, a cure as in complete restoration back to a "pre-PD state" seems very far away. Firstly because there is, to my knowledge, currently no way of actually knowing what that state is, in an individual and secondly, since no-one really knows what actually causes the disease, it is my understanding that it would be very difficult to actually measure it if that illusive cause was removed and to what extent. This might be perceived as pessimistic, but I am very optimistic regarding the future for PwPs. I feel confident that there are better treatments just around the corner and I also feel very strongly that the treatments currently available can be used in a more effective and efficient way if we as individual patients were able to take more responsibility in our own treatments. To achieve this, both we, the patients, as well as the healthcare professionals we interact with, need to change our attitudes.

Perry

To me a cure is a process of healing from the long term effects of mis-alignment of body functions (movement and others), and thus requires a combination of both medicine and activated self help (eg exercise) for the best results. You can read my blog about this at:

http://blog.michaeljfox.org/2012/05/route-cures-patient-centered-model/

There will be better treatments. For advanced PwP like me, GDNF is the last best choice, but at the rate that they are going, it may never reach the market. So I am trying to wait out enrollment in the NIH GDNF phase 1 study which will be going on for several years as it stands (the 1st several slots of 24 total are lined up, pending screening).

Ceregene's Neuturin [NTN] seem like the most likely of the most promising new therapies to reach the market 1st ~ 5+ years, if it actually works (it is not totally clear who it works for but probably not everyone) and the sham controlled studies succeed.

In the near term [5 to 10 years] most new therapies will involve neuro-surgery for gene therapy or cell transplants, so we need to make our voices heard on patient-friendly study designs (no sham surgery) and patient-centered regulatory policies to get them approved.

We also need to use the power of internet to educate PwP about activation for self help with peer group reinforcement (exercise, diet etc), as well as use of technology to create clinical databases from PwP-reported observations of daily living to discover better ways to manage meds and other non-medical therapies(eg dance, music, etc).

Tom

My sole mission is to make Parkinson extinct. In order to reach this goal communication and teamwork are key. It is these two attributes that will make more of a difference in Parkinson progress than any other factors. A cure will be found through having adequate funding, accurate measures, less red tape, more patients signing up for trials, pioneering spirit and the voices of people with Parkinson pushing things along every step of the way. In terms of my own future, I firmly believe that one day my condition will be reversed.

TREATMENTS COULD BE MORE EFFECTIVE AND EFFICIENT

WE NEED A BETTER FOCUS ON EDUCATING THE PUBLIC ABOUT PD

Dilys

I feel hopeful that there will be positive changes ahead. I think things are moving forward. Internationally, high profile people have begun the public conversations that are helping to lift the profile of Parkinson. Added to this, the technology to assist in research has progressed significantly in recent years. Having said that, I still think we have quite a way to go.

To talk of cure for Parkinsons is useful in unifying us toward a common vision but what cure means varies greatly from person to person. I think of it in terms of arresting the condition and eventually reversing the symptoms. Maybe this will happen in my lifetime but if it doesn't I still want and expect there to be ongoing refinement of our medication to help us live with this chronic condition.

As well as this quest for a cure, we need a deeper understanding by those in the health services of the many effects Parkinson has on our lives physically and socially. Complimenting this, I would like to see an international campaign bring together Parkinson organisations around the world to focus on educating the public about Parkinson. Better understanding by family, co workers, friends and employers would improve the lives of many.

Anders

Hopeful, but not romantically so. I don´t know what my life will be like. It is worrying. but completely normal. I exercise and try to keep the disease at bay while I hope for new treatments to come. But things happen so slowly !

I put some hope in 23andme.com and their efforts to see new patterns through their surveys and genetic testing. To bring a cure one needs to look beyond neurology and explore more of the so called "alternative treatments".

I personally don´t believe in a cure.

Fulvio

Honestly, I'm not confident I'll live enough to see the cure for PD. This is not an excuse to stop fighting and contributing to bring us one step further to a cure. Every day brings us closer. As people before us did, we are responsible to run our part of this relay race to hand the baton to the next runner.

Sorry but I broke my crystal ball the day I was diagnosed with PD.
I discovered it was useless, because it never warned me about it…

I wish I had the formula to solve this dilemma, but there is definitively something we are doing wrong if it is nearly 200 years since Dr. James Parkinson described the condition and we are still on the L-Dopa golden rule. In a perfect world, I mean perfect for a PwP, the drug treatment would be complemented by non-pharmaceutical therapies in order to preserve PwP physical and mental abilities as much as possible.

In the real world, we now see that the resources needed to care for people with neurological diseases (like AD, PD and MS) may be enough to bankrupt any Social Security system in the next 20 years.

Q6 Tom and Jon, we introduced you and Parkinson's Movement in the previous chapter, and in some ways you are the new kids on the block, as the most recent patient-driven org. Can you tell me a little about how Parkinson's Movement came about, and why? What are the aims of Parkinson's Movement?

Tom

Parkinson's Movement emerged from conversations with The Cure Parkinson's Trust's Advocacy Group in the Spring of 2010. This kernel of an idea sprouted at World Parkinson Congress, where fantastic like-minded and motivated advocates came together.

Jon

Making PM a reality took a little longer, but day by day more voices join the movement, and with more voices comes the potential to add pressure for change. PM is designed to unify and communicate the voices of people with Parkinson directly and bridge the cultural and communication divide between us and those who hold the keys to our future health. At the moment, we have such little control over the management of our healthcare and progress with new therapies.

Q7 Who makes a good advocate for Parkinson disease? In the past advocacy was done by sympathizers and charities/nonprofit orgs rather than the people who are living and working with PD in a more immediate sense, like patients, doctors and researchers.

Peggy

Someone who is willing to sacrifice part of their family life, someone who can empathize, walk the walk, talk the talk. You need to become a counsellor, a scientist, a researcher, a friend, and spend a long time in search of answers. A good advocate is someone who can see the big picture - you can't zero in on dopamine replacement and expect a cure for this disease to just happen.

Paula

There is no better advocate than a person that has it! That isn't to say that there aren't people with skills and organizations that are helping us. We must be able to speak for ourselves!

Israel

A good advocate for PD is a person who has the best interest of the PD community at heart. Thinking of and working for both the most unfortunate and those with the best care available. Non-profits seem to be changing to include the advocate because, I feel, they have seen how much of an impact an advocate can have when promoting the good that is being done. More people want to have a voice and share what they are able to do - to make a difference.

WE HAVE SO LITTLE CONTROL OVER MANAGING OUR HEALTH

MORE PEOPLE NEED TO BE ABLE TO SEE WHAT PD LOOKS LIKE

Linda

I think people who don't give up! They are persistent and they know that each individual voice is important and who research and keep themselves informed and have all the facts. Patients know more than anyone else what it is to live with PD and what patients need.

Sara

In my view, a good advocate in any disease is a person able to see beyond his or her own situation and more take an entire community into account and see to the needs and wishes of more than just yourself. Very important is to do this without taking too much liberty in interpreting for the other members of this community but actually listen to what they have to say and put yourself in their situation, or "shuffle in their slippers", as Jean Burns so fittingly puts it. And this is of course easier to do with a more direct experience of the disease.....

Jackie

I always tell folks that if they are out in public living with PD, they are advocates because they are allowing their community to see what Parkinson looks like.

I believe that while it is necessary to have organizations to interact with government agencies and coordinate efforts, we Parkies are our own most effective and most accurate advocates, (which is why I wrote this commentary, "Let Me Speak For Myself," published in the Washington Post: **http://www.washingtonpost.com/wp-dyn/content/article/2009/06/01/AR2009060102835.html**/)

I do think that in order to really get things moving, we need to go from being "advocates" to "activists." We need to go beyond traditional safe methods of asking for what we need to actions that effect change and grab attention - non-violently, of course!

Jin

I think patients would better widen the realm of what they are doing to include their friends by getting them involved their efforts to find a cure. Otherwise ordinary people have no chance to understand this disease well! Once they understand it more they'll become good supporters, too.

Perry

The best advocates:

First - PwP and their care partners.
Second - PwP and research teams
Third - Professional lobbyists

Jon

An inspirational advocate has an infectious enthusiasm. Advocates have a hunger to learn about their subject and a determination to see the bigger picture, to identify how they can add pressure to influence change.

Tom

I completely agree - but would add, good advocacy involves more listening than advocating. Advocacy is not about you, it's about everyone else.

Dilys

Who makes a good advocate? The answer is as diverse as those with the condition. It is the passion that people bring that is important. Along with passion there has to be skills and planning.

I think advocates need to have a good understanding of their condition and need to be able to speak with authority about their experience. I also think advocates need an analysis of power structures and a good understanding of strategies to effect change.

In the past people who did not have Parkinson have advocated on our behalf.

Alongside this we need a strong patient-driven model such as found in Parkinsons Movement. Advocacy is best when it is informed by the experience of people affected. There is a place for not for profit groups as they often have the infrastructure and the credibility along with the long established links which makes it easier to be heard by decision makers. However it is important that their work is informed and guided by those with Parkinson.

Anders

I think there is a need for all kinds of personalities and expertise.

Fresh thinking is welcome!

Fulvio

Young Onset PwP are passionate and have more energy to invest into advocacy.

PM PROVIDES A STRONG PATIENT DRIVEN MODEL OF ADVOCACY

Q8

We can see that people who come new to PD have very little awareness of what it is, and this needs to change, the public need to know about it in the same way they know about MS, Cancer, and heart disease. How can a movement like PM, and other patient advocate groups, large or small, help make that happen

Peggy

PM is doing global awareness, and making it very personal. They are looking at the big picture, and using patients as educators and researchers, and finding a place at the table. This is as relevant as the scientific research, and they are recognizing that now; they are using patients' anecdotal records to inform science. Patients are learning scientific methods in order to comprehend why the scientist has to have the evidence they need, and science is now seeing us as the most important stakeholder in this process.

Paula

Maybe they should do more teaching about it in university, or schools. You need more spokespeople who allow themselves to be seen with their symptoms showing. Movements like PM could make this happen. I don't know how you reach a big world. As people are getting PD younger even though it is thought of as an older person's disease, it may become more alarming (the thought of getting it), and get more attention. I think PM provides a variety of activities, things for people to do. Learn about PD, through a variety of interactive things, questions, blogs, polls. Their location in Europe makes it close to a number of countries - there is more opportunity to spread the word by travelling and talking to people in different places.

Israel

Just the fact that we are making people aware of the disease is no longer enough (and perhaps it never has been enough). Establishing our presence in social media will help greatly but also taking the time to educate those whom are interested in learning more will create the biggest impact. Knowledge is power and we've seen it with advocates that use their platform in a positive way, creating some unease in the research community because of the fact that we are knowledgeable about our situation and want to take an active role in our own care.

Linda

By doing what they are doing, educating the public - the website, and webinars, and on a local level through support groups and community wide activities.

Jackie

By getting more Parkies involved on the boards of organizations and by speaking out as we are able. We need to be the faces of PD in our communities so that the world can see what this disease does to us and our families. This is what people with cancer - especially breast cancer and heart disease - are doing.

SOCIAL MEDIA CAN BE USED TO RAISE AWARENESS OF PD

Tom

PM provides a platform or hub for those who wish to engage with their condition and actively do something about Parkinson to meet, exchange views and instigate change. There is no more compelling influence over the future of living with Parkinson than the opinions of those who experience it day to day. PM allows this voice to reach out beyond the spectrum of pure advocacy to the wider Parkinson community and informs science and brings passion and urgency to bear in our quest to find better treatments.

Dilys

I have noticed that most newly diagnosed people know very little about Parkinson so this needs to be addressed, because if we want to educate the public we need to first be educated ourselves. The question then is how to get people to want to be informed patients, that is, knowledgeable about their condition and aware of their own body and its responses? I think there is also a need for more universally shared understanding of how we are affected by Parkinson especially the non-motor effects.

Initiatives such as Parkinsons Movement give voice to the experiences and concerns of the - and are the way forward. PM's strength is in its position as a patient led project with a broad geographic focus. It uses the latest developments in information technology and has the potential to effect change by working at the interface of practitioners and the academic community with PwP.

Anders

Not sure.
Some people like Michael J. Fox mean a lot to the public understanding. Perhaps PM create public focus on certain particular persons with PD who can take "center stage' in the media. Like Tom Isaacs.

Do events that attract attention.

But this requires that PM has resources beyond what is the case today.

Fulvio

As I mentioned before, I believe that, first of all, people need to be informed.
A movement like PM should be able to accomplish the mission to establish an information platform targeting a specific and growing segment of PwP: YOPD and newly diagnosed. First of all because a web-based platform like PM will be more likely accessed by people with at least basic skills in using the internet.

The community of PwP using internet is growing in numbers.

This should contribute to maximizing the return on efforts invested in teaching and training.

Q9 Can you tell our readers why a global awareness of Parkinson disease is so important?

Peggy

We need to bring all these important stakeholders together into one unit that will be focused on the same path, reaching for the same end result. Science is often as much a business venture as a scientific exploration, global patient-centred approaches will soften this.

Paula

Researchers must share, and the research must be regulated to make progress. It is important to avoid dangerous unregulated treatments and people making money out of PwP.

Israel

Global awareness of PD is important because of the fact that this disease knows no bounds and does not discriminate. There is definite strength in numbers and by uniting globally as the PD community, we will not only be heard, but listened to in the process.

Linda

Because it is a global problem, it affects people from all over the world and part of that problem is that in the US and Europe we get the best of treatment, but in so many other places people are not treated, or are being used as guinea pigs in clinical trials, so there must be a way of getting awareness of treatments to all who need them.

Sara

I would like to say that we need a global awareness of health issues and the fact that we all need to take more responsibility when it comes to knowing how to remain healthy - or in our case, knowing how to best manage our disease.

Jackie

Because it's a global disease!

I want Parkies in Bangladesh to have the same opportunities for diagnosis, treatment and someday, cures as Parkies in the US or UK.

PWP AND EXPERTS IN PD ARE SPREAD ACROSS THE GLOBE

Jin
PD doesn't stop at any sex, age, or ethnic group any more!

We have to find a cure together. We can all help each other.

Tom
Parkinson needs to be a global health priority. For too long it has been a hidden disease, and only by putting a spotlight on Parkinson can we hope to change this and raise public awareness of the lack of innovation in the area, and the desperate need for it now.

The Health Economics argument is strong, as is the knowledge that scientifically we are getting close to the goal, and as such, with one concerted effort, we might be able to obliterate Parkinson once and for all.

Perry
Because PD and other serious illnesses don't recognize political boundaries.

Dilys
Global awareness helps us to move forward. Raising the profile internationally gives momentum to treatment and research. Global awareness for me also encompasses caring about those with Parkinson in different parts of the world.

While progress is noticeable in some countries, there are still major differences in the level of health care available from one country to another.

Anders
See what happened with AIDS. Excellent medicines.

I think there are SO many lonely people with PD. Their lives may better with a better understanding of PD in their society.

More awareness will bring a "cure" closer.

Fulvio
This one is easy to answer:
If no one knows you are there, you don't exist

THERE ARE STILL INEQUALITIES IN AVAILABILITY OF TREATMENTS

INVOLVING DECISIONMAKERS HELPS EDUCATE PEOPLE ON PD

Q10

Finally, I would like to ask you why it is important for our decision-makers, people in government, in healthcare facilities, educational establishments etc. to be aware of the implications of PD. Briefly, what do we need to do to reach them, and how are they useful in the battle against PD?

Peggy

Forty years ago, before levodopa was discovered, people were being institutionalized and often died after around nine years with the disease. We have come a long way from that, our lives are now greatly extended. We now have 80 million people in the US alone, who are at the average age of Parkinson onset. Because it is similar to the later stages of the normal aging process, everyone would get Parkinson if they lived long enough, into extremely old age. Caring for our aging population, who are now often called the baby boomers and who now live longer, will impact our socio-economic position. We won't be able to put them all in care homes. When you remove a PwP from society you remove the caregiver too. Society loses their combined income and gains the expense of caring for a complex disorder. Parkinson accelerates the aging process, so peoples needs are greater for a longer period of time. They are being treated for multiple issues that all fit under the PD umbrella. It costs a huge amount to do this, and they can no longer ignore it. The government needs a cure for PD just as much as we do.

They recognize the impact it is going to make.

Paula

An example here in the USA. We have a Parkinson Caucus, and we attempt to get as many signatures as we can when we go to Congress, but I have never heard of anything they've ever done! I think it exists in name only. Some Senators say 'I don't sign caucuses', so you know they don't care.

I don't really have much faith in government, but they do give us money. Pharma and government are business. I do not see the humanity.

Israel

The importance of involving decision-makers, etc. and making them aware can't be stressed enough. My congressman told me that he appreciated the work that I was doing because before I walked into his office to talk about PD research, funding, etc. he had never known anyone with PD. He also mentioned that the fact that I was so young at the time of onset and diagnosis provided a much stronger impact when letting people know what our fight was all about.

We often have the thought in mind that many more people know about PD - because of those around us who know what the disease is and the difficulties involved with it.

We need to start from scratch when explaining the disease to others and allow them to ask questions of us.

Linda

Nationally we need to improve education about PD in medical school and healthcare facilities, and locally look at each institution and see how we can educate the staff about the needs of PD patients.

On an individual level, if we come across hospital staff we need to talk to them and let them know what we need, such as getting medication on time and the importance of being able, to some extent, to have some control over our our own medication.

Sara

In my view, the knowledge of Young Onset PD is far from adequate presently, even among neurologists. This mean taking into account the completely different situation in life that people with Young Onset PD have to cope with. This includes diagnosing it as well as treating it effectively and efficiently.

I think that fact should be able to bring more immediate action to the treatment and research of PD, since the potential effects on economical aspects are considerably greater for people in working age than for older people.

Jackie

We need to reach decision makers if we are ever going to achieve any changes. Governments provide or deny funding for research, which, in turn, sends a strong message to private investors in research.The medical education community in general has little to no understanding of PD, yet every specialty in medicine deals with us at some point. The best time to reach the doctors, nurses, social workers, etc. is before they are loosed upon the world. If we can't reach them then, we need to teach them about PD's effects on the workplace and the tax base, but also on our bodies' teeth, bones, skin, gastrointestinal tract, eyes, etc.

Jin

We need to have them recognize how rapidly this disease is spreading, especially as people live to a higher average age. Unless we can stop it developing in people so young, we have to pay more to take care of more patients. So, we need to ask our law-makers and people in government to allocate more budget money for finding a cure.

Perry

Awareness is important because the cost of serious illness is high and growing as the population ages both in terms of human suffering and disability as well as direct and indirect medical and other economic costs.

THE COST OF PD IS GREAT - A CURE MAKES ECONOMIC SENSE

ADVOCATES CAN PRIORITSE THE HUMAN COST OF YEARS WITH PD

Jon

I am in many respects a scientific, not a political, animal. But this notwithstanding, it's obvious to me that appropriate decisions can only be made on the basis of appropriate information. Parkinson is a highly heterogeneous condition, with differing rates of progression and primary symptoms. Above all we need to make decision-makers rethink the classification of Parkinson as a movement disorder. Especially nowadays, with modern treatments, the longer term consequences - particularly cognitive, sleep and mood, and impulsivity - are becoming much more apparent.

The principal way of reaching people in government is via a cost. The economic burden of Parkinson is highly persuasive. This cannot be said for educational establishments where the primary focus of interest is likely to be the science behind the condition. Each group will need to be approached in a different way.

Parkinsons Movement has no magic bullet for achieving this but there is little doubt that the PM ambassadors will, in some way, be the pivot between patients and establishment. Each group should be approached in the appropriate language and context of their specialty.

Dilys

Until those with the power to effect change on the local and the national level realise the impact of this condition on our lives and on those near to us we will continue to be misunderstood and may not receive optimal care. A poor understanding of Parkinson means PwP are often faced with proving over and over their level of disability to social agencies, employers etc. Societal ignorance and an uninformed public compounds the daily difficulties that confront us.

Anders

A big question! Sorry!

Fulvio

I think I would rephrase the question!

It is not important for them to be aware of it!

It's important for US that they are aware of the implications of PD.

It doesn't matter whether we like it or not, these people have the power to decide where the money will go, and they don't have PD.

Once again, we need to inform them first.

Only once you have told, explained and shown those in power what living with PD means for the patient and the family will you have a chance that 'someone' will escalate the position of Parkinson on the decision makers priority agenda.

LUCY - A VISION FOR THE FUTURE

A cure means a chance again to live the way I visioned myself living.

It means sleep.
It means relaxation.
It means ease of movement.

A cure would bring us together only if it was available worldwide.

The countries that don't have Parkinson centres, specialists, or the funds available for people to be able to get care - this is sad - and we need to help each other, to work together.

I would feel bad for someone who lives in a country where they were not able to get this help.

We need to find the cure and advance in the way we help each other.

Lucy Roucis

Lucy is an actress and comic and can be seen performing 'stand up' in the film, **Love and Other Drugs**. After diagnosis as a YOPD, she became active in PHAMALY (Physically Handicapped Actors and Musical Artists League) where Parkinson is an asset because all members have a disability. She brings her talents to advocacy for Parkinson and disability awareness.

POSTSCRIPT

Dear Reader,
To close this tale, we offer you the real beginning - in a post Lindy Ashford wrote on the old BrainTalk forum in December 2005: "I would also like to see a body of reference developed by the PD community, that documents this [PD] in human terms, through the experiences and writings of real people. If you like, an anthology of experience..."

It took four years before the project began and four more years of work to achieve it. We leave you with this postscript describing what has happened to some of the authors in their personal journey with PD from 2009 to 2013.

This ending is another beginning. How will you act and what will you do with this information?

Sincerely,
The Editors and NeuroWriters (and Alice, of course.)

UPDATE: How we've changed

Peggy Willocks
How have I changed since we started writing this book? This has been one of the most difficult tasks that I have ever attempted, and I have done many in my advocacy career.

While writing this book my PD has advanced - more dyskinesia, more dystonia and pain, and (shudder) more cognitive interference. It has been a long-term project, where in my experience I have done quick tasks - write an article, present a speech, draw a cartoon, etc. Writing the book has been just like living with the disease - it's chronic - long-term! I have watched each of its contributors 'keep the faith.'

Two of our authors have passed away since we started, but their advocacy has been preserved as the book comes to fruition. This book is an anthology of HOPE.

Linda Herman:
Three years ago in 2010, I was in my 15th year with Parkinson.

For the first 10 years I was able to control my symptoms fairly well, with a cocktail of drugs that allowed me to live a fairly productive life. Although 10 years of ever-progressing PD forced me into early retirement, I kept busy and involved with my advocacy work with PAN, PDF, the Parkinson's Pipeline Project, New Yorkers for the Advancement of Medical Research, and my writing and researching.

I noticed all my symptoms were slowly worsening. Through my research, I believed that our best hopes for a cure were in GDNF and stem cell research. Both of these experimental treatments have faced challenges (mostly business and political issues) that have slowed the already slow drug development process. In the case of GDNF, clinical research was halted for close to 9 years.

I've often thought, 'What if..?'

My condition has worsened, as it has with many of my colleagues and peers, threatening our ability to speak, write, travel and make a difference.

It is time to pass the baton on to a new generation of PwP and pray that they will reach the finish line. I have accepted the fact that the cure will come too late for me, but I know it is coming and I remain hopeful that it will be here for our children and grandchildren.

In the meantime, I hope to lead the best life that I can with PD and continue to do what I can to fight the disease - like helping NeuroWriters create this book.

Pamela Kell
In 2009, my world had reduced to an unacceptably small place. I was without relevance or direction and daily turned more inward. I did not sleep and occasionally, very late at night, when I was assured I was alone, I even said aloud 'Why me?' By pure serendipity a woman I met casually, many years before, sent me a nice note to say she remembered me and was glad to see me posting on NeuroTalk again. That small, generous gesture began a miraculous journey that required involvement, commitment, diligence, responsibility and risk.

Today I am not as functional as I was in 2009. I am rarely able to spend a day, or even an hour, as I did in the beginning, wrapped in blissful, serene denial.

I became involved in this project and once again took on the trappings of a contributing adult in a world filled with impossible tasks. I have grown in spirit and I am the better for it in both mind and body. I have come to believe over the past two years that our lives are not measured in results but rather in how often and how hard we try.

Girija Muralidhar
In the three years of working on this book, I went through quite a transformation, from research scientist to research advocate, and from patient to patient advocate/activist.

It is almost 10 years since my diagnosis with PD. In the last two years the aches and pains associated with PD have slowed me down.

My priorities and limits are clear to me. I had to give up my lab and research career, as I could no longer work safely in a biology lab. It took me a while to come to terms with this difficult decision. I could not have done it without my PCC friends, who assured me that I would be OK and that I would find 'something' to do. Indeed, I have found my niche, in research and patient advocacy. As a researcher, I believed in science and as a patient advocate, I realized that science alone will not bring 'cures' for patients. The path of 'Brain to Bench to Body' is littered with obstacles; from limited funds for research, to failed clinical trials, to delayed FDA approvals. Clearing that path without compromising science or patient safety are my new goals. I cannot think of a better way to use my education and training. I know it is a long one…

Katherine Huseman

How have I changed in these three years? Physically I still do well for 12 years after diagnosis. But… I'm much more aware of my limits. I must plan rest and medication, which doesn't work as well or as long, and I've had problems with my eyes and hips that probably connect to PD.

Each day is a roller coaster, fueled by positive and negative levels of medicine, stress, sleep and unknown factors. Emotionally and philosophically my life is richer because of the people I've met through PCC, especially the authors of this book - they're more than a support group, they've become family.

When I began this journey my desire was for PwP to have a 'seat at the table'. Now I want even more respect from the medical community and others. So I'll borrow the words of the disability rights movement and say, 'Nothing about us, without us.' Let's talk.

May Griebel

Like several of our group, my PD symptoms have progressed, for me especially the dyskinesias caused by medication, which led me to have bilateral deep brain stimulators placed in August 2011.

My quality of life has greatly improved, but I had to retire about 18 month early, at least partially due to other medical conditions, such as significant spinal disease.

I sometimes feel that if I could lie along a tropical beach, with a cool drink and a good book, while people brought me fruit and met my every need, I might be symptom free.

Unfortunately (or maybe fortunately, since PD patients seem to do better if our every need is not met by someone else), that is not LIFE. So, like all of us, I drag myself out of bed each morning and go to exercise, or sing with a group at various care facilities, or meet a friend for lunch. Life goes on, and I am determined to live it.

Lindy Ashford

I was fortunate to fall among some of the brightest and most tenacious of PwP minds, first at BrainTalk, then Neurotalk, and much later at Parkinson's Movement. Little did I know when I first 'met' them online that they were the backbone of a lively patient activist movement. The way people coped

with their condition amazed me, many had progressed over years of living with PD and had the dyskinesias that PD drugs can gift us with. Their generosity in sharing a wealth of experience gave all comers a living resource of information to dip into and relate to.

Three years 'birthing' this book has brought changes to us all. My own PD has progressed and is harder to live with, but I have a road map to guide me, and good company.

Who could ask for more, except of course a treatment that would take away the inevitability of progression and give people with PD around the world a better future.

John Citron

In 2006, I was diagnosed as having possible atypical Parkinsonism. Initially medication worked. Today, if I come close to dosage time I am sore, stiff and generally feel unwell. Skipping a dose is out of the question. I now have more and more side effects, including the dreaded nausea and some dyskinesia if I take too much medication because it is difficult to regulate.

In July 2010, after a year as a full-time student, I returned to full-time work. I did quite well and received an employee award two years in a row. But with the ever-increasing fatigue, cognitive problems, balance issues and falls, I was put on notice due to lack of production. In September 2012, I applied for disability. I am now facing a new chapter, so to speak, in my life.

Perry Cohen

My active participation in this ambitious book project has come late in the process as reinforcement to make up for the loss of key contributors.

When the book group began, I was principally involved with several other projects related to methods and technology for patient-centered medical research. For example, I played a central role in the NIH sham surgery conference. I kept up with progress on the book through the work of my closest colleagues in the Parkinson Pipeline Project who have been heavily involved with the book.

At that time, I was at the top of my game as an authentic voice for the interests of patients, with invitations to present at international meetings, recognition of my expertise in national health policy forums and a growing appreciation of the value of patient perspectives in the process of research and medical care. But time marches on and PD has continued to take an ever increasing toll, so I have gone from saying that "I have PD and I can see the dark at the end of the tunnel" to saying "I am in the dark at the end of the tunnel." I have always thought that I would find a passage way through the tunnel, so I do maintain a degree of hope and expectation necessary to survive.

This optimism is severely challenged by the slow pace of science and the general disregard of movement specialist Neurologists for collaborating or even communicating with PwP.

I still think that PD is the best worst thing that ever happened to me.

Valerie Graham (page 56 update)

Editor's note: In the summer of 2011, guest author Valerie Graham had to have all her DBS hardware removed due to a staph infection. She said: "While I may have appeared to have been the poster child for DBS surgery, the reality is that my journey down the DBS pathway has been fraught with more complications than many, including the fact that I have had to have two electrodes re-implanted, four broken electrical leads replaced and two pulse generators replaced, not to mention scores of other problems. Having said all that, I remain a staunch supporter of the benefits that can potentially be derived from DBS and I remain a firm believer that DBS offers the best chance for improving the overall quality of one's life with Parkinson disease at this time." Her update continued: "I had my DBS re-implantation surgeries in 2012. On April 20th, April 27th and May 7th, to be precise. I am still (August, 2012) in the process of being programmed and am doing relatively well - to others, I am certain that it seems that I am doing amazingly well. But, from my perspective, though I am doing much better than when I was without neurostimulation, due to the staph infection, and have been able to reduce my meds considerably, I am not doing as well as I once was with DBS. Of course, it has been 10 years almost to the day since my first DBS surgery and it has been 20+ years since I was first diagnosed, so all things considered, I guess that I am doing better than most!"

YOU HAVE NO FUTURE! Bob Cummings

When our editor-in-chief asked us to write a few paragraphs covering our experiences since beginning this book two years ago, together with some additional commentary on what we expected for the future, I was immediately reminded of a story I have heard several times over the years. Many who have heard this story believe it to be just another Internet fable.

A Christmas party, held annually by a Southern California computer company, included a handwriting analyst, a psychic and a fortuneteller, as entertainment. One of the more hard-drinking revelers said he was going to sample all three. Choosing a simple question he asked, "What is my future?" and was told by all three, "You have no future." Within hours following the party's end, he was killed in an automobile accident!

As the only late onset PwP I am frequently reminded of the story and can readily identify with it. We know that for patients nearing the end stages of this disease there is no present cure, treatments are very limited and passing is usually not peaceful. So, it should be no surprise to the reader that I am not very optimistic about the future.

As for the past two years, the experience has been nothing short of superlative. My colleagues have been talented, dedicated, supportive, and among the best friends a man dealing with 11 female collaborators might expect. We have shared our lifestyles, our families, our successes and failures, trials and tribulations, mixing in generous doses of good humor and fun.

It has been a great ride!
1/25/12

Editor's Note: The Parkinsons Creative Collective is sad to inform the reader that Bob Cummings died on April 7, 2012. Bob was our Peripatetic Papa (his own definition of his role). He kept us on task with his determination, creativity and incredible sense of humor - but most of all, he was our friend.

MY WAY OUT: Paula Wittekind

Editor's note: Paula Wittekind sent the following piece to friends and family and also posted it for online friends on the NeuroTalk Forum in May 2012. There over 100 people replied and over 13,000 people read it. (yes, some were probably repeat visitors.)

After at least 25 years with Parkinson disease, one expects to slowly become less functional in every way.

Communication becomes slurred, muscles freeze, swallowing becomes difficult and - last but not least - there is a constant danger of falling. All of these symptoms can lead to to other health conditions that are also life-threatening.

Our insides become sluggish and backed up. Internal tremors are not always visible to the eye but they reveal themselves on machines.

How will our lives conclude with this illness? So many possibilities, but mine was revealed to me with an esophageal cancer diagnosis after what seems like a lifetime of painful food backup, bloating, and heartburn. I don't know or care if it was the PD that caused it. I used to smoke and drink, but I suspect the sludge that ferments and creeps through my digestive system wore out my esophagus.

When I woke up from the endoscopy my doctor said, "You have a tumor." I asked, "Is it cancer?" He said, "I think it is; you will need chemo and radiation." I said, "I finally got a way out."

It doesn't stop there. Lymph nodes are next and now it's just cancer as it is beyond the esophagus. Little sprinkles of it scattered on the PET SCAN - some here and some there.

"If you have symptoms," explained a very well respected oncologist, "you are already past stage 1; the survival rate drops to 30 per cent if it's in the muscles and down to 10 if it's in the lymph nodes." I also have a spot on my lung. Not identified yet but it is likely going to contribute to what is indeed a way out - like it or not.

That brings me to the reason for writing to you all. I am not afraid. Whether you realize it or not, Parkinson prepares you for death, especially as the years go by and you suffer losses all along the way that you can't get back - like carrying my new grandson while standing up - no balance.

I am not depressed, I'm relieved. I basically haven't felt well since I was 35.

I have become pretty cynical about the medical community and seem to see more waste, competition, repetition and dishonesty, than success and compassion.

I am not going to fight it. It will only destroy all the gains I've made from exercising. The oncologist said I have no cogwheeling and he's never seen someone as 'normal' as me after 23 years. After reading an article called **Doctors Die Differently** I learned that doctors don't take as much treatment as they prescribe. The oncologist said, "I probably wouldn't take the treatment. I think we have the same view about death. It will make your PD much worse and it's too far advanced." God bless him. He said he might suggest a little radiation to shrink the tumor to enable me to swallow. Therefore that's our goal. See if radiation can shrink the esophageal tumor so I can eat and travel.

I can cash in my life insurance if I have it verified that I have only one year to live. Where should I travel to first? My oncologist estimates I may have 2 to 6 months. When he said 2 to 6 months I realized how bad it really was. Again, no butterflies, no fear, just acceptance.

My faith guides me everyday - one at a time. "Fear no evil for thou art with me." I believe I am in the right hands.

Editor's Note: Paula did use her life insurance but couldn't travel; radiation had weakened her. Instead she rented a four-bedroom condo overlooking an inlet with dolphins playing in the water and glorious sunrises. She invited friends and family to visit and stay with her while she lived her final months in hospice care. She died surrounded by love on November 8, 2012.

And we leave you with Bob Dawson's words:

We all live long enough; it really is the quality of life that matters, to not stop marveling at the beauty of the universe, and the general craziness of everything.

And everything is funny, some of the time. It's a disease that teaches a lot. Not what we would have chosen; but it changes the world you live in and you see great and horrible things, the best and the worst. It's a strange adventure.

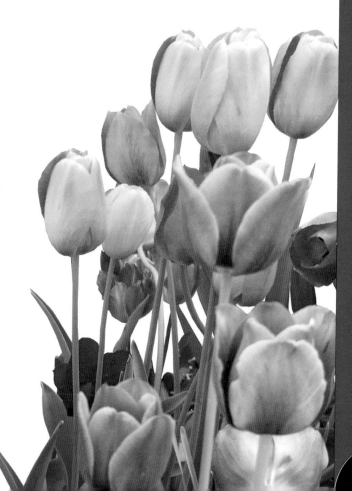

CHAPTER 1

These three web sites are good starting points, with comprehensive information on many aspects of PD, and links to other recommended resources:

Parkinson's Disease Foundation Resource List
http://www.pdf.org/en/resourcelink

National Institute of Neurological Disorders and Stroke (NiNDS)
http://www.ninds.nih.gov/disorders/parkinsons_disease/
parkinsons_disease.htm

WE MOVE: Comprehensive resource for movement disorder information and activities on the web.
http://www.wemove.org/

ESPECIALLY FOR THE NEWLY DIAGNOSED:

Christensen, Jackie Hunt. **The First year - Parkinson's disease: An Essential guide for the newly diagnosed.** Da Capo Press, 2005.(book)

Parkinson's Disease Foundation. **Diagnosis Parkinson's Disease: You are not alone** (video)
http://www.pdf.org/en/not_alone_DVD

MEDICAL GUIDES

Ahlskog, J. Eric. **The Parkinson's disease Treatment Book: Partnering with your doctor to get the most from your medications.** Oxford University Press, 2005. (book)

Lieberman, Abraham.**The Muhammad Ali Parkinson Center 100 Questions & Answers about Parkinson Disease**, Jones and Bartlett Publishers, Inc., 2010.(book)

Okun, Michael and Fernandez, Hubert. **Ask the Doctor about Parkinson's disease.** : Demos Health, 2009.(book)

Parashos, Sotirios, Wichmann, Rosemary, and Melby, Todd. **Navigating Life with Parkinson's disease.** Oxford University Press, 2012.(book)

Southeast Parkinson Disease Association. **Drugs contraindicated for Parkinson's disease patients.** Available online : http://www.sepda.org/id29.html

PATIENT LED AND PATIENT-CENTRIC GROUPS

Cure Parkinson's Trust
http://www.cureparkinsons.org.uk/

Davis Phinney Foundation
http://www.davisphinneyfoundation.org/

Parkinson's Movement
Parkinson's Movement @ Health Unlocked
http://parkinsonsmovement.healthunlocked.com

Parkinson Creative Collective
http://parkinsonscreativecollective.org/

Patients Like Me
http://www.patientslikeme.com/conditions/4-parkinson-s-disease

PD Plan for Life
http://www.pdplan4life.com/

NATIONAL AND INTERNATIONAL ORGANIZATIONS

American Parkinson's Disease Association (APDA)
http://www.apdaparkinson.org/

European Parkinson's Disease Association (EPDA)
http://www.epda.eu.com/

Michael J. Fox Foundation
htttp://www.michaeljfox.org

National Parkinson Foundation (NPF)
http://www.parkinson.org/

Parkinson's Action Network (PAN)
http://www.parkinsonsaction.org/

Parkinson Alliance
http://www.parkinsonalliance.org/index.php

Parkinson's Disease Foundation
www.pdf.org

Parkinson Society Canada
http://www.parkinson.ca

Parkinson's UK
http://www.parkinsons.org.uk/

Unity Walk (held every April in Central Park in NYC)
http://www.unitywalk.org/

DEEP BRAIN STIMULATION

Bronstein, Jeff M. et al. **Deep Brain Stimulation for Parkinson Disease: An Expert Consensus and Review of Key Issues.** Archives of Neurology, 2011 Feb;68(2):165, full text available at:
http://archneur.ama-assn.org/cgi/content/short/68/2/165

Christensen, Jackie Hunt. **Life with a battery-operated brain - A patient's guide to deep brain stimulation.** Langdon Street Press, 2009.(book)

DBS Surgery Yahoo group (online discussion group) - this discussion group also maintains a database of PWP's experiences with and ratings of DBS surgeons and their hospitals. Click on Databases from the home page
http://health.groups.yahoo.com/group/DBSsurgery/

or go directly to database
http://health.groups.yahoo.com/group/DBSsurgery/database

DBS-STN.org (affiliate of Parkinson's Alliance)
http://www.dbs-stn.org/

CHAPTER 2

(Non-motor symptoms/cognitive problems/pain/depression/fatigue/sleeping)

Clognition Website. Cognitive issues from the viewpoint of PWP; http://www.clognition.org/

A Guide to the Non-Motor Symptoms of Parkinson's Disease. The Parkinson Society Canada's guides are very informative and are available in patients' and doctors' versions. Available at: http://bit.ly/J5xhya

Non-Motor Symptoms in Parkinson's Disease: The Dark Side of the Moon. (Medscape article) Includes a lengthy list of references to medical journals.
http://www.medscape.com/viewarticle/734227

Parkinson's UK Non-Motor Symptoms Questionnaire - identifies non-motor symptoms you may have experienced, and should discuss with your doctor. access at:
http://www.parkinsons.org.uk/PDF/nms_questionnaire.pdf

Under-recognized Nonmotor Symptoms of Parkinson's Disease (PDF expert briefing). Webcast March 16, 2013. Available in Parkinson's Disease Foundation archives at: http://www.pdf.org/en/online_education_past

CHAPTER 3
(alternative treatments/ exercise/dance/creativity, nutrition)

THERAPIES

Lee Silverman Voice Treatment.
A therapy program to improve speech and voice, especially voice volume, for PWP (LSVT-Loud)
http://www.healthline.com/galecontent/lee-silverman-voice-treatment

Brooks, Megan. **"Training BIG" Improves Motor Performance in Parkinson's Disease.** Medscape neurology news, 2010. (article) full text at:
http://www.medscape.com/viewarticle/723803
Ramig, Lorraine, Fox, Cynthia, and Farley,Becky,

The Science and Practice of "Speaking LOUD" and "Moving BIG." (article) American Parkinsons Disease Association, Midwest Chapter, 2009.

Full text at
http://www.apdamidwest.org/APDA_Midwest/Speaking_LOUD.html

ALTERNATIVE TREATMENTS

National Center for Complementary and Alternative Medicine (NIH) – part of the NIH, the center funds and conducts research on alternative treatments.
http://nccam.nih.gov/

Mischley, L. **Natural Therapies for Parkinson's disease.** Coffeetown Press, 2009.(book)

Tumeric at a glance
http://nccam.nih.gov/health/turmeric/ataglance.htm

EXERCISE

Alberts J. et al. **It's not about the bike, It is about the pedaling: Forced exercise and Parkinson's Disease,** Exercise and Sport Sciences Review. 2011;39(4):177-186. Abstract and Introduction at:
http://www.medscape.com/viewarticle/751998
Future directions and summary at:
http://www.medscape.com/viewarticle/751998_2

Argue, John. **Parkinson's disease and The Art of Moving,** New Harbinger Publications, 2000. (book)

Dance for PD (DVD)
Features a complete class from the internationally acclaimed dance program developed by Mark Morris Dance Group/Brooklyn Parkinson Group. For more information contact
www.danceforpd.org or call 1-800-957-1046

Garbarini, Nicole J. **Tai Chi helps Parkinson's patients with balance and fall prevention** (article), NINDS, 2012.

Full text at:
http://www.ninds.nih.gov/news_and_events/news_articles/Li_TaiChi_and_PD.htm

Hacken,ME. **Tai Chi Improves Balance and Mobility in People with Parkinson Disease. Gait Posture.** 2008 October; 28(3): 456–460. Published online 2008 April 18. Available at
http://www.ncbi.nlm.nih.gov/pmc/articles/PMC2552999/?tool=pubmedYoga

Russell, Jackie. **Delay the Disease: Exercise and Parkinson's Disease** (Fitness program; DVD and book available), 2007.
http://delaythedisease.com/

Smith, M. **What Is the Impact of Exercise on Parkinson's Disease?** (web site). Livestrong.com,June 14, 2011. Available online at:
http://www.livestrong.com/article/323262-what-is-the-impact-of-exercise-on-parkinsons-disease/

Zid, David and Russell, Jackie. **Delay the disease – functional fitness for Parkinson's.** Delay the disease, 2012.
Delay the disease – Exercise and Parkinson's disease. 2007

NUTRITION

Holden, Kathrynne. **Cook well, stay well with Parkinson's disease.** Five star living, 2003.(book)

____**Eat well, stay well with Parkinson's disease.** Five star living, 1998. (book)

____**Parkinson's disease and Constipation : A Nutrition Audiotape and Guidebook for People with Parkinson's.** Five star living,[n.d.](book)

Leader, Gregory, Leader, Lucille. **Parkinsons Disease Reducing Symptoms with Nutrition and Drugs.** Revised Edition. Denor Press; 2nd Revised edition (2009)

TRADITIONAL EASTERN MEDICINE

Halpern, Marc. **What is Ayurvedic Medicine / About Ayurveda.** California College of Ayurved, 2013. (web site) - contains many articles on the philosophy and practices of this healing science from India. Full text at:
http://www.ayurvedacollege.com/college/what-is-ayurveda

Pan,W. et.al. **Traditional Chinese medicine improves activities of daily living in Parkinson's disease. Parkinsons disease.** 2011.Published online 2011 May 17.Full text available at: http://www.ncbi.nlm.nih.gov/pmc/articles/PMC3109418/?tool=pubmed

CHAPTER 4
HOSPITALS

Aware in Care National Parkinson Foundation's national program, "which aims to help people with Parkinson's disease get the best care possible during a hospital stay, including receiving their medications on time" A tool kit can be ordered from NPF on their web site or by calling : 1-800-4PD-INFO (473-4636) http://www.awareincare.org/

WORK AND DISABILITY ISSUES

Job Accommodations Network (JAN)
Advises and promotes accommodations in the workplace for people with disabilities.
http://askjan.org/

National Council on Independent Living
http://www.ncil.org/

Parkinson's Action Network. (PAN)
Social Security Disability Insurance:PAN has created an assessment form to be filled out with your doctor, so that your medical record adequately includes information on your disability when filing for SSDI.
Download form at: http://www.parkinsonsaction.org/federal-initiatives/ssdi-medicare/disability-insurance

LIVING WITH PD: BOOKS BY PWP

Atwell, Jim. **Wobbling home: A spiritual walk with Parkinson's**. Square Circle Press LLC, 2011.

Ball, John. **Living well, running hard: Lessons learned from living with Parkinson's disease.** iUniverse Publishing 2007.

Baumann, John. **DECIDE SUCCESS: You Ain't Dead Yet: Twelve Action Steps to Achieve The Success You Truly Desire**. JK Success Enterprises,2011.

Curren, Arthur. **Dumb Bells & Dopamine: A Parkinson's Success Story**. Author House, 2005.

Green, Dennis, Snyder, Joan Blessington and Kendell, Craig. **Voices From The Parking Lot: Parkinson's Insights And Perspectives.** The Parkinson's Alliance, 2000.

Havemann, Joel and Reich, Stephen. **A Life shaken**, 2010.

Isaacs, Tom. **Shake Well Before Using.**
Cure Parkinsons Press, 2007.

Murphy. Austin and Phinney, Davis. **The Happiness Of Pursuit: A Father's Courage, A Son's Love And Life's Steepest Climb**, 2011.

Petrick, Ben. **40,000 To One**. KMP Enterprises, 2012.

Robb, Karl. **A Soft Voice In A Noisy World: A Guide To Dealing And Healing With Parkinson's Disease**. RobbWorks, 2012.

Stamford, Jon. **A Piece Of My Mind**. Lulu.com, 2012.
_____ **A Slice Of Life**. Lulu.com, 2012.
_____ **Coming To Terms**. Lulu.com, 2012.

LIVING WITH PD: WEBSITES & BLOGS BY PWP

Parkinson's Disease: Wobbly Williams
http://www.wobblywilliams.com/

Parkinson's Movement
http://www.cureparkinsons.org.uk/sites/parkinsons-movement
PD Plan for Life
http://www.pdplan4life.com/

Some of our favorite bloggers:

Sheryl Jedlinski. **Living well with Parkinson's Disease**
http://livingwellwithparkinsonsdisease.com/about/

Bob Kuhn. **Positively Parkinson's**
http://positivelyparkinsons.blogspot.com/

Israel Robledo. **Blogs about PD Research advocates**
http://en.wordpress.com/tag/pd-research-advocate/

Marshall Davidson, MD, K. Guiffre MD. **Solid Information with a Personal Touch.**
www. dopadoc.com

Bob Dawson. **Dance to raise a question**
http://parkinsonsdance.blogspot.com/2005/07/chapter-49.html

Soania Mathur. **Canadian physician, YO PwP**
www.designingacure.com

Rick Everett. **A Matter of Balance**
http://amatterofbalance.wordpress.com/index/

Karl Robb. **A Soft Voice In A Noisy World Making the Best of A Life with Parkinson's Disease.**
http://pdpatient.wordpress.com/

CHAPTER 5

Advance health care directive.
Wikipedia, 2013. Available online:
http://en.wikipedia.org/wiki/Advance_health_care_directive

Dutton, J. **Legal Issues and Parkinson's: Delegating Decisions for Health Care.**
Parkinson's Disease Foundation, 2010. Available online:
http://www.pdf.org/en/fall10_legal

----- **Legal Issues: Planning Ahead When You are Living with Parkinson's.**
Expert briefing.(webinar) Available online:
http://www.pdf.org/en/parkinson_briefing_legal_issues

Gardner, J, and Wichmann, R. **Managing advanced Parkinson's disease.**
National Parkinson Foundation (NPF). Available online:
http://www3.parkinson.org/site/DocServer/Managing_Advanced_PD.pdf

Kondracke, Morton. **Saving Milly: love, politics and Parkinson's disease.** Ballantine Books, 2002

Living wills and advanced directives for medical decisions. Mayo Clinic. Available online:
http://www.mayoclinic.com/health/living-wills/HA00014

U S military veterans with Parkinson's (USMVP) .
Yahoogroups online discussion list. Read messages and join the group at: http://groups.yahoo.com/group/vets_parkinsons_agentorange/

CAREGIVERS

CARE (Caregivers Are really Essential) mailing list
A safe place for CGs to share information, ask questions and vent feelings with understanding support. Visit the website at http://www.pdcaregiver.org/ If you wish to join, please introduce yourself by email to Teresa Marcy <tmarcy@saintmarys.edu>, and she will send you instructions.

National Parkinson Foundation (NPF)
Improving care, Improving lives
http://www.parkinson.org/caregivers

Parkinson's Action Network. (PAN).
Online caregiver interview. You-Tube video series:
http://www.parkinsonsaction.org/for-caregivers

Parkinson Disease Foundation (PDF).
Tips for People with Parkinson and their Care Partner
http://www.pdf.org/pdf/fs_pd_partnership_08.pdf

CHAPTER 6

Fox, Michael J. **Lucky Man**: A Memoir. Hyperion, 2003.
_____ **Always looking up: The Adventures of an Incurable Optimist.** Hyperion, 2009.

Braintalk archives. The original online discussion group.
Later became NeuroTalk. Archives available 2006 – 2011, at: http://www.braintalkcommunities.org/forums/forumdisplay.php?f=214

Neurotalk Forum
http://neurotalk.psychcentral.com/forum34.html

Parkinsn List or Parkinson's Information exchange network. International mailing list. The most recent messages are under this url
http://www.parkinsons-information-exchange-network-online.com/parkmail1.5/2011d/maillist.html

People Living with Parkinson's (PLWP) Yahoo groups mailing list http://health.groups.yahoo.com/group/plwp2

World Parkinson Congress. International conference for and by the whole Parkinson's community – patients, doctors, researchers, organizations, etc. The 3rd WPC will be held in **Montreal, Canada, October 1-4, 2013**.
http://www.worldpdcongress.org/

CHAPTER 7

CLINICAL TRIALS
Getz, Kenneth. **The Gift of Participation: A Guide to Making Informed Decisions About Volunteering for a Clinical Trial.** Jerian Publishing, 2007. (book)

Parkinson's Disease Foundation. **Getting involved with Parkinson's research.** http://www.pdf.org/pdf/PAIRBooklet1.pdf

TO FIND A CLINICAL TRIAL TRY:
Clinicaltrials.gov
www.clinicaltrials.gov

Fox Trial finder
https://foxtrialfinder.michaeljfox.org/

SHAM SURGERY
Cohen, PD, et.al. **Examination of 'Failed' Clinical Trials Using Placebo Brain Surgery Controls.**
Parkinson Pipeline Project, presented at the 2009 American Society for Experimental Neurotherapeutics (ASENT) Annual Meeting; Washington, DC. Available online at : http://www.pdpipeline.org/advocacy/2009%20poster_update.html

Cohen, PD. **Sham Control Groups for Evaluation of Neurosurgery Delivered Therapeutics**: Patient Activists Views presented at the 2011 American Society for Experimental Neurotherapeutics (ASENT) Annual Meeting; Washington, DC.

Havemann, Joel. **Sham Surgeries, Real Risks.** Neurology Now,6(4), July/August, 2010. Available online at :http://www.aan.com/elibrary/neurologynow/?event=home.showArticle&id=ovid.com:/bib/ovftdb/01222928-201006040-00015

Sham Neurosurgical Procedures In Clinical Trials For Neurodegenerative Diseases: Scientific And Ethical Considerations. Conference at NIH, 2010.

The entire conference can be viewed on the NIH website.

DAY 1: http://videocast.nih.gov/summary.asp?Live=9474

DAY 2: http://videocast.nih.gov/Summary.asp?File=16059

DRUG DEVELOPMENT
Nelson, Nick. **Monkeys In The Middle**: How One Drug Company Kept a Parkinson's Disease Breakthrough Out of Reach (book). Booksurge, 2008

Parkinson Pipeline Project. **GDNF History**. collection of articles, web sites, legal documents, etc. related to the GDNF trial halt
http://www.pdpipeline.org/2011/GDNF/gdnf_table.htm

PATIENT-CENTERED MEDICINE & ORGANISATIONS
The Cure Parkinson's Trust
http://www.cureparkinsons.org.uk

e-Patients
http://e-patients.net/

Parkinson Pipeline Project
http://www.pdpipeline.org

Society for Participatory Medicine
http://participatorymedicine.org/
Cohen, PD, et.al. **Ethical Issues in Clinical Neuroscience Research: a Patient's Perspective**, Neurotherapeutics, 4(3) (July, 2007), 537-544.

ENVIRONMENTAL ISSUES
Collaborative on Health and the Environment.
Toxicant and Disease Database Parkinson's and Movement Disorders
http://www.healthandenvironment.org/tddb/disease/794

Neurodegenerative Diseases Working Group
http://www.healthandenvironment.org/initiatives/neuro

The Role Of The Environment In Parkinson's Disease
http://www.niehs.nih.gov/health/assets/docs_p_z/the_role_of_the_environment_in_parkinsons_disease.pdf

Spivey, A. **Rotenone and Paraquat Linked to Parkinson's Disease: Human Exposure Study Supports Years of Animal Studies.** Environmental Health Perspectives. 2011 June; 119(6):A259. http://www.ncbi.nlm.nih.gov/pmc/articles/PMC3114841/?tool=pubmed

JOURNAL CITATIONS

A set of current (free full text) pd research articles can be found at:

Cold Spring Harbor Perspectives in Medicine: PD
http://perspectivesinmedicine.org/site/misc/parkinsons_disease.xhtml

Inflammation and Autoimmunity

Tan EK. **Genetic marker linking inflammation with sporadic Parkinson's disease.** Ann Acad Med Singapore. 2011;40;(2)111-2. PMID: 21468470

Alpha-Synuclein

Leonidas Stefanis. **a-Synuclein in Parkinson's Disease**. Cold Spring Harbor Prospectives in Medicine. Feb 2010 2 (2). Full text at http://www.perspectivesinmedicine.org/content/2/2/a009399.abstract

Park MJ, Cheon SM, Bae HR, Kim SH, Kim JW. Elevated **Levels of a-Synuclein Oligomer in the Cerebrospinal Fluid of Drug-Naïve Patients with Parkinson's Disease.** J Clin Neurol. 2011;7;(4)215-22. PMID: 22259618

Prion (Protein Misfolding)

Hilker R, Brotchie JM, Chapman J. **Pros and cons of a prion-like pathogenesis in Parkinson's disease.** BMC Neurol. 2011;11;74. PMID: 21689433Prion (Protein Misfolding)

Hilker R, Brotchie JM, Chapman J. **Pros and cons of a prion-like pathogenesis in Parkinson's disease.** BMC Neurol. 2011;11;74. PMID: 21689433

Olanow CW, Prusiner SB. **Is Parkinson's disease a prion disorder?** Proc Natl Acad Sci U S A. 2009;106;(31)12571-2. PMID: 19666621

Braak's Staging of PD

Burke RE, Dauer WT, Vonsattel JP. **A critical evaluation of the Braak staging scheme for Parkinson's disease.** Ann Neurol. 2008;64;(5)485-91. PMID: 19067353

Iron Accumulation

Kell DB. **Towards a unifying, systems biology understanding of large-scale cellular death and destruction caused by poorly liganded iron: Parkinson's, Huntington's, Alzheimer's, prions, bactericides, chemical toxicology and others as examples.** Arch Toxicol. 2010;84;(11)825-89. PMID: 20967426

Mitochondria

Esteves AR, Arduíno DM, Silva DF, Oliveira CR, Cardoso SM. Mitochondrial Dysfunction: **The Road to Alpha-Synuclein Oligomerization in PD.** Parkinsons Dis. 2011;2011;693761. PMID: 21318163

Perier C, Vila M. **Mitochondrial biology and Parkinson's disease.** Cold Spring Harb Perspect Med. 2012;2;(2) a009332. PMID: 22355801

Block ML, Calderón-Garcidueñas L. **Air pollution: mechanisms of neuroinflammation and CNS disease**. Trends Neurosci. 2009;32;(9)506-16. PMID: 19716187

van der Mark M, Brouwer M, Kromhout H, Nijssen P, Huss A, Vermeulen R. **Is pesticide use related to Parkinson disease? Some clues to heterogeneity in study results.** Environ Health Perspect. 2011;120;(3)340-7. PMID: 22389202

Bondy SC. **Nanoparticles and colloids as contributing factors in neurodegenerative disease.** Int JEnviron Res Public Health. 2011;8;(6)2200-11. PMID: 21776226

The biochemistry of the basal ganglia and Parkinson's disease. G. Curzon. Postgrad Med J. 1977 December; 53(626): 719–725. http://www.ncbi.nlm.nih.gov/pmc/articles/PMC2496787/?page=1

Neurobiological mechanisms of the Placebo Effect. Benedetti, et al. Journal of Neuroscience. 25(45) http://www.jneurosci.org/cgi/content/full/25/45/10390

What Is the Impact of Exercise on Parkinson's Disease? http://www.livestrong.com/article/323262-what-is-the-impact-of-exercise-on-parkinsons-disease/ Study Indicates Cycling is Effective Therapy for Parkinson's Disease.Frontiers in Rehabililation. Fall 2008. J. Alberts bikelayne.com/media/uploads/Jay%20Article.pdf

LSVT

Neural correlates of efficacy of voice therapy in Parkinson's disease identified by performance-correlation analysis. Narayana S, Fox PT, Zhang W, Franklin C, Robin DA, Vogel D, Ramig LO. http://www.ncbi.nlm.nih.gov/pmc/articles/PMC2811230/?tool=pubmed

Green Tea

Mandel, SA, et. al. **Targeting multiple neurodegenerative diseases etiologies with multimodal-acting green tea catechins.** Journal of nutrition. August 2008, 138:1578S-1583Sfull text at: http://jn.nutrition.org/content/138/8/1578S.long

O. Weinreb, et al. **Neuroprotective molecular mechanisms of (-)-epigallocatechin-3-gallate: a reflective outcome of its antioxidant, iron chelating and neuritogenic properties.** Genes and Nutrition. 2009 Dec: 4 (4): 283-296.full text at: http://www.ncbi.nlm.nih.gov/pmc/articles/PMC2775893/?tool=pubmed

Tai Chi improves balance and mobility in people with Parkinson disease. Hackney ME, Earhart GM. http://www.ncbi.nlm.nih.gov/pmc/articles/PMC2552999/?tool=pubmedYoga

Mind-body interventions: applications in neurology Wahbeh H, Elsas SM, Oken BS. http://www.ncbi.nlm.nih.gov/pmc/articles/PMC2882072/?tool=pubmed

Wang, M. et al. **Curcumin reduces a-synuclein induced cytotoxicity in Parkinson's disease cell model.** BMC Neuroscience 2010, 11:57 full text at: http://www.biomedcentral.com/1471-2202/11/57

RESOURCES

Acknowledgements and Thanks

They say it takes a village to raise a child. It has taken a global, internet-connected community to produce this book. We must open with apologies: even in a book of this size and scope there are limits. If some worthy people or organizations are missing, it was probably due to space and time constraints. We also inadvertently may have missed an acknowledgement. If we have, please know that we are grateful for your contribution. We will correct any oversights in the next edition.

There are so many people to thank for content contributions: all the authors, photographers, artists and advocates who shared their stories and work so generously. Without you, this book would not have been possible, thank you!

Then there are those who read drafts of sections, chapters or even the whole work, sometimes multiple times and who offered editorial advice, even if we didn't always follow it. We thank them all and specially recognize: Hank Newell, Webb Hubble, Bill Rich, Bruce Parker and Lee Pugh.

For pre-publication materials and support, we thank David Kell and Brad Horton

For grants and funds to produce this work and provide copies to support groups, we most sincerely thank:

> The J.W. and Ida M. Jameson Foundation, The Rae Alice and Bernard Cohen Generations Fund of The Atlanta Jewish Federation, The Stein-Bellet Foundation Inc. and the GlassRatner Advisory & Capital Group LLC.

> The Cummings, Clark and Wittekind families for requesting that memorial gifts be directed to the project.

> Dr. Frank Nicklason of the Royal Hobart Hospital, Tasmania, Australia for giving us our first monetary contribution at WPC 2 in Scotland.

> American Parkinson Disease Association for distribution of this book to US support groups.

We also wish to thank all who have given donations to PCC - it has helped us put in print the voices of people with Parkinson (PwP).

For every other type of support, we are grateful and thank specifically:

> Doc John Grohol, Psych Central Founder, who re-established the internet link (originally BrainTalk Communities) to NeuroTalk, where this book was born. He believed in and encouraged us when the concept of the book was very far from reality and only a dream. Thank you, Doc John!

> Parkinson's Movement, under the direction of Jon Stamford, Ph.D. and The Cure Parkinson's Trust founded by Tom Isaacs, UK, for their support and promotion of the book and their efforts to unite the PwP community globally.

> All the PwP who have fought for improvements in managing PD, we thank you for showing us the way to LIVE with PD!

> The physicians and health care providers who practice participatory medicine, truly listening to us while providing patient-centered care.

> The World Parkinson Congress for providing the opportunity for the whole PD community to meet under one roof and exchange ideas.

> The technology and software that made it possible for us, as volunteers with home computers, to plan, create and collaborate globally. In particular, we thank Google for Mail and Drive; Skype for endless calls and the supporting cast of unknown designers and developers whose work enabled ours.

Finally, we offer a special note of gratitude to our families and friends who had plans postponed, dinners delayed and many things deferred while we devoted ourselves to 'THE BOOK.' (A very special thank you to Leo Ashford, who was there through it all and did much at late hours.) Thank you all for being with us and helping us stay focused. We hope you will still recognize us when we resume 'normal life' or as normal as life ever is with PD.

A PARKINSON GLOSSARY
A patient's guide to the scientific language of Parkinson

Acetylcholine: A neurotransmitter that is also involved in controlling smooth movement in the brain. Loss of dopamine causes the rigidity seen in Parkinson patients due to decrease in basal ganglia control.

Agonists: a chemical that can combine with a receptor on a cell to produce a physiological reaction.

Akinesia: Inability to move spontaneously

alpha synuclein (SNCA): a protein postulated to play a central role in the pathogenesis of Parkinson disease, Alzheimer disease, and other neurodegenerative disorders.

amantadine: can be used as a single therapy or with L-DOPA to decrease the L-DOPA created motor fluctuations and L-DOPA related dyskinesis. Can also be used as an antiviral.

amygdala: Located deep in the medial temperal lobe in complex mammals. Involved in fear, anxiety in particular in the formation of memories involved in emotion.

anticholinergics: Helps to restrict the action of acetylcholine by blocking binding at the receptor. Examples of such are below:
- benztropine mesylate,
- biperiden hydrochloride,
- orphenadrine citrate,
- procyclidine hydrochloride,
- trihexyphenidyl hydrochloride.

antagonists: Any compound that decreases the binding of an agonist to a receptor, by either blocking the activation site or changing the conformation of the receptor.

ataxia: Inability to coordinate voluntary muscle movements; unsteady movements and staggering gait.

ATP13A2 (PARK 9): A gene which may be involved in early onset Parkinson. Codes for an enzyme; ATPase 13A2.

Autonomic nervous system (ANS): consisting of sympathetic and parasympathetic aspects and controls involuntary actions, in particular the heart, smooth muscle and glands.

autosomal: When referring to chromosomes all the chromosomes that are non sex related chromosomes are autosomal.

autosomal recessive: Suggests that in order for a particular trait to be expressed both parents have to have the particular allele or gene, therefore the presence of another allele will not allow this allele to be expressed. In the case of Parkinson the Parkin gene is autosomal recessive.

axon: nerve fibers that carry electrical impulses through the brain and spinal cord; they are surrounded by a protective sheath called myelin; in multiple sclerosis the axon can be damaged.

basal ganglia: Clusters of neurons, which include the caudate nucleus, putamen, globus pallidus and substantia nigra, that are located deep in the brain and play an important role in movement. Cell death in the substantia nigra contributes to Parkinsonian signs.

benserazide as co beneldopa (BAN), brand names- Madopar (UK): Catalyses L-DOPA to dopamine 5-HTTP to serotonin and tryptophan to tryptamine. Therefore in Parkinson patients speeds up break down of L-DOPA.

blood brain barrier: The separating membrane between the cerebrospinal fluid (CSF) and the blood a tight physical barrier that keeps immune cells out of the brain, normally.

bradykinesia: Decrease in motor activity. It is associated with basal ganglia diseases, mental disorders and prolonged inactivity due to illness.

brain stem: the part of the brain continuous with the spinal cord and comprising the medulla oblongata, pons, midbrain and parts of the hypothalamus. Damage to this area may cause non-motor dysfunctions such as sleep disorders and autonomic dysfunction.

calcium: calcium is important for signalling and is involved in energy formation in mitochondria. Calcium overload in substantia nigra kills cells.

carbidopa: A drug given with levodopa to decrease its metabolism via inhibition of Dopa decarboxylase.

caudate nucleus: Located in the basal ganglia important in learning and memory.

cerebellum: Part of the hind brain controls learnt actions such as riding a bike, actions that feel second nature.

cerebrospinal fluid (CSF): a water cushion surrounding the brain and spinal cord protecting them from physical impact.

chronic: describing a disease of long duration involving very slow changes. Such disease is often of gradual onset. The term does not imply anything about the severity of a disease.

Computed tomography (CT): is a medical imaging method employing tomography created by computer processing. Digital geometry processing is used to generate a three-dimensional image of the inside of an object from a large series of two-dimensional X-ray images taken around a single axis of rotation.

COMT (catechol-O-methyltransferase): Is an enzyme that breaks down dopamine, adrenaline and noradrenaline.

cytokines: are any of a number of small proteins that are secreted by specific cells of the immune system and that carry signals locally between cells, and thus have an effect on other cells. Higher levels of proinflammatory cytokines are found in Parkinson brains. Unlike growth factors they have no specific role in cell proliferation are and are primarily linked to blood and immune cells. They have also been known to be involved in apoptosis.

deep brain stimulation (DBS): Involves the implantation of a medical device that acts as a brain pacemaker sending electrical impulse to specific areas. In Parkinson patients the device is attached to either the subthalamic nucleus or the globus pallidus.

dementia: A decline in cognitive function due to damage or disease in the brain beyond what might be expected from normal aging. Areas particularly affected include memory, attention, judgement, language and problem solving.

dendrite: (from Greek déndron, "tree") are the branched projections of a neuron that act to conduct the electrochemical stimulation received from other neural cells to the cell body, or soma, of the neuron from which the dendrites project.

depression: A state of low mood. Some consider it a dysfunction, while others see it as an adaptive defense mechanism.

DJ-1: Mutations in this gene have been proved to cause an autosomal recessive form of Parkinson disease in this gene. It may also have an affect in the idiopathic form of the disease. The function of the protein created by DJ-1 is unknown still.

Dopa decarboxylase inhibitors: Such as carbidopa, act to decrease the breakdown of levodopa in the body allowing more to reach the brain where it is converted to dopamine. Particularly useful for Parkinson patients when used alongside levodopa.

dopamine: Acts as one of the brain's messengers to signal movement and maintain balance and coordination

dopamine agonists: Such as; bromocriptine mesylate (Parlodel), pergolide, pramipexole (Mirapex), ropinirole hydrochloride (Requip), piribedil, cabergoline, apomorphine (Apokyn) and lisuride. Act as dopamine, but is not actually dopamine. These are used in the early stages of Parkinson disease or in the late stages when levodopa is no longer as effective.

dopaminergic pathways: Split into four major groups the nigrostriatal, mesocortical, mesolimbic and tuberoinfundibular.
　Nigrostriatal- Connects the substantia nigra to the striatum. Involved heavily in Parkinson.
　Mesocortical and mesolimbic from Ventral Tegmental Area to Nucleus Accumbens, Amygdala & Hippocampus and Prefrontal Cortex. Involved in memory, motivation, emotional response, reward and addiction. Can cause hallucinations and schizophrenia if not functioning properly
　Tuberoinfundibular- from hypothalamus to pituitary gland involved in hormonal regulation, maternal behavior (nurturing), pregnancy and sensory processes

dysarthria: Impaired speech function.

dyskinesia: Abnormality in performing voluntary muscle movements

dysphagia: Difficulty in swallowing.

embryonic stem (ES) cells: see stem cells

entacapone: A Parkinson drug that is used alongside levodopa and carbidopa. Inhibits COMT decreasing breakdown of levodopa, dopamine, adrenaline and noradrenaline.

functional magnetic resonance imaging (fMRi): An imaging technique designed specifically for the brain. It measures rate at which oxygen is removed from the blood to the cells, Therefore suggesting the activity of a particular area of the brain.

GABA: (gamma amino butyric acid) the principal inhibitory neurotransmitter in human brain. GABA neurons project from the striatum to the substantia nigra and are involved in motor control.

GDNF: see growth factors

gene therapy: Gene therapy is the insertion of genes into an individual's cells and tissues to treat hereditary diseases where deleterious mutant alleles can be replaced with functional ones..

genotype: The collection of genetic material in an organism that gives rise to its characteristics.

glia: Glial cells, commonly called neuroglia or simply glia (Greek for "glue"), are non-neuronal cells that maintain homeostasis, form myelin, and provide support and protection for the brain's neurons.

globus pallidus: A major part of the basal ganglia involved in movement control. Split into two main parts the internal globus pallidus (GPi), the external globus pallidus (GPe). Deep brain stimualtion of the GPi is shown to have an increase in motor function in PD patients.

Glutamate: the main excitatory neurotransmitter in the human brain. A major projection from the cerebral cortex to the striatum modulates motor activity

growth factors: Useful for regulating a number of cell processes, in particular cell growth, proliferation and differentiation. Some growth factors are being looked at to try to promote the survival of the neural cells that are degenerating in PD.
　Glial cell line dervied nerve growth factor (GDNF): has showed positive results in regards to cell proliferation and has been shown to reduce the tremors caused by levodopa.
　Fibroblast growth factor (FGF): Possible genetic link to Parkinson disease on the FGF20 gene found in Japanese people.
　Vascular endothelial growth factor-B (VEGF-B): Has been shown to have neuroprotective affects in Parkinson disease and is released in neurodegenerative challenges to the brain.

hippocampus: a complex neural structure (shaped like a sea horse) located on the floor of each lateral ventricle; intimately involved in motivation and emotion as part of the limbic system; has a central role in the formation of memories.

hyperkinesia: Abnormal increase in movement and/or muscle activity.

hypokinesia: Abnormal decrease in movement and/or muscle activity.

hypothalamic pituitary adrenal axis (HPA): Made up of the hypothalamus, pituitary gland and the adrenal cortex, these three components are the primary components of the endocrine system and have a wide range of functions from stimulating the stress response to control of digestion, the immune system, mood, sexuality and energy storage and consumption.

hypothalamus: Located at the bottom of the brain and links the limbic system to the pituitary gland.

idiopathic: Arising from an unknown cause.

Leucine rich repeat kinase 2 (LRRK2): Created by LRRK2 gene which when mutated can lead to Parkinson. Four different LRRK2 gene variants are found in Parkinson patients compared to just one in the general population.

Levodopa: A precursor to dopamine that can pass through the blood brain barrier and then be converted into dopamine the neurotransmitter that is lacking in Parkinson disease.

Lewy bodies: Abnormal aggregates of proteins found in both Parkinson and Alzheimer disease.

MAO (monoamine oxidase): Two subtypes, MAO-A and MAO-B, catalyse the breakdown of amines so replacing the amine group with an oxygen molecule.

MAO A inhibitors: inhibitor of the MAO A enzyme which is responsible for the metabolism of dietary tyramine. MAO-A inhibitors can cause tyramine-induced hypertension.

MAO B inhibitors: e.g. selegiline, rasagiline. Inhibit the break down of dopamine via monoamine oxidase B, better for treatment of PD than the normal non-selective MAO inhibitors as less adverse effects from tyramine-induced hypertension.

n-methyl-4-phenyl-1,2,3,6-tetrahydropyridine (MPTP): A neurotoxin created after by failed effort to synthesize a recreational drug. It causes irreversible Parkinson disease after conversion to MPP+ by MAO B. The MPTP acts by killing the dopaminergic neurons in the substantia nigra.

microglia: The first immune defence mechanism in the brain and central nervous system.

motor skills: The degree of control or coordination given to the skeletal muscles.

magnetic resonance imaging (MRI): is primarily a noninvasive medical imaging technique used in radiology to visualize detailed internal structure and limited function of the body. MRI provides much greater contrast between the different soft tissues of the body than computed tomography (CT) does, making it especially useful in neurological (brain), musculoskeletal, cardiovascular, and oncological (cancer) imaging.

multiple system atrophy (MSA): is a degenerative neurological disorder related to Parkinson but more severe, with problems of movement, balance and autonomic function.

neuromelanin: Formed as a byproduct of dopamine it is believed to bind heavily with iron. Gives the substantia nigra its black appearance.

neuromodulator: A substance other than a neurotransmitter, released by a neuron at a synapse and either enhancing or dampening their activities.

neuroprotection: The term neuroprotection refers to mechanisms within the nervous system which protect neurons from apoptosis or degeneration, for example following a brain injury or as a result of chronic neurodegenerative diseases.

neurotransmitter: A chemical messenger in the nervous system that permits communication between two neuronal cells, normally across a synapse. Examples include; dopamine, acetylcholine, adrenaline, noradrenaline, serotonin, glutamate, GABA, etc.

nicotine: acts as an agonist at nicotinic receptors. NIcotine is thought to decrease chances of developing Parkinson disease.

paradoxical kinesis: the movement of a person who previously could not, usually in response to an extreme stress stimulus, cases of this are reported in Parkinson disease.

parkin: Parkin is a protein which in humans is encoded by the PARK2 gene. The precise function of this protein is unknown; however, parkin is also the gene involved in the creation of the Parkin protein, and is the causative gene for autosomal recessive Parkinson disease.

Parkinsonism: A group of neurological diseases whose main features include slowness and paucity of spontaneous movement (bradykinesia), tremors and rigidity of the muscles.

Parkinsonian gait: A type of stooped, shuffling movement that is common in Parkinson.

PINK-1: A gene that encodes serine/threonine kinase, an enzyme found in mitochondria that stops stress related cell destruction. PINK-1 mutations have an involvement in early onset Parkinson disease. Lack of PINK-1 causes an overload of calcium in mitochondria and indirectly cell death. The substantia nigra is shown to be particularly sensitive to PINK-1 mutations.

Positron emission tomography (PET): A medical imaging technique which detects the gamma rays produced by positrons emitted from injected radionuclides, such as radioactive glucose.

reactive oxygen species (ROS): are chemically-reactive molecules containing oxygen that may trigger cell death. Examples include oxygen ions and peroxides.

receptor: a protein structure, embedded in either the plasma membrane or the cytoplasm of a cell, to which specific kinds of signaling molecules may attach.

Sodium channel: voltage gated channels in nerve cell membranes that allow the generation of action potentials. Sodium channels may be a target for new drugs in Parkinson.

SPECT: Single photon emission computed tomography is a nuclear medicine tomographic imaging technique using gamma rays and able to provide 3D information for instance on brain chemistry.

stem cells: found in all multicellular organisms and are characterized by their ability to differentiate into a diverse range of specialized cell types. Stem cells are a potential line of treatment in Parkinson, either directly replacing the old nigrostriatal neuronal cells or creating growth factor releasing cells. Problems have arisen due to the inability to stop growth which may cause tumour growth.

striatum: Part of the basal ganglia, it is a large cluster of nerve cells, consisting of the caudate nucleus and the putamen, that controls movement, balance, and walking; the neurons of the striatum require dopamine to function.

substantia nigra: Latin for black substance. Is a brain structure located in the midbrain that plays an important role in reward, addiction, and movement. Parts of the substantia nigra appear darker than neighboring areas due to high levels of melanin in dopaminergic neurons. The substantia nigra is part of the basal ganglia; the other parts of the basal ganglia include the striatum (caudate nucleus, putamen, and nucleus accumbens), globus pallidus, and

subthalamic nucleus. Made up of the pars compacta and the pars reticulata.
  ▢ Pars compacta: Primarily involved in Parkinson, are mainly dopaminergic and black due to the high concentration of melatonin.
  ▢ Pars reticulata: Mainly GABAergic neurons.

subthalamic nucleus (STN): The subthalamic nucleus is a small lens-shaped nucleus involved in movement control. As suggested by its name, the subthalamic nucleus is located ventral to the thalamus. It is also dorsal to the substantia nigra and medial to the internal capsule.

shuffle gait: Short, uncertain steps, with minimal flexion and toes dragging. Often presents in Parkinson disease.

synapse: the junction between two neurons (axon to dendrite) or between a neuron and a muscle; nerve impulses cross a synapse through the action of neurotransmitters.

synaptic plasticity: the ability of the connection, or synapse, between two neurons to change in strength.

tau proteins: proteins that stabilize microtubules. They are abundant in neurons in the central nervous system and are less common elsewhere. When tau proteins are defective, and no longer stabilize microtubules properly, they can result in dementias, such as Alzheimer disease.

tauopathies: are a class of neurodegenerative diseases resulting from the pathological aggregation of tau protein in so-called neurofibrillary tangles (NFT) in the human brain.

thalamus: is a midline paired symmetrical structure situated between the cerebral cortex and midbrain, both in terms of location and neurological connections.

T.R.A.P.: Acronym for four primary PD symptoms:
  ▢ Tremor: Shaking of limb (usually hand) while at rest
  ▢ Rigidity: Muscle stiffness and resistance to movement
  ▢ Akinesia/bradykinesia: see above
  ▢ Postural instability: See ataxia

transcription factors: Proteins in eukaryotes that regulate the trancription of other genes

translation: The process of ribosomal reading of mRNA molecules in the cytoplasm and attaching correct amino acids at the right points to allow the formation of a protein molecule

tyramine-induced hypertension: Due to an increase in tyramine in the blood which forces noradrenaline out of vesicles and into circulation causing high blood pressure.

Ubiquitin: Involved in the degradation of certain proteins, it sticks to proteins that need to be degraded and the process of ubiquitination later breaks down the protein with various enzymes. In Parkinson disease excess proteins form causing the eventual death of the cell.

vesicle: A organelle in a cell that seperates other molecules from the rest of the cell. They can transport neurotransmitters to the cell surface and release them to stimulate other cells. This occurs in synaptic transmission.

Glossary compiled by Jon Stamford, PhD
Reprinted with permission.

INDEX

GLOBAL DECLARATION ON PARKINSON'S DISEASE

Reproduced with kind permission of European Parkinson's Disease Association

www.epda.eu.com/global-declaration

WE, THE WORKING GROUP ON PARKINSON'S DISEASE FORMED BY THE WORLD HEALTH ORGANISATION IN GENEVA ON 27 & 28 MAY 1997, CALL ON WORLD GOVERNMENTS & ALL HEALTHCARE PROVIDERS TO JOIN US IN TAKING STRONG & DECISIVE ACTION TO MEET THE OBJECTIVES & RECOMMENDATIONS ON THE EDUCATIONAL MANAGEMENT AND PUBLIC HEALTH IMPLICATIONS OF PARKINSON'S DISEASE AS AGREED AT THAT MEETING.

Parkinson's disease is a neurodegenerative disorder which is globally distributed, affecting all cultures and races.

THE OVERALL PREVALENCE IN THE WORLD IS ESTIMATED TO 6·3 MILLION.

MORE THAN 1:10 PEOPLE WITH PARKINSON'S ARE DIAGNOSED BEFORE THE AGE OF 50 YEARS.

Although Parkinson's disease is a complex disorder of unknown cause, for more than 40 years it has been recognised that loss of dopamine cells in the brain is responsible for the commonly observed disorders of movement. As yet the cure remains elusive. Parkinson's disease affects every aspect of daily living. In the modern era a range of treatments have been available to control symptoms and extend life span. These include medication, surgery, and physical therapies.

EFFECTIVE AND APPROPRIATE MANAGEMENT STRATEGIES COULD IMPROVE THE QUALITY OF LIFE OF THOSE WITH PARKINSON'S AND REDUCE COST AND IMPACT ON THE GLOBAL COMMUNITY.

Specifically, we urge every government to:

Support the World Charter for people with Parkinson's disease launched 11 April 1997. Which states that People with Parkinson's have the right to:
- Be referred to a doctor with a special interest in Parkinson's disease;
- Receive an accurate diagnosis;
- Have access to support services;
- Receive continuous care; and
- Take part in managing the illness.

Increase public awareness of Parkinson's disease as a priority health challenge thereby reducing its stigma and remove discrimination against people with Parkinson's disease in the workplace.

Improve the lives of people impacted by Parkinson's disease by ensuring that they receive appropriate treatment and strong medical education in support of the WHO 'Health for All' initiative.

Encourage all health authorities worldwide to support the WHO 'Health for All' concept and implement a Parkinson's disease programme consistent with resources available at each stage of industrial development to achieve co-ordination of effort by health workers within the three-tier model of service delivery.

Arrange care across the full spectrum of the illness structured in accordance with the results of cost effectiveness studies.

Encourage partnership between neuroscientists and health workers to devise ways to improve access to needed care and treatment for all people with Parkinson's disease and foster practice guidelines to assist health care workers in the management of medication side effects especially among the elderly.

Support a partnership between doctors and other health care workers with voluntary (non governmental) organisations representing patient interests to promote better understanding of Parkinson's disease.

Reach out to all ethnic and cultural groups of patients and to overcome negative attitudes in society towards chronic neurological and psychiatric illness and provide practical assistance for countries with underdeveloped Parkinson's services.

Encourage research into Parkinson's disease and the development of multidisciplinary teams to improve its management.

WRIT BY PETER HALLIDAY CALLIGRAPHER OCTOBER 2003

WE THE UNDERSIGNED SUPPORT THE GLOBAL DECLARATION ON PARKINSON'S DISEASE

Muhammad Ali (USA)
Kasturba Ali (USA)
Janet Reno (USA)
The Rt Hon Tony Benton (UK) High Commissioner to USA
John Bovis
John Bovis, GOBE MEP (UK)
Desmond M Tutu Archbishop Emeritus USA
Mary Baker Parkinson (member UK)
Ruth Martin
Marvin Bartholomew (member USA)
Matthew Kuhn (USA)
Alexandra Avago
Oscar Gershanik (Argentina)
Aleksander Vinka (Australia)
Wolfgang Oertel (Germany)
Anon Singhal (India)
Jean Jacques Hauw (Japan)
Ashok Kundu (Jordan)
Alla Gucke (Russia)
Eduardo Tolosa (Spain)
Mary C Baker OBE VC Chair
Leslie Findley (UK)
William Keller (USA)
Lizzie Graham Coordinator UK
Philip Thompson (Australia)
Mundar Siyi (India)
Alan J Bonilla (France)
S U He (China)
Eldad Melamed (Israel)
Jin-soo Kim (Korea)
Kailash Bhatia (UK)
David J Brooks (UK)
N Ray Chaudhuri (UK)
Roger Barker (UK)
Niall P Quinn (UK)
Anthony Schapira (UK)
Mahlon DeLong
Paul Greene (USA)
Mark Hallett (USA)
Irene Litvan (USA)
Bala Manyam (USA)
John C Nutt (USA)
Kapil Sethi (USA)
Lisa Shulman (USA)
M Hauy
Mark Stacy (USA)
Andrew Perlman (USA)
Kalyan Bhattacharyya (India)
Paresh Doshi (India)
Asha Kishore (Trivandrum)
Uday Muthane (Bangalore)

Letters of Support from: Rt Hon Tony Blair Prime Minister UK; Michael J Fox, USA; Danie Naveh MK Minister of Health Israel; The Hon John Howard Prime Minister Australia.

You can order this book online directly from the publisher:

www.parkinsonscreativecollective.org

or from Amazon

Alternatively you can order by mail by sending your request to:

Parkinsons Creative Collective
PO Box 22416
Little Rock, AR 72211

Please include a check for the number of books that you would like to order.
(Arkansas residents, add the appropriate Arkansas sales tax.)

For 1 to 2 books, shipped to a single U.S. address, the price is $35.00 each,
which includes free shipping and handling.

For shipping costs beyond the U.S. and discounts for larger quantity purchases
and related shipping and handling charges, please see the PCC website or contact PCC.

Printed by Horton & Horton Printing Company, Mabelvale, Arkansas